A-Level
Maths
Exam Board: AQA

You wouldn't enter a pie-eating competition without eating a few pies first, and the same goes for your A-Level Maths exams — practice is key!

This book has heaps of exam-style questions covering every topic from the A-Level course — it's loaded with practice to get you into tip-top exam shape. We've included questions to build your problem-solving skills and extra challenge questions to really test your knowledge.

Not only that, we also provide step-by-step solutions and full mark schemes for every question, right here in this book! Plus a full set of practice exam papers, too. So what are you waiting for? Let's get stuck in...

A-Level revision? It has to be CGP!

Contents

✓ Use the tick boxes to check off the topics you've completed.

Section Four — Problem Solving

Published by CGP

Editors:
Michael Bushell, Liam Dyer, Sammy El-Bahrawy, Sean McParland, David Ryan, Ben Train

Contributors:
Kevin Bennett, Paul Garrett, Aleksander Goodier, John Fletcher, Paul Freeman, Charlotte Young

ISBN: 978 1 78294 741 7

With thanks to Glenn Rogers for the proofreading.
With thanks to Emily Smith for the copyright research.

Clipart from Corel®
Printed by Elanders Ltd, Newcastle upon Tyne

Based on the classic CGP style created by Richard Parsons.

Exam Advice

Good exam technique can make a big difference to your mark, so make sure you read this stuff carefully.

Get familiar with the **Exam Structure**

Papers 2 and 3 are split into Section A (Pure Maths) and Section B (Mechanics/Statistics) — worth 50 marks each.

For **A-level Mathematics**, you'll be sitting **three papers**.

Paper 1 (Pure Maths) **2 hours** **100** marks	**33.33%** of your A-level	Tests the topics covered in **Section One** of this book.
Paper 2 (Pure Maths and Mechanics) **2 hours** **100** marks	**33.33%** of your A-level	Tests the topics covered in **Section One & Three** of this book.
Paper 3 (Pure Maths and Statistics) **2 hours** **100** marks	**33.33%** of your A-level	Tests the topics covered in **Sections One & Two** of this book.

Some formulas are given in the **Formula Booklet**

In the exam you'll be given a **formula booklet** that lists some of the formulas you might need. The ones relevant for A-level are shown on page 174 of this book.

You don't need to learn these formulas but you do need to know **how to use** them.

Manage Your Time sensibly

1) The **number of marks** tells you roughly **how long** to spend on a question — you've got just over a minute per mark in the exam. If you get stuck on a question for too long, it may be best to **move on** so you don't run out of time for the others.
2) You don't have to work through the paper **in order** — you could leave questions on topics you find harder until last.

Get **Familiar** with the **Large Data Set**

Throughout the A-Level Maths course you'll be working with a **large data set**. This is a **spreadsheet** containing information about a selection of **vehicles** registered in England. The large data set will only be used in Paper 3 for A-level Maths.

Questions in this paper might:
- Assume that you're familiar with the **terminology** and **contexts** of the data.
- Use **summary statistics** based on the large data set — this might reduce the time needed for some calculations.
- Include **statistical diagrams** based on the large data set.
- Be based on a **sample** from the large data set.

You might be expected to know specific details about the large data set — e.g. cars first registered in 2002 generally have higher carbon dioxide emissions than cars first registered in 2016.

Watch out for **Modelling** and **Problem-Solving** questions

The A-level Maths course has a few **overarching themes** — **proof**, **problem solving** and **modelling**. The first topic in this book covers proof (and there are other proof questions dotted throughout the book). Problem solving and modelling questions appear throughout the book, and are stamped so they're easy to spot.

PROBLEM SOLVING **Problem-solving** questions involve skills such as **combining** different areas of maths or **interpreting information** given to identify what's being asked for. They can be quite tricky, so for extra practice, **Section Four** of this book contains just this type of question, covering topics from throughout the course.

MODELLING **Modelling** questions involve using maths to represent **real-life situations**. You might be asked to think about the **validity** of the model (how realistic it is) or to interpret values **in context**.

The most **challenging** questions in this book are marked with a box behind their question number, e.g. **1**

Proof

Welcome one and all to this wondrous (if I do say so myself) A-Level practice book. First up is a real tough cookie — proof. But, if you prove yourself worthy on this section, you'll be well on your way to success...

1 Statement A says that $x^3 + 1 > 65$. Statement B says that $x > 4$.

Which option best describes the relationship between A and B? Circle your answer.

$A \Rightarrow B$ $A \Leftarrow B$ $A \Leftrightarrow B$ No connection between A and B

(1 mark)

2 Prove the following statement:

For all integers n, $n^3 - 16n$ is a multiple of 3.

(3 marks)

3 Prove that the product of any two distinct prime numbers has exactly four factors. PROBLEM SOLVING

(3 marks)

4 Prove that $n^3 + 2n^2 + 12n$ always has a factor of 8 when n is even.

(3 marks)

5 Riyad claims that, "if x and y are both irrational, then $\frac{x}{y}$ is also irrational".

a) Disprove Riyad's claim with a counter-example.

(1 mark)

Riyad goes on to claim that "any non-zero rational number multiplied by any irrational number is irrational."

b) Prove Riyad's claim by contradiction.

(3 marks)

Proof

6 Let x be an irrational number. Prove by contradiction that $\sqrt[4]{x}$ is irrational.

(3 marks)

7 A student makes the following statement:

PROBLEM SOLVING

"For an integer x, if x^3 is even, then x is even."

She attempts to prove the claim as follows:

"Let $x = 2k$. Then $x^3 = (2k)^3 = 8k^3 = 2(4k^3)$ which must be even, therefore the claim is true."

a) Explain why the student's proof is not valid.

....

....

(1 mark)

b) Prove the student's statement.

(4 marks)

8 Prove algebraically that if a four-digit number is a multiple of 3 then the sum of its digits is also a multiple of 3.

PROBLEM SOLVING

(4 marks)

EXAM TIP — When you're doing a proof in an exam, it's really important that it's laid out in a clear and logical manner. If it's a proof by contradiction, state the assumption you've made and then show how this assumption leads to a contradiction. Once you have the contradiction, don't just stop — finish with a concluding line starting "hence" or "therefore".	Score / 26

Algebra and Functions — 1

Algebra is a pretty important part of maths — so it's a good idea to get to grips with it now. First up, Algebra and Functions — 1, where you can practise all things surd-like and fraction-y. The excitement is almost palpable.

1 Simplify $\frac{a^6 \times a^3}{\sqrt{a^4}} \div a^{\frac{1}{2}}$. Give your answer in the form $a^{\frac{p}{q}}$.

....

(2 marks)

2 Find the value of x such that:

a) $27^x = 3$

$x =$ ....

(1 mark)

b) $27^x = 81$

$x =$ ....

(1 mark)

3 Fully simplify $\frac{(3ab^3)^2 \times 2a^6}{6a^4b}$. Circle your answer.

$\frac{3a^8b^2}{2}$ $3a^4b^5$ a^5b^4 $\frac{3a^4b^5}{2}$

(1 mark)

4 Show that $\frac{(5+4\sqrt{x})^2}{2x}$ can be written as $\frac{25}{2}x^{-1} + Px^{-\frac{1}{2}} + Q$, where P and Q are integers.

(3 marks)

Algebra and Functions — 1

5 Express $(5\sqrt{5}+2\sqrt{3})^2$ in the form $a+b\sqrt{c}$, where a, b and c are integers. Fully justify your answer.

....

(4 marks)

6 Show that $\dfrac{1}{(4\sqrt{7}-\sqrt{2})^2}$ can be written in the form $\dfrac{a+4\sqrt{b}}{c}$, where a, b and c are integers.

(3 marks)

7 Show that $\dfrac{14(1-\sqrt{2})}{1+\sqrt{8}}$ can be simplified to $6\sqrt{2}-10$.

(4 marks)

8 Express $\dfrac{(x^2-9)(3x^2-10x-8)}{(6x+4)(x^2-7x+12)}$ as a fraction in its simplest form.

....

(3 marks)

Algebra and Functions — 1

9 For this question, give all answers as fractions in their simplest form.

a) Simplify $\frac{x^2 + 5x - 14}{2x^2 - 4x}$.

....

(2 marks)

b) Using your answer to part a) or otherwise, write $\frac{x^2 + 5x - 14}{2x^2 - 4x} + \frac{14}{x(x-4)}$ as a single fraction.

....

(3 marks)

10 Express $\frac{1}{x(2x-3)}$ in partial fractions. Circle your answer.

$\frac{1}{3(2x-3)} + \frac{2}{3x}$ $\qquad$ $\frac{3}{2(2x-3)} - \frac{1}{2x}$ $\qquad$ $\frac{1}{(2x-3)} + \frac{1}{3x}$ $\qquad$ $\frac{2}{3(2x-3)} - \frac{1}{3x}$

(1 mark)

11 Express $\frac{6x-1}{x^2 + 4x + 4}$ in partial fractions.

You'll have to factorise the denominator first.

....

(4 marks)

EXAM TIP

In an exam, you might not always be asked to write an expression as partial fractions, but if the denominator is a product of two linear factors, it's usually a good place to start. There's so much algebra to cover in A-Level Maths, I've decided to split it up into a few parts. This is the end of Part 1. Next, with crushing inevitability, comes Part 2...

Score

32

Algebra and Functions — 2

Algebra and Functions Part 2 will take you on a whistle-stop tour of quadratic equations, make a slight detour into the world of simultaneous equations and inequalities and finish with everyone's favourite — cubics.

1 Given that the equation $3jx - jx^2 + 1 = 0$, where j is a constant, has no real roots, find the range of possible values of j. Fully justify your answer.

....

(3 marks)

2 $f(x) = \dfrac{1}{x^2 - 7x + 17}$

a) Express $x^2 - 7x + 17$ in the form $(x - m)^2 + n$, where m and n are constants.

....

(3 marks)

b) Hence find the maximum value of $f(x)$.

....

(2 marks)

3 The curve $y = 3kx^2 + kx + 2$ intersects the line $y = kx + 27$. Given that the equation $3kx^2 + kx + 2 = 0$ has two distinct real roots, find the possible values of k. Fully justify your answer. PROBLEM SOLVING

....

(5 marks)

4 Solve the equation $x^6 = 7x^3 + 8$ using a suitable algebraic method. PROBLEM SOLVING

....

(4 marks)

Algebra and Functions — 2

5 A scientist working at a remote Arctic research station monitors the temperature during the hours of daylight. For a day with 9 hours of sunlight, she models the temperature using the function $T = 10h - h^2 - 27$, where T is the temperature in °C and h is the time in hours since sunrise.

a) **(i)** Express $T = 10h - h^2 - 27$ in the form $T = -(m - h)^2 + n$, where m and n are integers.

....

(3 marks)

(ii) Hence show that T is always negative according to this model.

(1 mark)

b) **(i)** State the maximum temperature predicted by this model, and state the number of hours after sunrise at which it will occur.

Temperature = ... °C, time = ... hours after sunrise

(2 marks)

(ii) Sketch the graph of $T = 10h - h^2 - 27$ on the axes below. Mark clearly on your graph the temperature at sunrise.

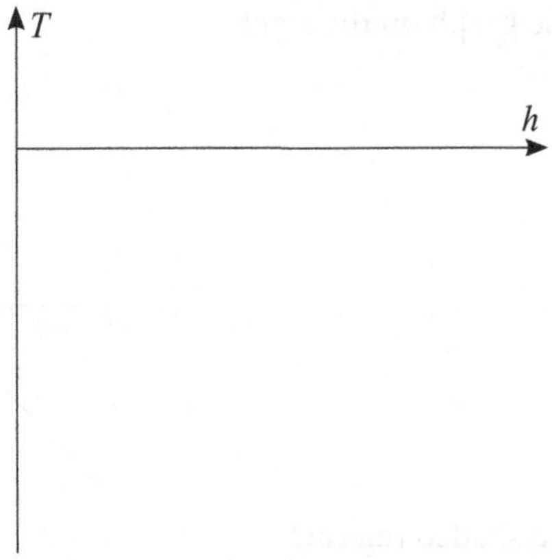

(2 marks)

6 Use algebra to solve the simultaneous equations $y + x = 7$ and $y = x^2 + 3x - 5$.

x = ... y = ... or x = ... y = ...

(4 marks)

Algebra and Functions — 2

7 The curve C has equation $y = -x^2 + 3$ and the line l has equation $y = -dx + 4$, where d is a positive constant. l is a tangent to C.

PROBLEM SOLVING

a) Find the coordinates of the point of intersection of C and l.

....

(5 marks)

b) Sketch the graphs of C and l on the axes on the right, clearly showing where the graphs intersect the x- and y- axes.

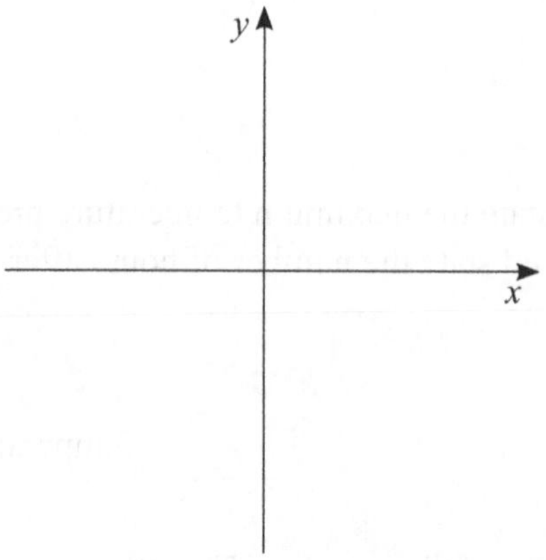

(5 marks)

8 Consider the shaded region on the graph on the right.

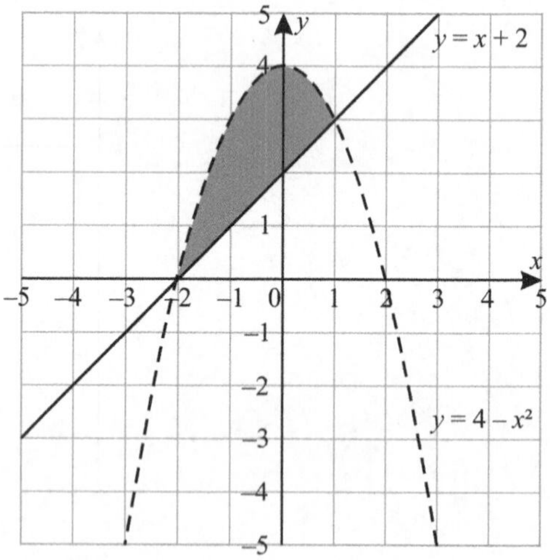

Which two inequalities define the shaded region? Circle your answer.

$y \geq x + 2$ and $y \leq 4 - x^2$	$y \geq x + 2$ and $y < 4 - x^2$	$y > x + 2$ and $y < 4 - x^2$	$y > x + 2$ and $y \leq 4 - x^2$

(1 mark)

9 Solve the inequality $x^2 - 8x + 15 > 0$. Give your answer in set notation.

Use of a calculator is not acceptable.

....

(4 marks)

Algebra and Functions — 2

10 $(x-1)(x^2+x+1) = 2x^2 - 17$

a) Rewrite the equation above in the form $f(x) = 0$, where $f(x)$ is of the form $f(x) = ax^3 + bx^2 + cx + d$.

....

(2 marks)

b) Show that $(x + 2)$ is a factor of $f(x)$.

Use the factor theorem.

(2 marks)

c) Hence write $f(x)$ as the product of a linear factor and a quadratic factor.

....

(2 marks)

d) By completing the square, or otherwise, show that $f(x) = 0$ has only one root.

(2 marks)

11 A function is defined by $f(x) = x^3 - 4x^2 - ax + 10$. $(x - 1)$ is a factor of $f(x)$.
Find the value of a and hence use algebra to solve the equation $x^3 - 4x^2 - ax + 10 = 0$.

PROBLEM SOLVING

$a =$ .... $x =$ ....

(6 marks)

EXAM TIP

Quadratics have a habit of popping up in exam questions where you least expect them (like in exponentials, trig equations or mechanics, not to mention in simultaneous equations, inequalities and cubics) — so make sure you can handle them. It's worth practising your factorising skills, in case the question won't let you just use your calculator to find the solutions.

Score

58

Algebra and Functions — 3

All the artists amongst you will love this section — you get to sketch some beautiful graphs. For all you non-artists, don't panic — there's also some equally beautiful algebra in the form of modulus, composite and inverse functions.

1 $f(x) = |2x + 3|$ and $g(x) = |5x - 4|$.

a) On the same axes, draw the graphs of $y = f(x)$ and $y = g(x)$, showing clearly where each graph meets the coordinate axes.

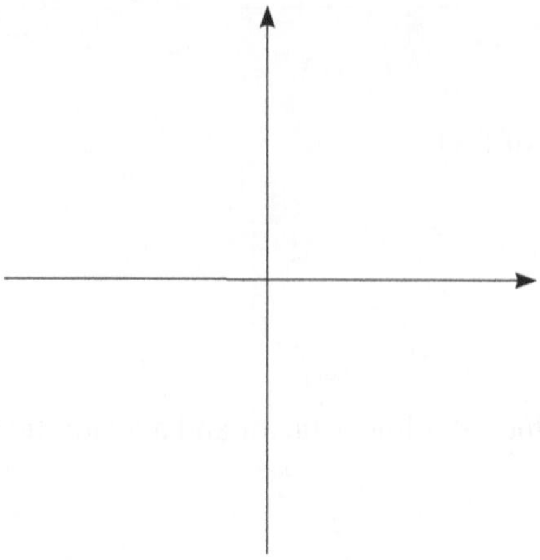

(2 marks)

b) Hence or otherwise solve the equation $f(x) = g(x)$.

....

(4 marks)

2 $f(x) = |4x + 5|$.

a) Find the possible values of $f(x)$ if $|x| = 2$.

....

(3 marks)

b) Find the values of x for which $f(x) \leq 2 - x$.

....

(3 marks)

c) Find the possible values of a constant A for which the equation $f(x) + 2 = A$ has two distinct roots.

....

(2 marks)

Algebra and Functions — 3

3 Sketch the curve of $y = (x-2)^2(x+3)^2$ on the axes provided.
Show clearly any points of intersection with the x- and y-axes.

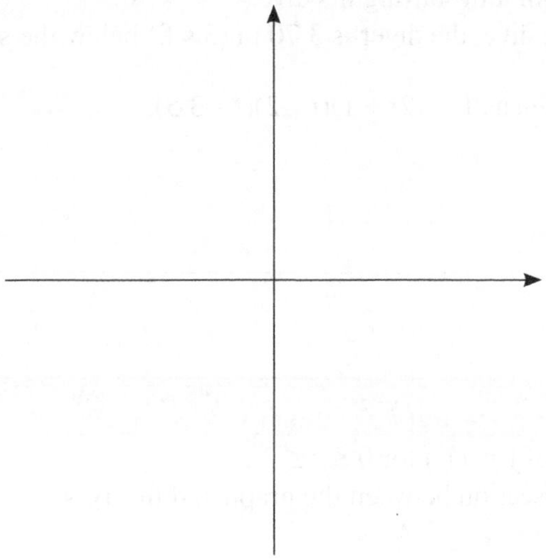

(3 marks)

4 The graph of $y = x^3 - 2x^2 + px$, for some constant p, crosses the x-axis at the points $(1-\sqrt{3}, 0)$, $(0, 0)$ and $(1+\sqrt{3}, 0)$.

a) Sketch the graph of $y = x^3 - 2x^2 + px$, showing clearly any points of intersection with the axes.

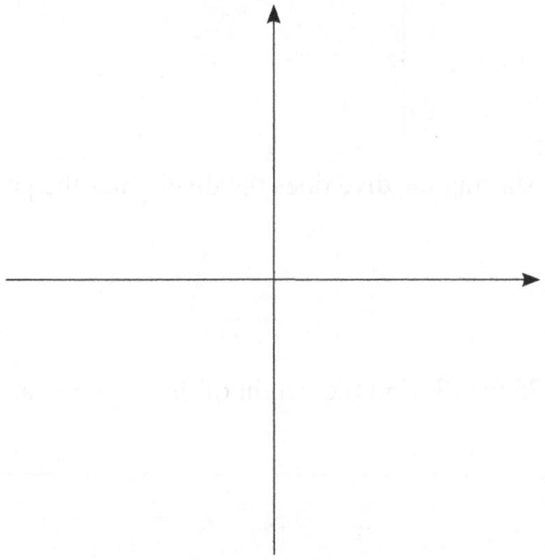

(2 marks)

b) Find the value of p.

It'll help to factorise the original function first.

....

(2 marks)

Algebra and Functions — 3

5 A diver's position is modelled by the function $V = 2t^3 - 10t^2 + 8.5t + 7$, $0 \leq t \leq 3.5$.

- V is the vertical height of the diver's head above the surface of the pool, in metres.
- t is the time in seconds from him starting his dive.
- At the deepest point of the dive, the diver is 3.70 m (3 s.f.) below the surface of the pool.

a) Show that V can be written as $V = (2t + 1)(t - 2)(t - 3.5)$.

(2 marks)

b) Hence sketch the graph of $y = V(t)$ for $0 \leq t \leq 3.5$.
Label any points of intersection between the graph and the axes.

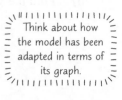

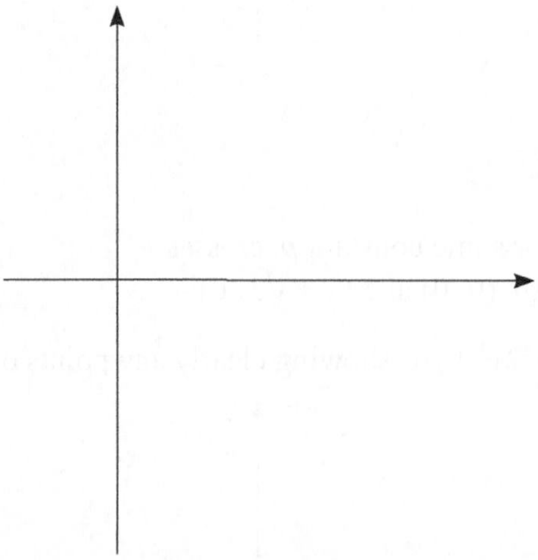

(3 marks)

c) How many seconds after starting the dive does the diver enter the pool?

.... s

(1 mark)

d) Given that the diver is 1.75 m tall, find the height of the diving board above the surface of the pool.

.... m

(2 marks)

e) The same diver then dives from a higher diving board. Darren suggests adapting the model for this diving board. The adapted model is $V = 2t^3 - 10t^2 + 8.5t + 10$.
Comment on the validity of this adapted model, giving reasons for your comments.

Think about how the model has been adapted in terms of its graph.

....

....

....

(2 marks)

Algebra and Functions — 3

6 Figure 1 shows a sketch of the function $y = f(x)$.
The function crosses the x-axis at $(-1, 0)$, $(1, 0)$ and $(2, 0)$, and crosses the y-axis at $(0, 2)$.

Figure 1

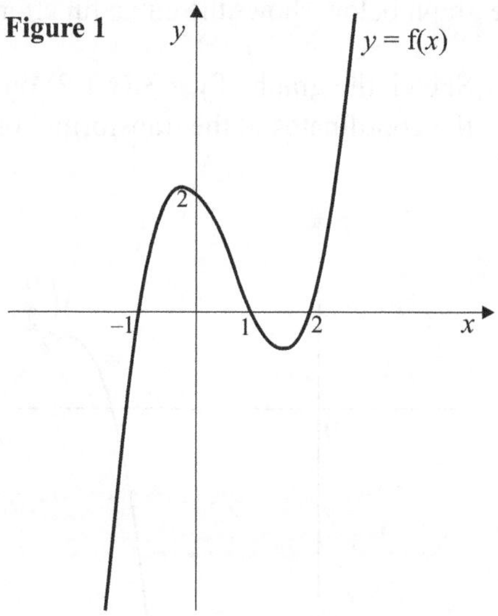

Sketch the transformation $y = 2f(x - 4)$ on the axes below.
Label any known points of intersection with the x- or y-axes.

Do one transformation at a time to help keep track of what's going on.

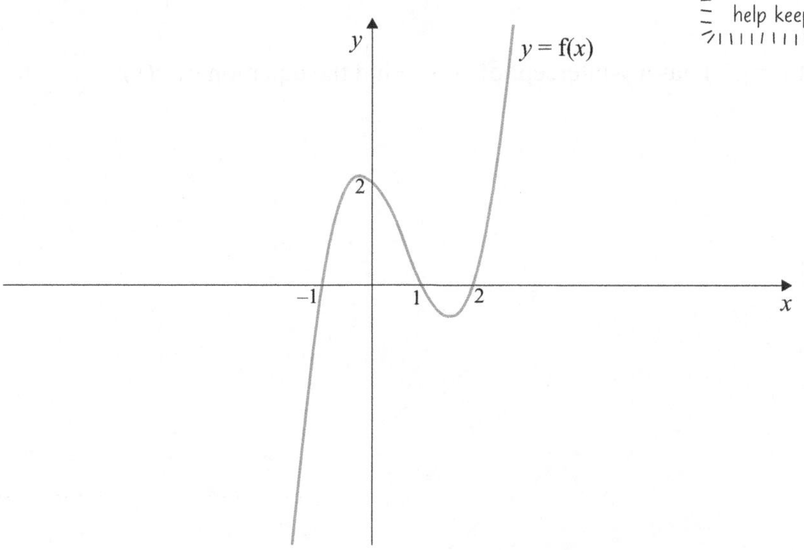

(3 marks)

7 Sketch the graph of $y = 3 + \frac{1}{x - 4}$, clearly indicating the equations of the asymptotes.

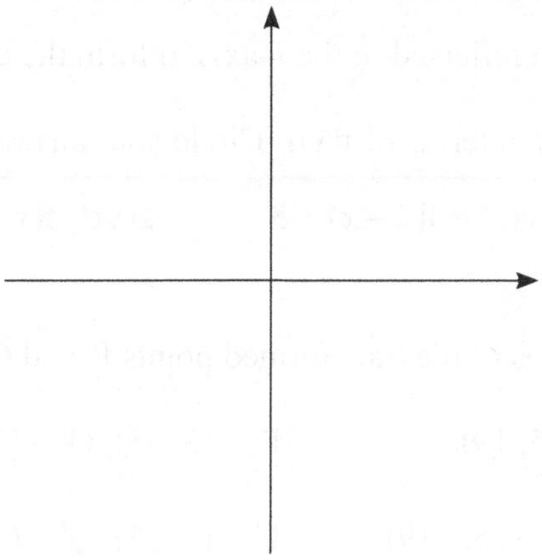

(3 marks)

Algebra and Functions — 3

8 The graph below shows the cubic function $y = f(x)$, $x \in \mathbb{R}$, that passes through points $A\left(\frac{9}{2}, \frac{1}{24}\right)$ and $B(5, 0)$.

a) Sketch the graph of $y = 3f(x + 2)$ on the axes on the right, clearly showing the coordinates of the transformations of A and B. Label your graph g(x).

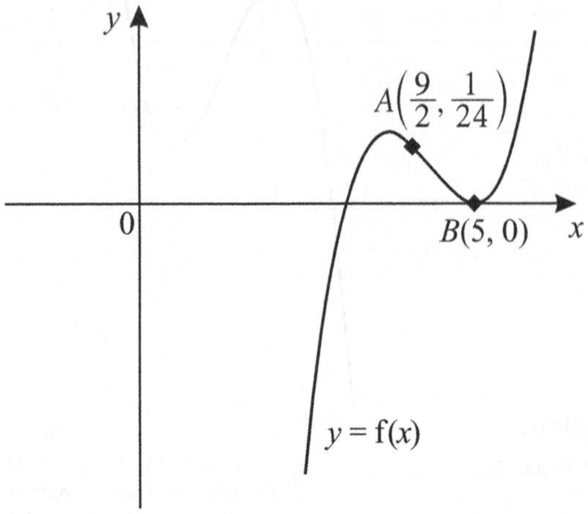

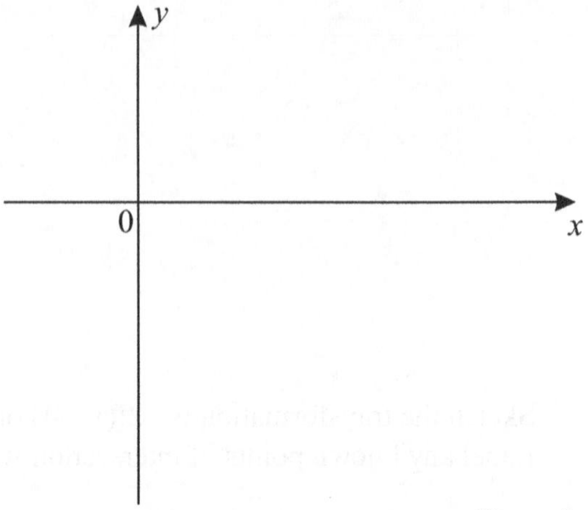

(3 marks)

b) The graph of $y = g(x)$ has a y-intercept of -18. Find the equation of g(x). PROBLEM SOLVING

....

(4 marks)

9 The graph of $y = f(x)$ passes through points P(1, 2) and Q(3, 16). The graph is first translated by vector $\begin{pmatrix} 2 \\ 3 \end{pmatrix}$ and then reflected in the y-axis to form the graph of $y = g(x)$.

a) What is the equation of g(x) in terms of f(x)? Circle your answer.

$g(x) = f(3 - x) + 2$ $\quad$ $g(x) = f(2 - x) + 3$ $\quad$ $g(x) = f(x - 2) + 3$ $\quad$ $g(x) = f(2 + x) - 3$

(1 mark)

b) What are the new coordinates of the transformed points P' and Q'? Circle your answer.

P' = (3, 5), Q' = (5, 19) $\quad$ P' = (3, –5), Q' = (5, –19)

P' = (–3, –5), Q' = (–5, –19) $\quad$ P' = (–3, 5), Q' = (–5, 19)

(1 mark)

Algebra and Functions — 3

10 The functions f and g are defined as follows: $f(x) = 2^x,\ x \in \mathbb{R}$ and $g(x) = \sqrt{3x+1},\ x \geq -\frac{1}{3}$.

a) **(i)** Find $gf(x)$.

....

(1 mark)

(ii) Hence solve $gf(x) = 5$.

....

(2 marks)

b) Find $g^{-1}(x)$ and state its domain and range.

....

(3 marks)

11 The functions f and g are defined as follows: $f(x) = \frac{1}{x^2},\ x \in \mathbb{R},\ x \neq 0$ and $g(x) = x^2 - k,\ x \in \mathbb{R}$, where k is a positive integer.

a) State the range of g. Give your answer in terms of k.

....

(1 mark)

b) Neither f nor g have an inverse. Explain why.

....

(1 mark)

c) **(i)** Given that $gf(1) = -8$, find the value of k and hence find $fg(x)$, and write down the domain of the composite function fg.

....

(5 marks)

(ii) Hence solve $fg(x) = \frac{1}{256}$.

....

(4 marks)

EXAM TIP

Don't worry, graph sketches don't have to be perfect — as long as they're generally the correct shape, and any turning points and intersections are in the right places (and labelled if the question asks for it), you should get all the marks. It's always a good idea to sketch graphs in pencil in case you make a mistake (and make sure you have a rubber to hand just in case).

Score

63

Coordinate Geometry

Up, down, up, triangle, circle, circle, down, triangle... I'm afraid when it comes to coordinate geometry and circle equations, there are no cheat codes. So pens at the ready — you've got to do this the hard way.

1 The line l has equation $y - 3x + 1 = 0$.

a) Find the gradient of a line perpendicular to l. Circle your answer.

3 $\qquad -3 \qquad \frac{1}{3} \qquad -\frac{1}{3}$

(1 mark)

b) Line j is parallel to l and passes through the point (4, 5). What is the equation of line j? Circle your answer.

$y = \frac{1}{3}x + 8 \qquad y = 7 - 3x \qquad y = 3x - 7 \qquad y = 8 - \frac{1}{3}x$

(1 mark)

2 The point A lies at the intersection of the lines l_1 and l_2, where the equation of l_1 is $x - y + 1 = 0$ and the equation of l_2 is $2x + y - 8 = 0$.

a) Use algebra to find the coordinates of point A.

....

(3 marks)

b) The points B and C have coordinates (6, –4) and $\left(-\frac{4}{3}, -\frac{1}{3}\right)$ respectively, and D is the midpoint of AC. Find the equation of the line through B and D in the form $ax + by + c = 0$, where a, b and c are integers.

....

(5 marks)

c) Show that the triangle ABD is a right-angled triangle. PROBLEM SOLVING

(3 marks)

Coordinate Geometry

3 The diagram shows a square ABCD, where point B has coordinates $(3, k)$.
The line through points B and C has equation $-3x + 5y = 16$.

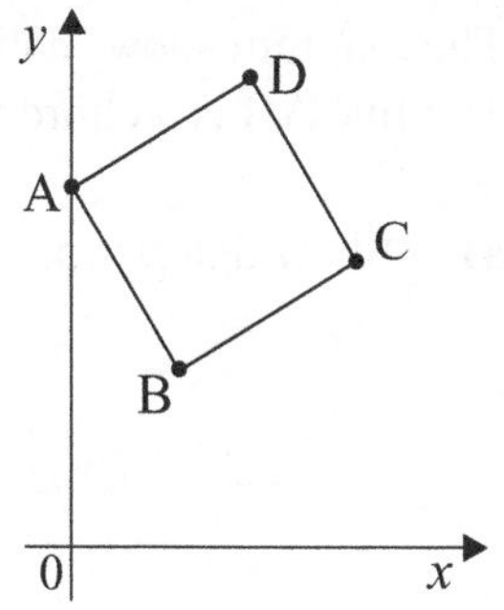

a) Show that the line with equation $5x + 3y - 6 = 0$ is parallel to the line through points A and B.

(3 marks)

b) Find the area of square ABCD.

....

(5 marks)

4 The route followed by an ant is modelled by the equation of a circle.
The points A(2, 1) and B(0, –5) lie along the route, where the line AB is a diameter of the circle.

a) Show that the point (4, –1) also lies along the ant's route.

(5 marks)

b) Show that the equation of the ant's route can be written in the form $x^2 + y^2 - 2x + 4y - 5 = 0$.

(2 marks)

c) The ant eventually leaves the route and travels at a tangent to the circle from point A.
Find the equation of the line the ant is now on, giving your answer in the form $y = mx + c$.

....

(3 marks)

Coordinate Geometry

5 The diagram shows a circle with centre P. The line AB is a chord with midpoint M.

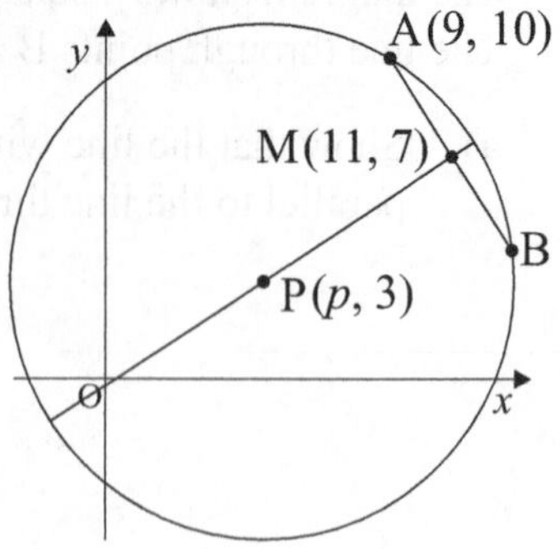

a) Show that $p = 5$. PROBLEM SOLVING

The diagram shows a chord, so think about which circle property might apply.

(5 marks)

b) Find the equation of the circle.

....

(3 marks)

6 The boundary of a forest is modelled as a circle with the equation $x^2 - 6x + y^2 - 4y = 0$, which crosses the y-axis at the origin and at the point A. x and y measure distance in kilometres. MODELLING

a) Find the coordinates of point A.

....

(2 marks)

b) Write the equation that models the boundary of the forest in the form $(x - a)^2 + (y - b)^2 = c$.

....

(3 marks)

c) Write down the radius and the coordinates of the centre of the forest.

radius = ..., centre = ...

(2 marks)

d) A straight path runs tangentially to the boundary of the forest at point A. It meets the x-axis at point B. Find the exact distance AB.

....

(6 marks)

Coordinate Geometry

7 A circle has parametric equations $x = 5 \sin\theta + 2$, $y = 5 \cos\theta - 3$.

a) Find the coordinates of the centre of the circle. Circle your answer.

(2, 3) (3, 2) (2, –3) (–3, 2)

(1 mark)

b) What is the radius of the circle? Circle your answer.

5 $\sqrt{5}$ 25 $\frac{1}{5}$

(1 mark)

8 The curve on the right has parametric equations $x = 3 \sin\theta$, $y = 4 \cos\theta$.

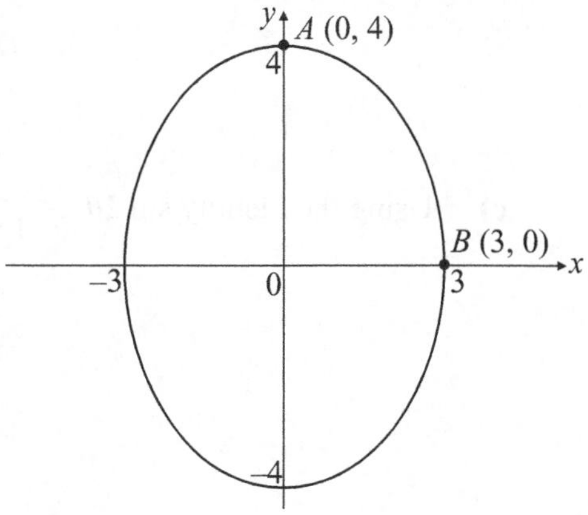

a) For $0 \le \theta \le \frac{\pi}{2}$, find the values of θ that correspond to the points A and B.

....

(2 marks)

b) Show that $y^2 = (4 + \frac{4x}{3})(4 - \frac{4x}{3})$.

PROBLEM SOLVING

You'll need to use a trig identity for this one...

(3 marks)

9 Part of the path of a boat sailing around an island is modelled on a shipping chart with the parametric equations $x = t^2 - 7t + 12$, $y = t - 1$, where t is time in hours.

MODELLING PROBLEM SOLVING

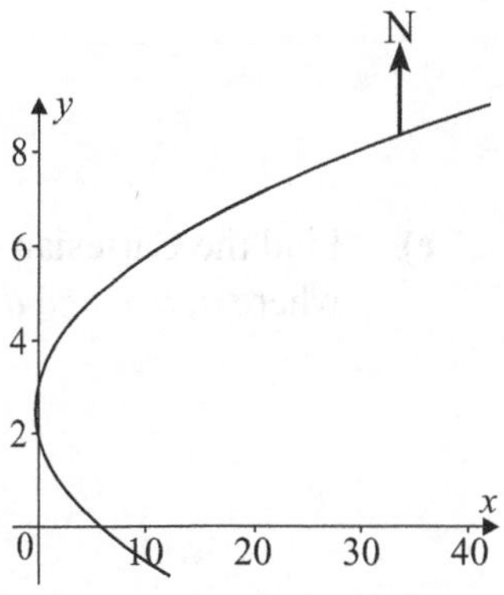

In this model, the western tip of the island has coordinates (12, 2). Calculate the length of time that the boat is further west than the tip of the island.

.... hours

(3 marks)

Coordinate Geometry

10 The curve C is defined by the parametric equations:

$$x = 1 - \tan\theta,\ y = \frac{1}{2}\sin 2\theta, \quad -\frac{\pi}{2} < \theta < \frac{\pi}{2}.$$

a) P is the point on curve C where $\theta = \frac{\pi}{3}$. Find the exact coordinates of P.

....

(2 marks)

b) Point Q on curve C has coordinates $(2, -\frac{1}{2})$. Find the value of θ at Q.

....

(2 marks)

c) Using the identity $\sin 2\theta \equiv \frac{2\tan\theta}{1 + \tan^2\theta}$, show that the Cartesian equation of C is $y = \frac{1 - x}{x^2 - 2x + 2}$.

(3 marks)

11 A curve C has parametric equations $y = t^3 + t$, $x = 4t - 2$.

a) Find the coordinates of the point where the curve C crosses the y-axis.

....

(2 marks)

b) Find the coordinates of the points where the curve C intersects the line $y = \frac{1}{2}x + 1$.

....

(4 marks)

c) Find the Cartesian equation of the curve C in the form $y = ax^3 + bx^2 + cx + d$, where a, b, c and d are fractions.

$y =$ ....

(3 marks)

EXAM TIP

Working with parametric equations can be a real chore. When converting to Cartesian form, it's not always obvious how to rearrange the parametric equations, so you might have to try a couple of different ways — it's best to start with the equation that gives the simplest expression for t. Also, make sure you're up to snuff with your trig identities, as they'll come in handy.

Score

78

Sequences and Series — 1

Time to test your knowledge of arithmetic and geometric sequences. Get ready for common differences, common ratios, recurrence relations, sums to infinity, sums to not-quite-infinity, sigma notation... I know you're gonna love it.

1 An arithmetic sequence has first term a and common difference d.
The value of the 12th term is 79, and the value of the 16th term is 103.

a) Find the values of a and d.

$u = a + (n-1)d$. $103 = a + 15d$.
$79 = a + 11d$ $d = 6$
$103 = a + 15d$.
$-\ 79 = a + 11d$.
$24 = + 4d$.

$a =$ 13. $d =$ 6.

(3 marks)

b) Determine the value of k such that $u_{k+6} = 2u_k - 1$.

$k =$ ....

(2 marks)

2 A sequence is defined by the recurrence relation: $h_{n+1} = 2h_n + 2$ when $n \geq 1$.

a) Given that $h_1 = 5$, find the values of h_2, h_3, and h_4.

....

(2 marks)

b) Calculate the value of $\sum_{r=3}^{6} h_r$.

....

(3 marks)

3 An arithmetic series has first term 21 and mth term 108.
The sum of the terms up to and including the mth term is 1935.

Determine the 23rd term in the series.

The formula for S_n is given in the formula booklet (see p.174).

....

(3 marks)

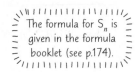

Sequences and Series — 1

4 A tower can be constructed using a set of blocks. The first block has a height of a cm. Each other block has height d cm, and is stacked directly on top of the previous block.

MODELLING

a) Let H_n be the total height of all towers that can be made with n blocks or fewer. Given that $H_{60} = H_5 \times H_6$, show that $2a^2 - 4a + 9ad - 118d + 10d^2 = 0$.

(3 marks)

b) A tower becomes unstable if its height exceeds 224 cm. Given that the first block has a height of 2 cm, determine the maximum number of blocks that may be used to build a stable tower.

PROBLEM SOLVING

.... blocks

(3 marks)

5 The first term of a geometric sequence is 18 and the common ratio is –1.

What type of sequence is this? Circle your answer.

Convergent sequence   Divergent sequence   Periodic sequence   Decreasing sequence

(1 mark)

6 A geometric series has third term $u_3 = \frac{5}{2}$ and sixth term $u_6 = \frac{5}{16}$.

a) Find the formula for the nth term of the series.

....

(4 marks)

b) Find $\sum_{i=1}^{10} u_i$. Give your answer as a fraction in its simplest terms.

....

(2 marks)

c) Show that the sum to infinity of the series is 20.

(2 marks)

Sequences and Series — 1

7 A geometric series has the first term 5 and is defined by: $u_{n+1} = 5 \times 1.7^n$.

a) Can the sum to infinity of this sequence be found? Explain your answer.

....

(1 mark)

b) Find the value of the 3rd and 8th terms.

$u_3 =$ .... $u_8 =$ ....

(2 marks)

8 In a geometric series with n^{th} term u_n, $a = 20$ and $r = \frac{3}{4}$.

Find values for the following, giving your answers to 3 significant figures where necessary:

a) S_∞

....

(2 marks)

b) the smallest value of n for which $S_n > 79.76$. PROBLEM SOLVING

....

(5 marks)

9 To raise money for charity, Alex, Chris and Heather were sponsored £1 for each kilometre they ran over a 10-day period. They receive sponsorship proportionally for partial kilometres completed. MODELLING

Alex ran 3 km every day. Chris ran 2 km on day 1 and on each subsequent day ran 20% further than the day before. Heather ran 1 km on day 1, and on each subsequent day ran 50% further than the previous day.

a) How far did Heather run on day 5, to the nearest 10 metres?

.... km

(2 marks)

b) Show that day 10 is the first day that Chris runs further than 10 km.

(3 marks)

c) Find the total amount raised by the end of the 10 days, to the nearest penny.

....

(4 marks)

Sequences and Series — 1

10 $a + ar + ar^2 + ar^3 + \ldots$ is a geometric series.
The second term of the series is –2 and the sum to infinity of the series is –9.

PROBLEM SOLVING

a) Show that $9r^2 - 9r + 2 = 0$.

(3 marks)

b) Hence find the possible values of a.

....

(3 marks)

11 The first three terms of a sequence are defined as $u_1 = x$, $u_2 = x^2$, and $u_3 = 9x$, where $x > 0$.

PROBLEM SOLVING

Use algebra to find an expression for the nth term, u_n, in terms of n, if the sequence is said to be:

a) a geometric sequence,

....

(3 marks)

b) an arithmetic sequence.

....

(4 marks)

EXAM TIP

This is a top tip straight from the mouth of the examiners themselves, so you'd best listen up. There are a few different formulae to contend with here, so make sure you don't get flustered in the exam and get them muddled up. Don't get your u_n and your S_n mixed up or accidentally find the sum to infinity when you don't mean to — you're just throwing away marks that way.

Score

60

Sequences and Series — 2

OK, now it's time for something a little different. The next few pages cover variations of binomial expansions — including cases where the power is a positive integer, a negative integer or even a fraction.

1 The binomial expansion of $(j + kx)^6$ is $j^6 + ax + bx^2 + cx^3 + ...$

a) Given that $c = 20\ 000$, show that $jk = 10$ (where both j and k are positive integers).

(3 marks)

b) Given that $a = 37\ 500$, find the values of j and k.

$j =$ ...., $k =$ ....

(4 marks)

c) Find b.

$b =$ ....

(2 marks)

2 Find the coefficient of x^5 in the expansion of $(1 - 3x)^{-8}$. Circle your answer.

–192 456   192 456   –792   13 608

(1 mark)

3 $f(x) = (2 + 4x)^{-4}$ and $g(x) = (1 + ax)^{-5}$.

a) Find the binomial expansion of $f(x)$ up to and including the x^3 term.

....

(4 marks)

b) Given that the coefficients of x^2 in the expansions of $f(x)$ and $g(x)$ are equal, and $a > 0$, find the value of a.

$a =$ ....

(3 marks)

Sequences and Series — 2

4 $f(x) = (27 + 4x)^{\frac{1}{3}}$, for $|x| < \frac{27}{4}$

a) Using the binomial expansion of f(x), up to and including the x^2 term, find an approximation to $\sqrt[3]{26.2}$. Give your answer to 6 decimal places.

....

(6 marks)

b) What is the percentage error in this approximation? Give your answer to 3 significant figures.

.... %

(2 marks)

5 $f(x) = \sqrt{\frac{1+3x}{1-5x}}$

a) **(i)** Use the binomial expansion in increasing powers of x to show that $f(x) \approx 1 + 4x + 12x^2$.

(5 marks)

(ii) For what values of x is your expansion valid?

....

(2 marks)

b) Using the above expansion with $x = \frac{1}{15}$, show that $\sqrt{1.8} \approx \frac{33}{25}$.

(2 marks)

Sequences and Series — 2

6 $f(x) = \dfrac{2 - 18x}{(5 + 4x)(1 - 2x)^2}$

a) Given that f(x) can be expressed in the form $f(x) = \dfrac{A}{(5 + 4x)} + \dfrac{B}{(1 - 2x)} + \dfrac{C}{(1 - 2x)^2}$, find the values of A, B and C.

If you're not sure how to handle this question, you probably need to brush up on partial fractions.

$A =$ .... $B =$ .... $C =$ ....

(4 marks)

b) Hence find the binomial expansion of f(x), up to and including the term in x^2.

....

(6 marks)

c) Claire states that the expansion above is valid for $\frac{1}{2} < x < \frac{5}{4}$.
Explain the error that Claire has made and state the correct range.

....

....

....

(2 marks)

EXAM TIP

As well as being happy with doing the expansions, make sure you're confident with the other things examiners often ask — such as approximations and ranges of validity. When you have several expansions you should calculate the valid ranges of each expansion, then the overall expansion will be valid for the narrowest of the two (or more) ranges.

Score

46

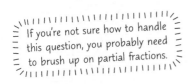

Trigonometry

You'd think that there's only so much you can do with a three-sided shape, right? Well, think again...
It's time to delve deeper into the twisted triangular world of trig, and discover new ways of measuring angles.

1 The diagram shows a sector of a circle of radius r cm and angle 120°.
The length of the arc of the sector is 40 cm.

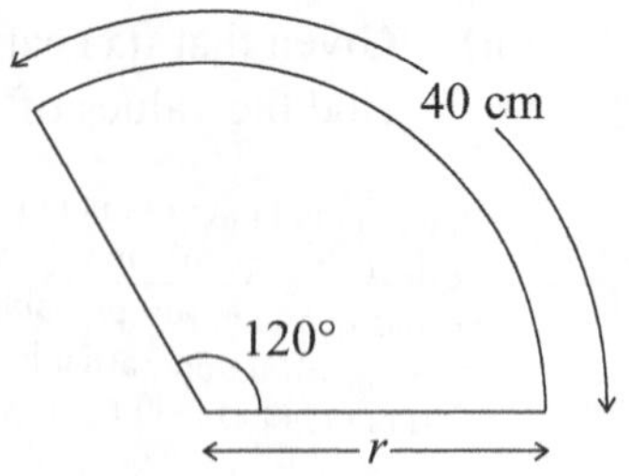

Find the area of the sector to the nearest square centimetre.

.... cm^2

(5 marks)

2 A new symmetrical mini-stage is to be built according to the design below.
The design consists of a rectangle of length q metres and width $2r$ metres,
two sectors of radius r and angle θ radians (shaded), and an isosceles triangle.

MODELLING

a) Find, in terms of r, q and θ, expressions for the perimeter P, and the area A, of the stage.

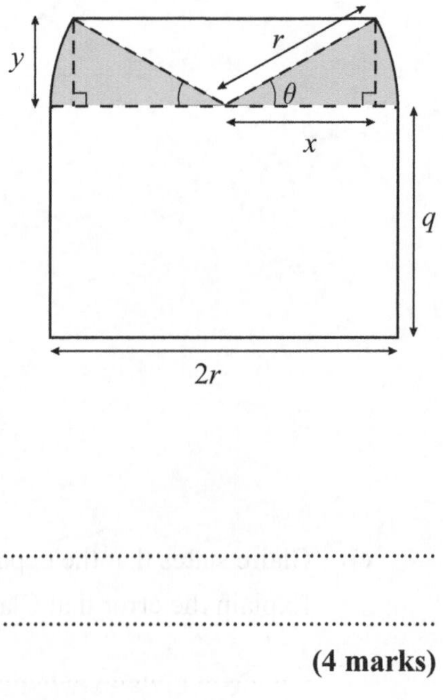

$P =$ ....

$A =$ ....

(4 marks)

b) Given that the perimeter of the stage is to be 40 m and $\theta = \frac{\pi}{3}$,

show that A is given by $A = 40r - kr^2$, where $k = 3 - \frac{\sqrt{3}}{4} + \frac{\pi}{3}$.

(4 marks)

Trigonometry

3 Sketch the graphs of $y = \sin x$ and $y = \sin \frac{x}{2}$ in the range $0 \leq x \leq 4\pi$ on the same set of axes, showing the points at which the graphs cross the x-axis.

(3 marks)

4 A sheep pen is modelled as a triangle with side lengths of 50 m, 70 m and 90 m.

MODELLING

a) Find the area of the sheep pen to the nearest square metre. Fully justify your answer.

.... m^2

(5 marks)

b) Comment on the accuracy of the model.

....

....

(1 mark)

5 Solve $\sin x = -\frac{\sqrt{2}}{2}$ in the range $\frac{\pi}{2} \leq x \leq \frac{3\pi}{2}$. Circle your answer.

$x = \frac{7\pi}{4}$ $x = \frac{3\pi}{2}$ $x = \frac{5\pi}{4}$ $x = \frac{3\pi}{4}$

(1 mark)

6 Find all the values of x, in the interval $0° \leq x \leq 180°$, for which $7 - 3\cos x = 9\sin^2 x$.

Solutions to this question based entirely on graphical or numerical methods are not acceptable.

....

(5 marks)

Trigonometry

7 Adam and Bethan have each attempted to solve the equation $\sin 2t = \sqrt{2}\cos 2t$ for the range $-90° < t < 90°$. Their working is shown below.

PROBLEM SOLVING

Adam
$\sin 2t = \sqrt{2}\cos 2t$
$\tan 2t = \sqrt{2}$
$\tan t = \frac{\sqrt{2}}{2}$
$t = 35.26...°$

Bethan
$\sin 2t = \sqrt{2}\cos 2t$
$\sin^2 2t = 2\cos^2 2t$
$1 - \cos^2 2t = 2\cos^2 2t$
$\cos^2 2t = \frac{1}{3}$
$\cos 2t = \pm\frac{1}{\sqrt{3}}$
$t = \pm 27.36...°$

a) Show that Adam's solution is incorrect.

(1 mark)

b) Identify an error made by Adam.

....

....

(1 mark)

c) Bethan's teacher explains that one of her solutions is incorrect.
Identify and explain the error Bethan has made.

....

....

(2 marks)

8 The function $f(\theta) = \tan^2\theta + \frac{\tan\theta}{\cos\theta}$ is defined for $0 \leq \theta \leq 2\pi, \theta \neq \frac{\pi}{2}, \frac{3\pi}{2}$.

a) Show that the equation $\tan^2\theta + \frac{\tan\theta}{\cos\theta} = 1$ can be written in the form $2\sin^2\theta + \sin\theta - 1 = 0$.

(3 marks)

b) Hence find all solutions to the equation $f(\theta) = 1$ in the interval $0 \leq \theta \leq 2\pi$.

....

(4 marks)

Trigonometry

9 The diagram on the right shows the graph of $y = \arccos x$, where y is in radians. A and B are the end points of the graph.

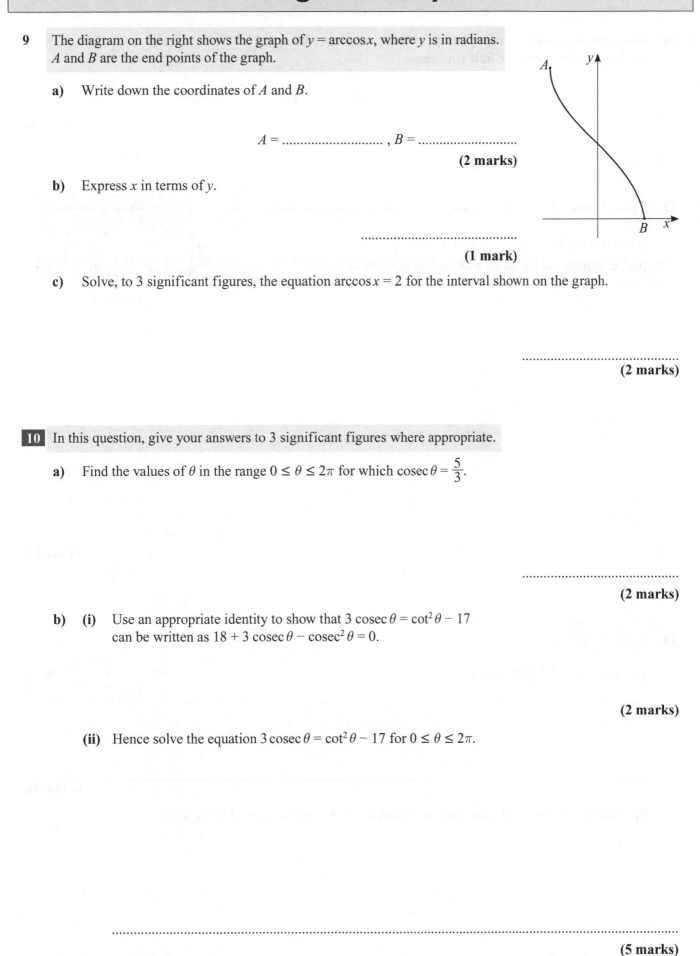

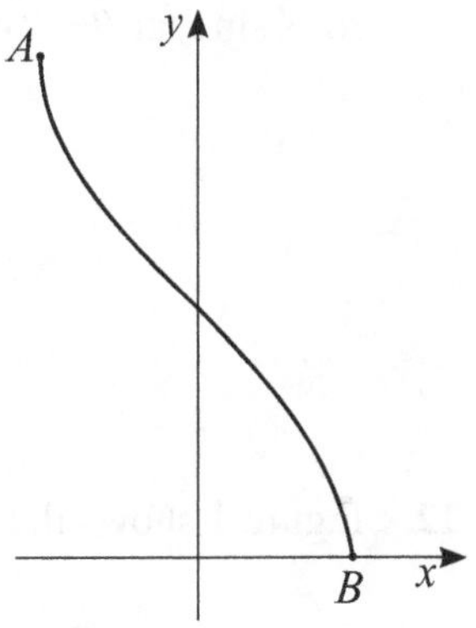

a) Write down the coordinates of A and B.

$A =$ ...., $B =$ ....

(2 marks)

b) Express x in terms of y.

....

(1 mark)

c) Solve, to 3 significant figures, the equation $\arccos x = 2$ for the interval shown on the graph.

....

(2 marks)

10 In this question, give your answers to 3 significant figures where appropriate.

a) Find the values of θ in the range $0 \leq \theta \leq 2\pi$ for which $\text{cosec}\,\theta = \frac{5}{3}$.

....

(2 marks)

b) **(i)** Use an appropriate identity to show that $3\,\text{cosec}\,\theta = \cot^2\theta - 17$ can be written as $18 + 3\,\text{cosec}\,\theta - \text{cosec}^2\theta = 0$.

(2 marks)

(ii) Hence solve the equation $3\,\text{cosec}\,\theta = \cot^2\theta - 17$ for $0 \leq \theta \leq 2\pi$.

....

(5 marks)

Trigonometry

11 Given that θ is small and measured in radians, find an approximation for $4\sin\theta\tan\theta + 2\cos\theta$. Circle your answer.

$4 + 2\theta^2$ $\quad$ $2 + 3\theta^2$ $\quad$ $6\theta^2$ $\quad$ $2 + 5\theta^2$

(1 mark)

12 Figure 1 shows the design of a flag that is a cm tall and b cm wide.

PROBLEM SOLVING

Given that $\tan 2\theta = \dfrac{1}{1+\tan\theta}$, and $0 < \theta < \dfrac{\pi}{2}$,
find an expression for the area of the flag in terms of a.

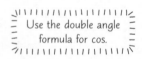

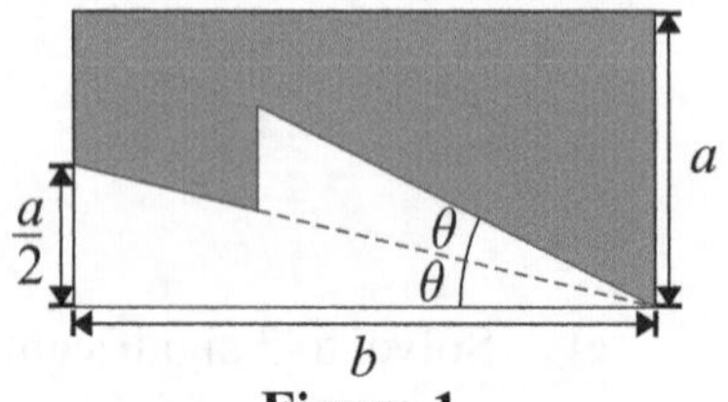

Figure 1

....

(4 marks)

13 $f(x) = \dfrac{1+\cos x}{2}$.

a) Show that $\dfrac{1+\cos x}{2} = \cos^2\dfrac{x}{2}$.

Use the double angle formula for cos.

(2 marks)

b) Hence find the exact values of x for which $f(x) = 0.75$ in the interval $0 \leq x \leq 2\pi$.

....

(2 marks)

Trigonometry

14 An engineer uses a microphone connected to a computer to record a sound wave. The computer displays the sound wave on a graph of amplitude against time, as shown in Figure 2.

MODELLING PROBLEM SOLVING

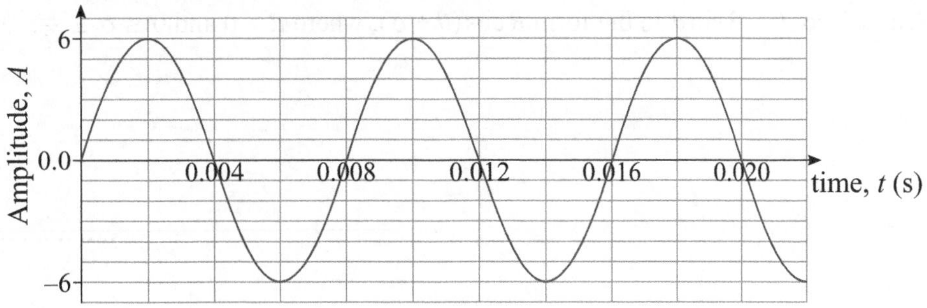

Figure 2

a) Show that the sound wave can be modelled by the equation $A = 6\sin(250\pi t)$.

(3 marks)

The engineer wants to combine the recorded sound wave with a second sound wave that can be modelled by the equation $A = 2\sqrt{3}\cos(250\pi t)$.

She forms an expression to model the combined sound waves by finding the sum of the two equations for the separate sound waves.

b) Determine a model for the combined sound waves in the form $A = R\sin(x + \alpha)$, where R and α are constants to be found. $R > 0$, $0 \leq \alpha < \frac{\pi}{2}$.

(4 marks)

15 By writing $\sin 2\theta$ in terms of $\sin\theta$ and $\cos\theta$, solve the equation $3\sin 2\theta\tan\theta = 5$, for $0 \leq \theta \leq 2\pi$. Give your answers to 3 significant figures.

(6 marks)

Trigonometry

16 A garden sprinkler system is set up to water a flower bed. The distance, d feet, the water sprays at time θ minutes can be modelled by the function $d = \sqrt{2}\cos\theta - 3\sin\theta$, where distance to the left of the sprinkler is modelled as negative and distance to the right of the sprinkler is modelled as positive.

MODELLING

a) Write $\sqrt{2}\cos\theta - 3\sin\theta$ in the form $R\cos(\theta + \alpha)$, where $R > 0$ and $0 \leq \alpha \leq \frac{\pi}{2}$.

(3 marks)

b) Find the times at which the water sprays 3 feet to the right of the sprinkler within the first 6 minutes after being switched on. Give your answers in minutes and seconds, to the nearest second.

PROBLEM SOLVING

(4 marks)

c) The distance (d) in feet that water is sprayed by an industrial sprinkler for a farmer's field is modelled by the function $d = (\sqrt{2}\cos\theta - 3\sin\theta)^4$. θ is the time in minutes.
Find the maximum distances to the left and right of this sprinkler that the water reaches.

PROBLEM SOLVING

(2 marks)

d) Give one possible explanation for the minimum distance found in part c) in the context of this model.

(1 mark)

17 Show that $2\tan A \operatorname{cosec} 2A \equiv 1 + 1\tan^2 A$.

(3 marks)

EXAM TIP

Be very careful with degrees and radians. If the question gives the range in radians, you must give your answer in radians, otherwise you'll lose marks. Make sure your calculator is set to radians when appropriate too. There are some bits of trig that you have to use radians for — like the small angle approximations and arc length and sector area. Better get used to them.

Score

88

Exponentials and Logarithms

Exponentials and logs might seem a bit tricky at first, but once you get used to them and they get used to you, you'll wonder what you ever worried about. Plus, they're really handy for modelling real-life situations.

1 Given that $p > 0$, what is the value of $\log_p(p^4) + \log_p(\sqrt{p}) - \log_p\left(\frac{1}{\sqrt{p}}\right)$? Circle your answer.

5 3 4 4.5

(1 mark)

2 Solve the equation $5^{(z^2 - 9)} = 2^{(z - 3)}$, giving your answers to 3 significant figures where appropriate.

Fully justify your answer. Solutions relying entirely on calculator methods are not acceptable.

....

(5 marks)

3 Solve the equation $3^{2x} - 9(3^x) + 14 = 0$, giving each solution to an appropriate degree of accuracy.

Fully justify your answer. Solutions relying entirely on calculator methods are not acceptable.

This should remind you of a quadratic equation...

....

(5 marks)

4 The curve with equation $y = \ln(4x - 3)$ is shown on the graph to the right.

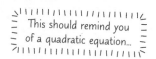

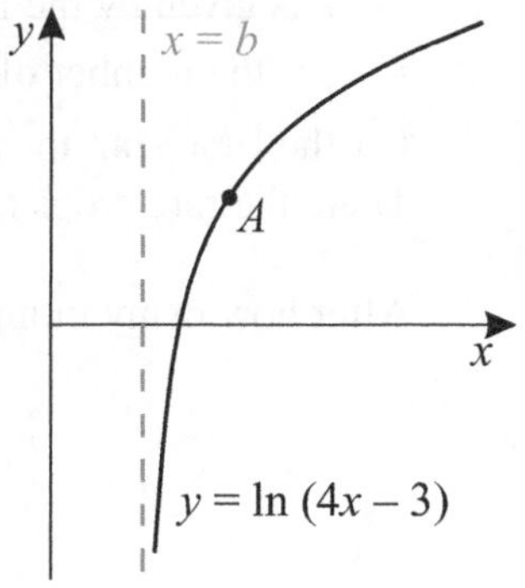

a) The point A with coordinate $(a, 1)$ lies on the curve.
Find a to 2 decimal places.

a = ...

(2 marks)

b) The curve only exists for $x > b$. State the value of b.

b = ...

(2 marks)

Exponentials and Logarithms

5 The curve below has equation $y = Ae^{bx}$.

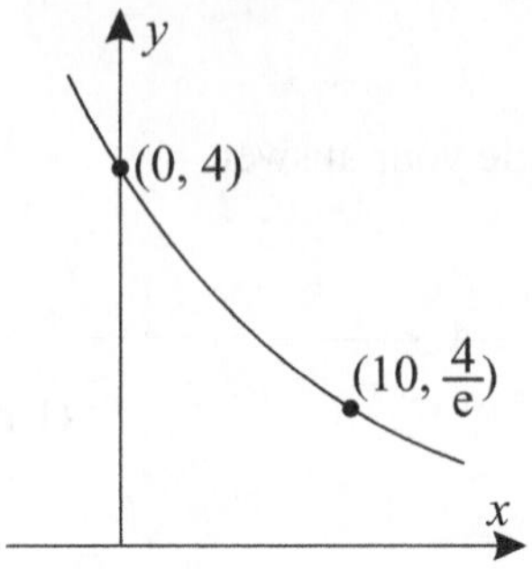

a) Find the values of A and b.

$A =$ .... $b =$ ....

(3 marks)

b) Find the exact coordinates of the point with gradient –1.

....

(5 marks)

6 The sketch on the right shows the function $y = e^{ax} + b$, where a and b are constants.

Find the values of a and b, and the equation of the asymptote shown on the sketch.

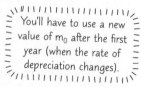

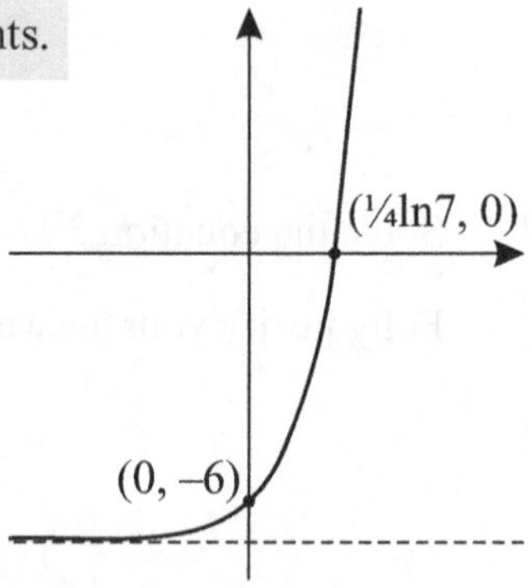

....

(4 marks)

7 Nadiya buys a motorbike for £8000.
The motorbike's value, £m, is modelled by the function $m = m_0e^{kt}$, where:

- m_0 is the initial value of the motorbike
- k is given by the formula $k = \frac{1}{12}\ln\left(1 - \frac{r}{100}\right)$, where r% is the rate of depreciation per year
- t is the number of months

For the first year, the motorbike depreciates by 8% per year.
Then, the rate drops to 4% per year for each subsequent year.

MODELLING

PROBLEM SOLVING

After how many months will the motorbike be worth less than half its original value?

You'll have to use a new value of m_0 after the first year (when the rate of depreciation changes).

....

(5 marks)

Exponentials and Logarithms

8 In 2010, a bird of prey species was introduced into a country.
The bird of prey hunts an endangered species of bird, as well as other animals.

- The population, P, of the endangered species is modelled by the equation $P = 5700e^{-0.15t}$.
- The population, Q, of the bird of prey is modelled by the equation $Q = 2100 - 1500e^{-0.15t}$.

Where $t \geq 0$ is time in years, and $t = 0$ represents the beginning of the year 2010.

MODELLING

a) Find the year in which the population of the bird of prey is first predicted to exceed the population of the endangered species according to these models.

....

(4 marks)

b) The graph showing the predicted population of the bird of prey is shown on the right. Add a curve to the graph to show the predicted population of the endangered species of bird over the same time period.

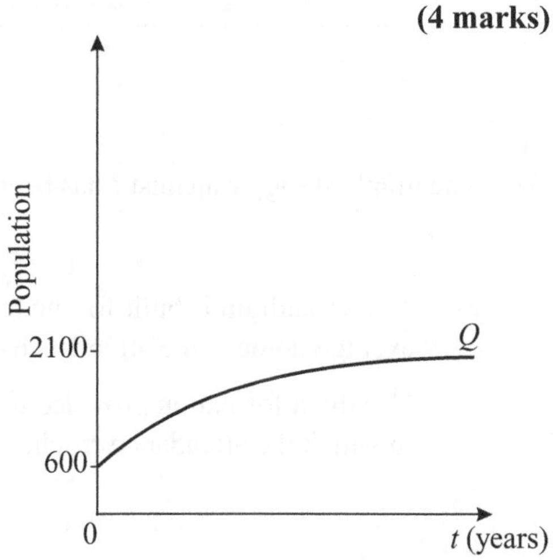

(2 marks)

c) Comment on the validity of each population model.

....

....

....

....

(2 marks)

d) Predict the year that the population of the endangered species will drop to below 1000.

....

(3 marks)

e) When this population drops below 1000, conservationists start enacting a plan to save the species. Suggest one refinement that could be made to the model to take this into account.

....

....

(1 mark)

Exponentials and Logarithms

9 The number of supporters of a local football team has tended to increase in recent years. The attendance can be modelled by an equation of the form $y = ab^t$, where y is the average home game attendance in hundreds, t is the number of years after the 2010/11 season, and a and b are constants to be determined.

a) Show that $y = ab^t$ can be written in the form $\log_{10}y = t\log_{10}b + \log_{10}a$.

(2 marks)

b) Interpret the value of a in the context of the model.

....

....

(1 mark)

The graph of $\log_{10}y$ against t has been plotted below. A line of best fit has been drawn on the graph.

c) A new stadium is built for the team when the average home game attendance exceeds 10 000.

Use the information provided to predict the season in which the attendance reaches this value.

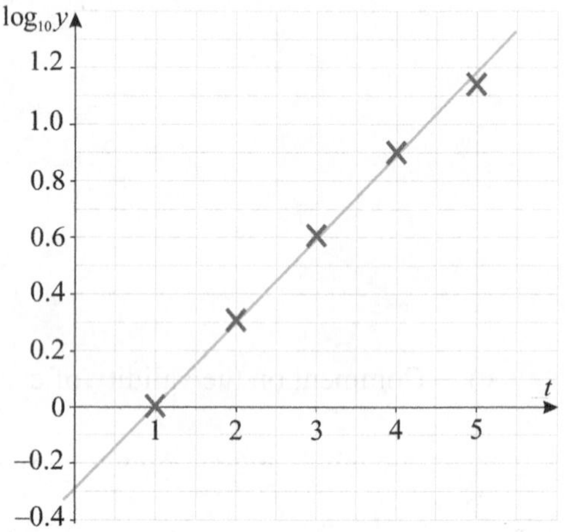

....

(5 marks)

d) Comment on the reliability of your answer from part c) in the context of this model.

....

....

(2 marks)

EXAM TIP

If you're asked to comment on the validity of models, or asked for limitations or refinements, think about anything that stops the model being realistic. For example, it might predict that a quantity will continue to rise until it becomes infinitely big, which might not be likely in a real-life situation — so you could refine the model by introducing an upper limit.

Score

54

Differentiation — 1

Differentiation can tell you all sorts of useful things about the gradient of a curve. The following questions use simple functions in powers of x — you'll find trickier functions in 'Differentiation 2'.

1 The curve C is given by the equation $y = 5x^2 - 4\sqrt{x} + 12$.

Find the gradient of the tangent to the curve at the point where $x = 4$. Circle your answer.

51 36 (39) 38

$y = 5x^2 - 4x^{\frac{1}{2}} + 12$

$\frac{dy}{dx} = 10x - 2x^{-\frac{1}{2}}$ When $x = 4$ $\frac{dy}{dx} = 39$

(1 mark)

2 The vertical displacement of a seabird from the sea's surface, y metres, at time t seconds is modelled by the equation $y = t^3 - 7t^2 + 8t + 9$. The vertical velocity of the seabird is given by $\frac{dy}{dt}$.

MODELLING

Use algebra to determine the times at which the seabird's vertical velocity is 0.

$\frac{dy}{dt} = 3t^2 - 14t + 8 = 0$ $S = -14$ $P = 24$ $-12, -2$

When $\frac{dy}{dt} = 0$ $3t^2 - 12t$ $-2t + 8$ $3t(t-4)$ $-2(t-4)$

$(3t - 2)(t - 4) = 0$ ....

$t = \frac{2}{3}$ $t = 4$

(3 marks)

3 A curve has equation $y = kx^2 - 8x - 5$, for a constant k. The point R lies on the curve and has an x-coordinate of 2. The normal to the curve at point R is parallel to the line with equation $4y + x = 24$.

PROBLEM SOLVING

a) Find the value of k.

$4y + x = 24$

$4y = 24 - x$

$y = 6 - \frac{1}{4}x$

grad of normal at R $= -\frac{1}{4}$ Grad tan $= 4$

$y = kx^2 - 8x - 5$

$\frac{dy}{dx} = 2kx - 8$ $4k - 8 = 4$

$x = 2$, $\frac{dy}{dx} = 4$ $4k = 12$ $k = 3$

$k =$ ....

(5 marks)

b) The tangent to the curve at R meets the curve $y = 4x - \frac{1}{x^3} - 9$ at the point S. Find the coordinates of S.

....

(5 marks)

Differentiation — 1

4 For $f(x) = 8x^2 - 1$, prove from first principles that $f'(x) = 16x$.

$y = 8x^2 - 1$

$\frac{dy}{dx} = 16x$

(4 marks)

5 The function $f(x) = 2x^4 + 27x$ has one stationary point.

a) Find the coordinates of the stationary point.

....

(4 marks)

b) Find the range of values of x for which the function is increasing and the range of values of x for which it is decreasing.

Increasing for: ...., decreasing for: ....

(2 marks)

c) Hence sketch the curve $y = f(x)$, showing where it crosses the axes and the position of its stationary point.

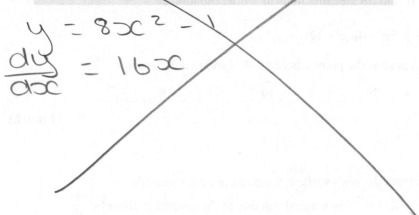

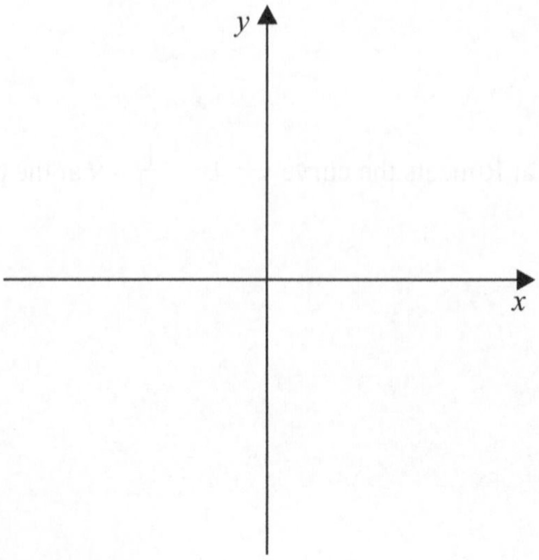

(3 marks)

Differentiation — 1

6 The diagram shows part of the graph of $y = x^4 + 3x^3 - 6x^2$.
Find the range of values of x for which the graph is concave.

Start by differentiating twice to find $\frac{d^2y}{dx^2}$.

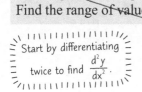

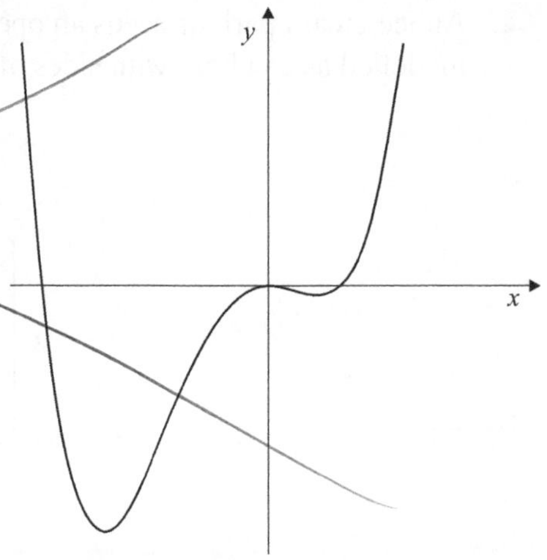

....

(4 marks)

7 The function $f(x) = 3x^3 + 9x^2 + 25x$ has one point of inflection.

a) Show that the point of inflection is at $x = -1$.

(5 marks)

b) Explain whether or not this point of inflection is a stationary point.

....

....

(2 marks)

c) Joe claims that the function $f(x) = 3x^3 + 9x^2 + 25x$ is an increasing function for all values of x.
Show that Joe is correct.

(2 marks)

Differentiation — 1

8 An ice cream parlour needs an open-top stainless steel container with a capacity of 40 litres, modelled as a cuboid with sides of length x cm, x cm and y cm, as shown in Figure 1.

MODELLING PROBLEM SOLVING

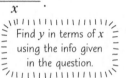

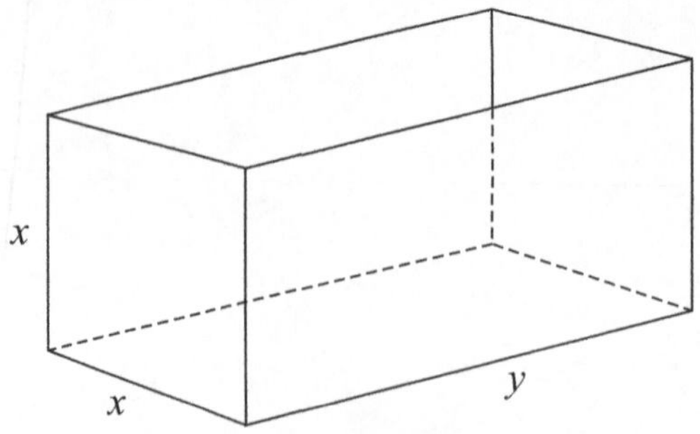

Figure 1

a) Show that the external surface area, A cm^2, of the container is given by $A = 2x^2 + \dfrac{120\,000}{x}$.

Find y in terms of x using the info given in the question.

(4 marks)

b) Find the value of x to 3 s.f. at which A is stationary, and show that this is a minimum value of A.

(6 marks)

c) Calculate the minimum area of stainless steel needed to make the container. Give your answer to 3 s.f.

.... cm^2

(2 marks)

d) Comment on the validity of this model.

....

....

(1 mark)

EXAM TIP

Remember, tangents have the same gradient as the curve and normals are perpendicular to the curve. To find stationary points, differentiate the expression and set equal to zero. And one more thing... $f''(x) > 0$ means the gradient is increasing (the curve is convex), $f''(x) < 0$ means the the gradient is decreasing (the curve is concave) and $f''(x) = 0$ at a point of inflection. Phew.

Score

53

Differentiation — 2

As promised, more differentiation. Make sure you use the correct rule for each type of function and you'll be fine.

1 Using algebraic differentiation, find $\frac{dy}{dx}$ at the given point for each of the following:

a) $y = \frac{1}{\sqrt{2x - x^2}}$, (1, 1)

....

(4 marks)

b) $x = (4y + 10)^3$, (8, –2)

....

(4 marks)

2 The diagram shows a container in the shape of a regular tetrahedron, which is being filled with water. After t minutes, the water in the container can be modelled as a regular tetrahedron with edge length a cm and vertical height x cm, and the volume of water in the container is V cm^3.

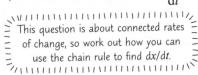

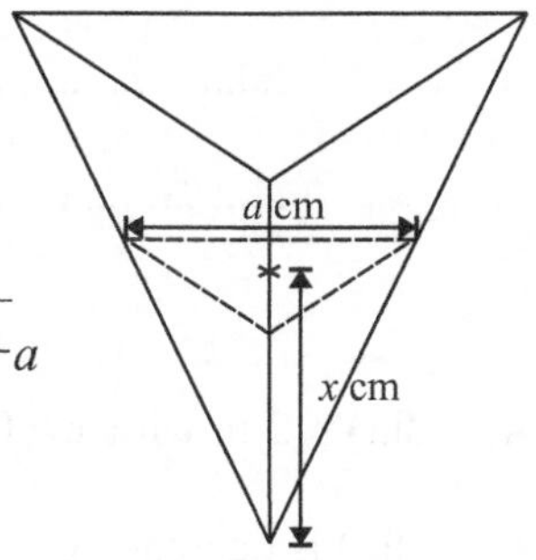

a) Given that a regular tetrahedron with edge length a has vertical height $h = \sqrt{\frac{2}{3}}a$ and volume $\frac{\sqrt{2}}{12}a^3$, show that the volume of water in the container after t minutes is given by $V = \frac{\sqrt{3}}{8}x^3$.

(2 marks)

Water is being poured into the container at a constant rate of 240 cm^3 min^{-1}.

b) Find the exact value of $\frac{dx}{dt}$ when the vertical height of the water in the container is 8 cm.

This question is about connected rates of change, so work out how you can use the chain rule to find dx/dt.

....

(5 marks)

The value of $\frac{dx}{dt}$ is measured when $x = 12$ and found to be $\frac{32}{9\sqrt{3}}$. This is less than the value expected if $\frac{dV}{dt} = 240$ cm^3 min^{-1}. It is discovered that water has been leaking out of the container at a constant rate.

c) Find $\frac{dV}{dt}$ if $\frac{dx}{dt} = \frac{32}{9\sqrt{3}}$ when $x = 12$.

....

(3 marks)

Differentiation — 2

3 A curve has the equation $y = e^{2x} - 5e^{x} + 3x$.

a) Find $\frac{dy}{dx}$.

....

(2 marks)

b) Show that the stationary points on the curve occur when $x = 0$ and $x = \ln \frac{3}{2}$.

(4 marks)

c) Determine the nature of each of the stationary points.

....

....

(3 marks)

4 $f(x) = 2 \ln x$ for $x > 0$. Which statement below is true? Circle your answer.

$f(x)$ is decreasing $f(x)$ is concave $f(x)$ is convex $f(x)$ has a point of inflection

(1 mark)

5 The shape of a canyon is modelled by the equation $y = \ln x\,(5x - 2)^3$, where $0.4 \leq x \leq 1$. y is the vertical displacement, in kilometres, and x is the horizontal displacement in kilometres.

MODELLING

a) Show that $\frac{dy}{dx} = (5x - 2)^2\left(a \ln x + b + \frac{c}{x}\right)$, where a, b and c are constants to be found.

(4 marks)

b) A bridge is built across the canyon. It meets one side of the canyon at $x = 0.9$ km, at a normal to the canyon's slope. Determine the gradient of the bridge at this point.

Gradient = ...

(2 marks)

Differentiation — 2

6 A curve has the equation $y = 4x^2 \ln x$, $x > 0$.

a) Determine an expression for $\frac{d^2y}{dx^2}$.

You need to use the product rule twice.

....

(4 marks)

b) Find the ranges of values of x for which the curve is concave and convex.

Concave for: ...., Convex for: ....

(4 marks)

7 What is the derivative of $\tan^2 x$? Circle your answer.

$2 \tan x \sec x$ $\tan^2 x \sec^2 x$ $2x \tan x \sec x$ $2 \tan x \sec^2 x$

(1 mark)

8 The diagram shows part of the curve $y = \frac{4x - 1}{\tan x}$, $0 < x < \pi$.

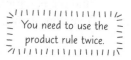

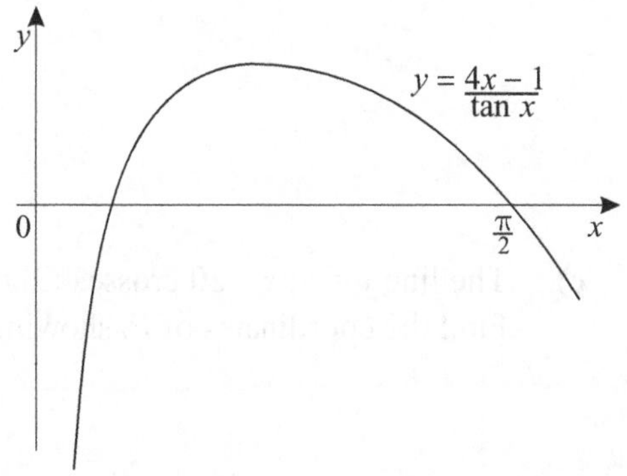

a) Show that an expression for $\frac{dy}{dx}$ is:

$$\frac{dy}{dx} = 4 \cot x - (4x - 1) \operatorname{cosec}^2 x$$

(3 marks)

b) The curve has a maximum in the range $0 < x < \frac{\pi}{2}$.
Show that at the maximum point, $2 \sin 2x - 4x + 1 = 0$.

(4 marks)

Differentiation — 2

9 A curve is defined by the parametric equations $x = t^2 + 1$, $y = t^3 + 2t$.

Find the equation of the tangent to the curve at the point where $t = 1$.
Give your answer in the form $y = mx + c$.

....

(5 marks)

10 The curve C is defined by the parametric equations $x = \frac{\sin\theta}{2} - 3$, $y = 5 - \cos 2\theta$.

a) Find an expression for $\frac{dy}{dx}$ in terms of θ.

....

(2 marks)

b) Hence find the equation of the tangent to C at the point where $\theta = \frac{\pi}{6}$.
Give your answer in the form $ax + by + c = 0$.

....

(3 marks)

c) The line $y = -8x - 20$ crosses C at point P.
Find the coordinates of P, showing your working clearly. PROBLEM SOLVING

....

(6 marks)

d) Find a Cartesian equation for C in the form $y = f(x)$.

....

(3 marks)

Differentiation — 2

11 For $y = \cos^{-1} x$, show that $\frac{dy}{dx} = -\frac{1}{\sqrt{1-x^2}}$.

(4 marks)

12 A curve has the equation $x^3 + x^2y = y^2 - 1$.

PROBLEM SOLVING

a) Find an expression for $\frac{dy}{dx}$.

....

(4 marks)

The points P and Q lie on the curve. P has coordinates $(1, a)$ and Q has coordinates $(1, b)$.

b) Find the values of a and b, given that $a > b$.

....

(2 marks)

c) Find the equation of the normal to the curve at Q.
Give your answer in the form $y = mx + c$.

....

(3 marks)

Differentiation — 2

13 The curve C is given by the equation $y^2 - 6xy + 9y + 2x = 7 - 9x^2$.

PROBLEM SOLVING

a) Find an expression for $\frac{dy}{dx}$.

....

(3 marks)

b) There is a vertical tangent to the curve C. Use your answer to part a) to determine the equation of the vertical tangent to the curve.

The vertical tangent here will occur at the point when dy/dx is undefined.

....

(3 marks)

14 A curve has the equation $\sin \pi x - \cos\left(\frac{\pi y}{2}\right) = 0.5$, for $0 \le x \le 2$, $0 \le y \le 2$.

Find the coordinates of the stationary point on this curve.

....

(7 marks)

EXAM TIP

Differentiation questions can get quite tricky. First of all, make sure you're using the correct rule, then set out your working clearly and take care when you're simplifying expressions. The actual differentiation is often just the first step in answering a question. So after you've done all that hard work, make sure you interpret your answer correctly to find what you're asked for.

Score

95

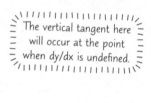

Integration — 1

Integration starts off pretty easy, but then gets really hard really quickly. Just keep your wits about you, and watch out for places where you can use clever tricks (like when the numerator is the derivative of the denominator).

1 Find $\int\left(2\sqrt{x}+\frac{1}{x^3}\right)\mathrm{d}x$. Circle your answer.

$\frac{1}{\sqrt{x}}-\frac{3}{x^4}+C$ $\quad\frac{3}{2}\sqrt[3]{x^2}-\frac{1}{2x^4}+C$ $\quad\frac{3}{4}\sqrt{x^3}-\frac{2}{x^2}+C$ $\quad\frac{4}{3}\sqrt{x^3}-\frac{1}{2x^2}+C$

(1 mark)

2 Given that $y=\frac{x^2+3}{\sqrt[3]{x}}$, find $\int y^2\,\mathrm{d}x$.

....

(4 marks)

3 The curve C has the equation $y=\mathrm{f}(x)$, $x>0$. $\mathrm{f}'(x)$ is given as $2x+5\sqrt{x}+\frac{6}{x^2}$.

A point P on curve C has the coordinates (3, 7). Find $\mathrm{f}(x)$, giving your answer in its simplest form.

....

(6 marks)

4 Region A is bounded by the curve $y=\frac{2}{\sqrt{x^3}}$ $(x>0)$, the x-axis and the lines $x=2$ and $x=4$. PROBLEM SOLVING

Show that the area of A is $2\sqrt{2}-2$.

(5 marks)

Integration — 1

5 Evaluate $\int_{p}^{4p}\left(\frac{1}{\sqrt{x}} - 4x^3\right) dx$, where $p > 0$, leaving your answer in terms of p.

....

(4 marks)

6 The curve $y = 2x^3 - 3x^2 - 11x + 6$ is shown below. It crosses the x-axis at $(-2, 0)$, $(0.5, 0)$ and $(3, 0)$.

Using algebraic integration, find the area of the shaded region bounded by the curve, the x-axis and the lines $x = -1$ and $x = 2$.

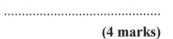

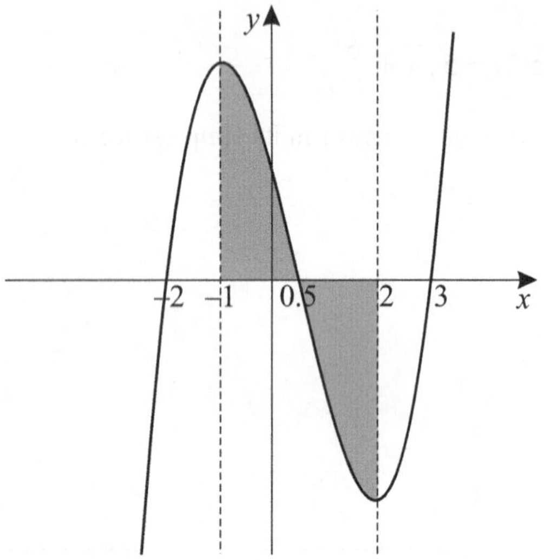

....

(6 marks)

7 Find the possible values of k that satisfy $\int_{\sqrt{2}}^{2}(8x^3 - 2kx)\, dx = 2k^2$, where k is a constant.

PROBLEM SOLVING

....

(5 marks)

Integration — 1

8 The graph on the right shows part of a curve with equation $y = \dfrac{2}{3(\sqrt[3]{5x-2})}$.

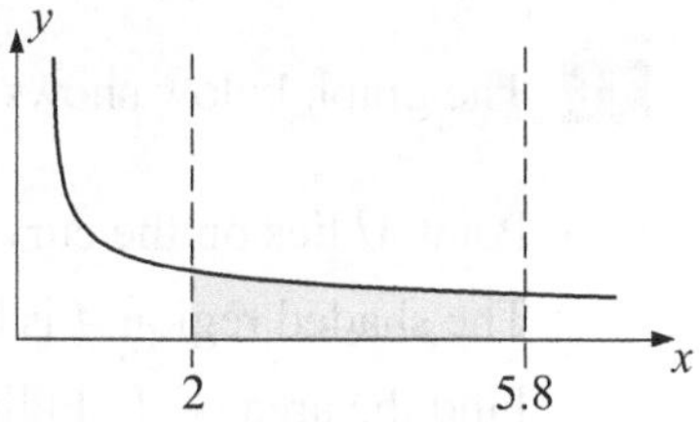

Find the exact area of the shaded region bounded by the curve, the x-axis, and the lines $x = 2$ and $x = 5.8$. Fully justify your answer.

....

(4 marks)

9 The graph on the right shows the curves $y = \dfrac{8}{x^2}$ and $y = 9 - x^2$ for $x, y \geq 0$.

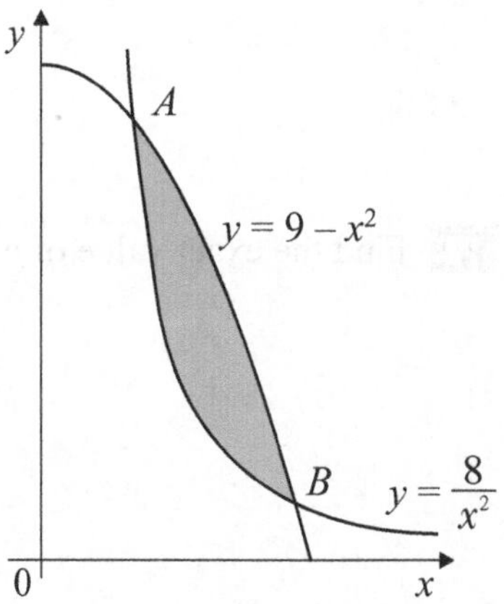

a) Show that the shaded area can be given by $\int_m^n \mathrm{f}(x)\,\mathrm{d}x$, where m and n are constants to be found and $\mathrm{f}(x)$ is a function of x.

(4 marks)

b) Hence show that the shaded area can be written in the form $a + b\sqrt{2}$, where a and b are fractions.

(4 marks)

10 Jason wants to work out the area between the curves $y = x^2 + 2$ and $y = x^3 - 2x + 2$ which intersect at (0, 2) and (2, 5). What calculation should he do? Circle your answer.

$\int_0^2 (2x + x^2 - x^3)\,\mathrm{d}x$ $\quad$ $\int_0^2 (x^3 - x^2 - 2x)\,\mathrm{d}x$ $\quad$ $\int_0^2 (x^3 + x^2 - 2x + 4)\,\mathrm{d}x$ $\quad$ $\int_0^2 (x^2 - x^3 - 4)\,\mathrm{d}x$

(1 mark)

Integration — 1

11 The graph below shows the curve C, which has equation $y = \sqrt{x} - \frac{1}{2}x^2 + 1\ (x \geq 0)$.

PROBLEM SOLVING

Point M lies on the curve and has coordinates $\left(1, \frac{3}{2}\right)$, and line N is the normal to the curve at point M.
The shaded region A is bounded by the y-axis, the curve and the normal to the curve at M.
Find the area of A. Fully justify your answer.

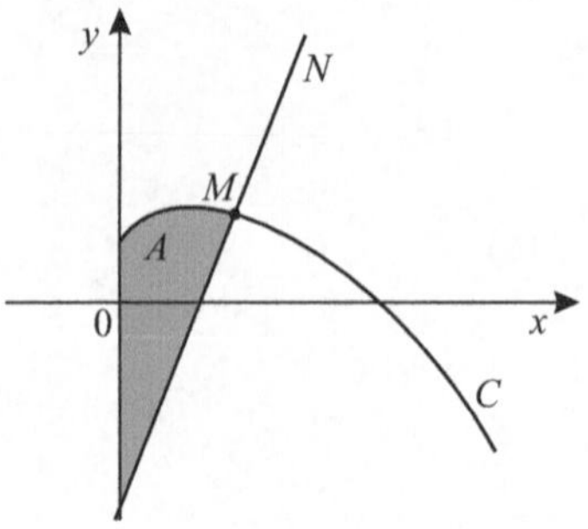

....

(7 marks)

12 Find the exact value of p given that $\int_{2p}^{6p} \frac{x^3 + 4x^2}{x^3}\,dx = 4 \ln 12$.

PROBLEM SOLVING

$p =$ ....

(4 marks)

13 A function is defined as $g(x) = \dfrac{4x - 10}{4x^2 + 4x - 3}$.

a) Write $g(x)$ in the form $\dfrac{A}{Cx + D} + \dfrac{B}{Ex + F}$, where A to F are constants to be found.

....

(4 marks)

b) Hence find $\int_{-1}^{0} g(x)\,dx$. Give your answer in the form $\ln k$, where k is an integer.

....

(3 marks)

EXAM TIP

Make sure you're completely happy with integrating powers — including the ones that give you a natural log (ln) when you integrate. It's usually best to write roots and fractions as powers of x — it makes it much easier to integrate (and means you're less likely to make a mistake). To find tricky areas, try splitting them into different bits and finding each bit separately.

Score

62

Integration — 2

As is typical with Hollywood blockbusters, after the box office success of Integration 1, here comes the sequel — Integration 2: Integration With A Vengeance. Just remember, in calculus, no one can hear you scream...

1 Use algebraic integration to find the exact value of $\int_{\frac{\pi}{12}}^{\frac{\pi}{8}} \sin 2x \, dx$.

....

(3 marks)

2 $f(x) = \sec^2 x \, e^{\tan x}$ is defined for $-\frac{\pi}{2} < x < \frac{\pi}{2}$.

a) Find $\int f(x) \, dx$.

....

(2 marks)

b) Show that $\int_0^{\frac{\pi}{3}} \left(f(x) + 3\tan^2\left(\frac{x}{2}\right) + 3 \right) dx$ can be written in the form $e^{\sqrt{3}} + a\sqrt{3} + b$, where a and b are constants to be found.

PROBLEM SOLVING

(5 marks)

3 Using the substitution $u = \ln x$, find $\int_1^2 \left(\frac{\ln x}{\sqrt{x}} \right)^2 dx$ to 3 significant figures. Fully justify your answer.

Don't forget to change the limits of integration when you make the substitution.

....

(5 marks)

Integration — 2

4 Oded calculates the value of $\int_{\sqrt{2}}^{2} 4x(x^2 - 2)^4 \, dx$ using the substitution $u = x^2 - 2$.

What are the limits he should use after making the substitution? Circle your answer.

$\sqrt{2}$ and 2 -2 and 2   0 and 2 $\sqrt{2}$ and $\sqrt{6}$

(1 mark)

5 The diagram to the right shows the graph of $y = \frac{x}{1 - x^2}$, for $0 \le x < 1$.

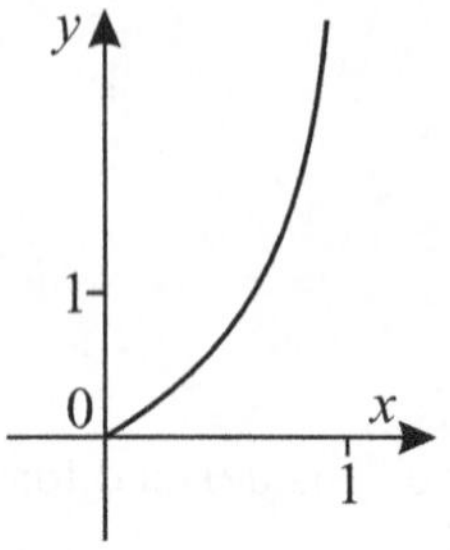

a) Find $\int \frac{x}{1 - x^2} \, dx$ using the substitution $x = \sin \theta$.

....

(6 marks)

b) Hence show that the area bounded by the graphs of $y = \frac{x}{1 - x^2}$, $y = -x^2 + 2$, the y-axis and the line $x = \frac{1}{2}$ is $\ln \frac{\sqrt{3}}{2} + \frac{23}{24}$.

(4 marks)

6 The graph to the right shows the curve C, which has parametric equations $x = -2 \cos t$ and $y = 3 \cos t \sin t$ (for $t \ge 0$). The shaded region A is bounded by the curve C and the x-axis.

PROBLEM SOLVING

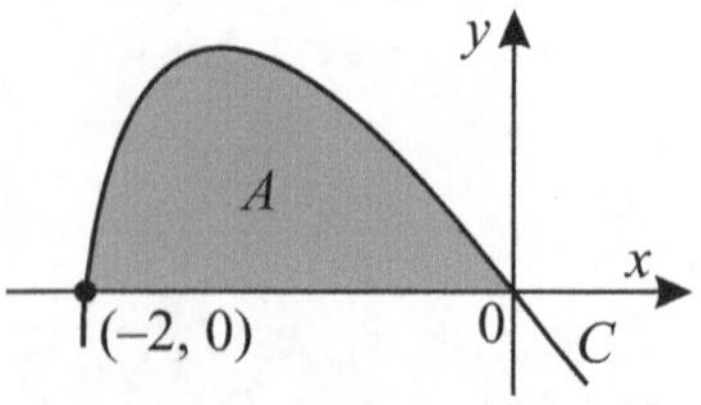

Use algebraic integration to find the area of A.

Use the chain rule to integrate parametric equations — and don't forget to change the limits.

....

(6 marks)

Integration — 2

7 The rate at which water flows into a container is modelled as $4te^{-2t}$ ml s^{-1}, where $t \geq 0$ is the time in seconds.

PROBLEM SOLVING MODELLING

a) Find an expression for the total amount of water that has flowed into the container after x seconds. Give your answer in its simplest form.

Use integration by parts for questions 7 and 8.

....

(5 marks)

After 6 seconds the container is sealed so that no more water can flow in.

b) Determine exactly how much more water flowed into the container during the first second than after it.

....

(2 marks)

8 Calculate the exact value of $\int_1^4 \frac{\ln x}{2x^2}\, dx$. Fully justify your answer.

....

(6 marks)

Integration — 2

9 An ecologist is monitoring the population of newts in a colony. The rate of increase of the population is directly proportional to the square root of the current number of newts in the colony. When there were 36 newts in the colony, the rate of change was calculated to be 0.36.

MODELLING

a) Formulate a differential equation to model the rate of change, in terms of the variables N (number of newts), t (time in weeks).

....

(4 marks)

b) After more research, the ecologist decides that the differential equation $\frac{dN}{dt} = \frac{kN}{\sqrt{t}}$, for a positive constant k, is a better model for the population.
When the ecologist began the survey, the initial population of newts in the colony was 25.

(i) Solve the differential equation, leaving your answer in terms of k and t.

....

(3 marks)

(ii) Given that the value of k is 0.05, calculate how long (to the nearest week) it will take for the population to double.

....

(3 marks)

10 A supermarket sets up an advertising campaign to increase sales on the cheese counter. After the start of the campaign, the number of kilograms of cheese sold each day, S, increases over time, t days. The increase in sales is modelled by the differential equation $\frac{dS}{dt} = k\sqrt{S}$ $(k > 0)$.

MODELLING

a) At the start of the campaign, the supermarket was selling 81 kg of cheese a day. Use this information to solve the differential equation, giving S in terms of k and t.

....

(3 marks)

b) Given that $\frac{dS}{dt} = 18$ at the start of the campaign, calculate the number of kg sold on the fifth day after the start of the campaign ($t = 5$).

....

(3 marks)

c) How many days will it take before the sales reach 225 kg a day? PROBLEM SOLVING

....

(2 marks)

Integration — 2

11 A solid hemisphere of radius r cm and surface area S cm^2 is decreasing in size.

a) The rate of decrease of r, over time t minutes, is directly proportional to rt.

(i) Formulate a differential equation in terms of r, t and a positive constant k.

....

(2 marks)

(ii) Show that $\frac{dS}{dt} = -2ktS$.

(4 marks)

b) The total surface area of the hemisphere is 200 cm^2 at time $t = 10$ minutes and 50 cm^2 at time $t = 30$ mins.

(i) Find the particular solution of the equation $\frac{dS}{dt} = -2ktS$.
Give the values of any constants to 3 significant figures.

....

(5 marks)

(ii) Hence find the initial surface area of the hemisphere to 3 significant figures.

....

(1 mark)

c) A solid sphere with the same initial radius as the hemisphere is also decreasing in size. Maddy decides to use the differential equation given in part a) (ii) to model the surface area of the sphere. Explain why this will not be appropriate.

PROBLEM SOLVING

....

....

(1 mark)

EXAM TIP

Does your brain hurt? Mine does. You're given the formula for integration by parts in the formula booklet, so you can always look it up if you're struggling to remember it — but make sure you know exactly how to use it. Questions on differential equations can look pretty nasty, but once you've separated the variables, it shouldn't be too hard to integrate each side.

Score

76

Numerical Methods

There are two main parts to numerical methods — finding roots using iteration (including my personal favourite, the Newton-Raphson method) and numerical integration (which is also pretty darn exciting if you ask me).

1 Circle the interval in which the graph of $y = x^6 - 4x^5 - 3x^3 - 2x + 3$ has a root.

$-0.5 < x < 0$ $\quad$ $0 < x < 0.5$ $\quad$ $0.5 < x < 1.0$ $\quad$ $1.0 < x < 1.5$

(1 mark)

2 The graph below shows the function $f(x) = 4(x^2 - 1)$, $x \geq 0$, and its inverse function $f^{-1}(x)$.

a) By finding an expression for $f^{-1}(x)$ and considering how the graphs are related, show that $\sqrt{\frac{x}{4} + 1} - x = 0$ at the point where the graphs meet.

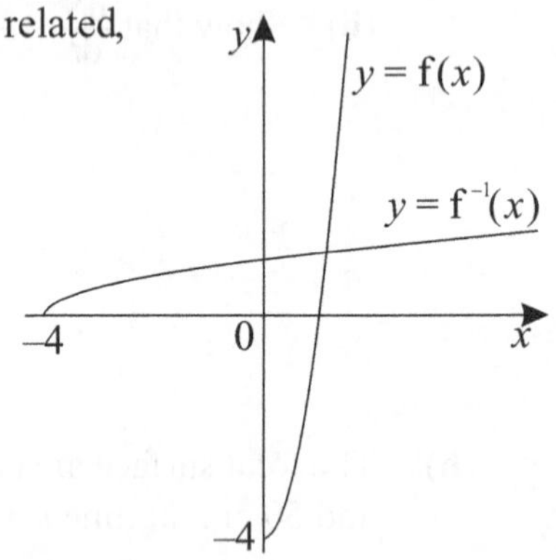

(4 marks)

b) Show that the equation $\sqrt{\frac{x}{4} + 1} - x = 0$ has a root in the interval $1 < x < 2$.

(2 marks)

c) Starting with $x_0 = 1$, use the iteration formula:

$$x_{n+1} = \sqrt{\frac{x_n}{4} + 1}$$

to find x_4 to 3 significant figures as an approximation for the x-coordinate of the point of intersection.

....

(3 marks)

d) Does the equation from part a) have any other roots? Explain your answer.

Look at the graph above...

....

....

(1 mark)

Numerical Methods

3 The sketch below shows the intersection of the curve $y = 6^x$ with the line $y = x + 2$ at the point P.

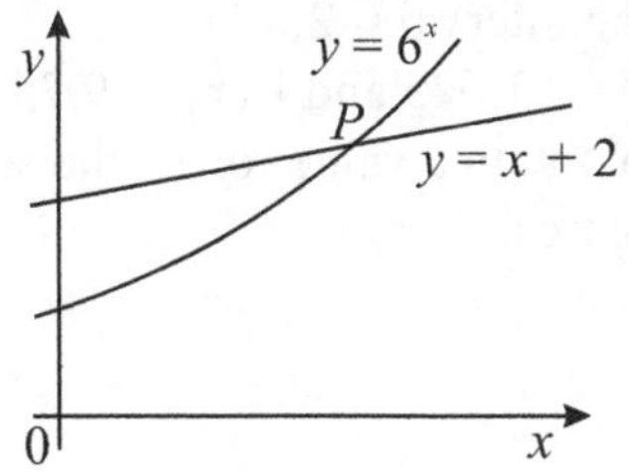

a) Show that a root of the equation $6^x - x - 2 = 0$ lies in the interval [0.5, 1].

(2 marks)

b) Show that the Newton-Raphson iteration formula for finding the x-coordinate of P can be written as:

$$x_{n+1} = \frac{6^{x_n}(x_n \ln 6 - 1) + 2}{6^{x_n} \ln 6 - 1}$$

Remember — the derivative of a^x is $a^x \ln a$.

(4 marks)

c) Using the Newton-Raphson formula with a starting value of $x_0 = 0.5$, find x_3 to 4 significant figures as an approximation for the x-coordinate of P.

....

(2 marks)

d) By considering an appropriate interval, verify that this value is accurate to 4 significant figures.

(3 marks)

e) k is chosen as a different starting value. The gradient of the tangent at $x = k$ is 0. Explain why the Newton-Raphson method will fail for this starting value.

....

....

(1 mark)

Numerical Methods

4 $f(x) = x^3 - x^2 + 4$

a) The equation $f(x) = 0$ has a root in the interval $(-2, -1)$.
For the starting value $x_0 = -1.5$, $f(x_0) = -1.625$ and $f'(x_0) = 9.75$.
Use the Newton-Raphson method to obtain a value for x_1, the second approximation for the root.
Give your answer to 4 significant figures.

....

(2 marks)

b) Show that the root, $b = -1.315$, is correct to 4 significant figures.

(3 marks)

c) Explain why the Newton-Raphson method fails when $x_0 = \frac{2}{3}$. PROBLEM SOLVING

....

....

(2 marks)

5 The diagram on the right shows the graph of $y = 2^{x^2}$.

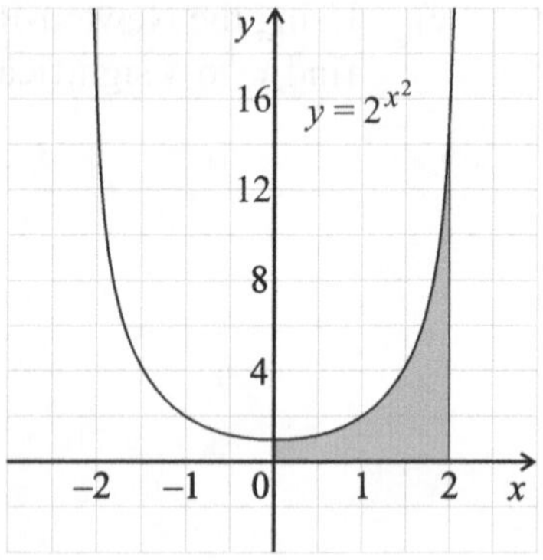

a) Use the trapezium rule with 4 intervals to find an estimate for the area of the region bounded by the axes, the curve and the line $x = 2$.
Give your answer to 3 significant figures.

....

(4 marks)

b) Given that the curve is convex for all values of x, explain whether the estimate in a) is an overestimate or an underestimate.

....

....

(1 mark)

c) Suggest one way to find a more accurate estimate for this area using the trapezium rule.

....

....

(1 mark)

Numerical Methods

6 Figure 1 shows the graph of $y = x \sin x$. The region R is bounded by the curve and the x-axis ($0 \le x \le \pi$).

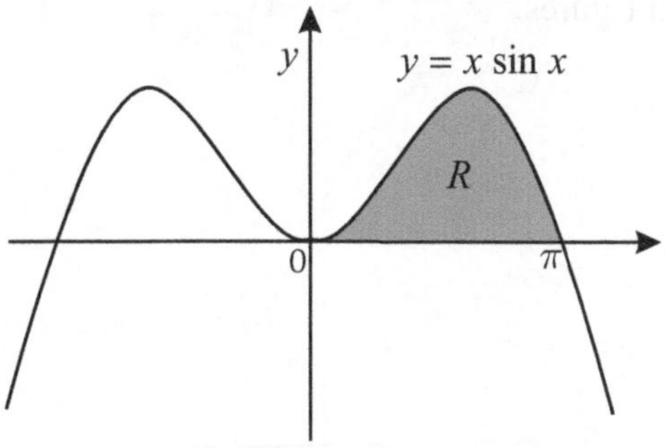

Figure 1

a) Fill in the missing values of y in the table below.
Give your answers to 5 significant figures.

x	0	$\frac{\pi}{4}$	$\frac{\pi}{2}$	$\frac{3\pi}{4}$	π
y	0	0.55536			0

(1 mark)

b) Hence find an approximation for the area of R, using the trapezium rule and all the values in the table.
Give your answer to 4 significant figures.

....

(3 marks)

c) Find the exact area of R using integration by parts.

....

(6 marks)

d) Hence find the percentage error of the approximation found in part b).
Give your answer to 2 significant figures.

Leave the answer from part b) in your calculator to get a more accurate value.

....

(2 marks)

Numerical Methods

7 Use the trapezium rule with 6 ordinates to estimate $\int_{1.5}^{4}(3x-\sqrt{2^x})\,dx$.
Give your answer to 4 significant figures.

PROBLEM SOLVING

....

(4 marks)

8 The graph below shows the curve $y = \frac{3\ln x}{x^2}$, $x > 0$.
The shaded region R is bounded by the curve, the line $x = 2.5$ and the line $x = 3$.

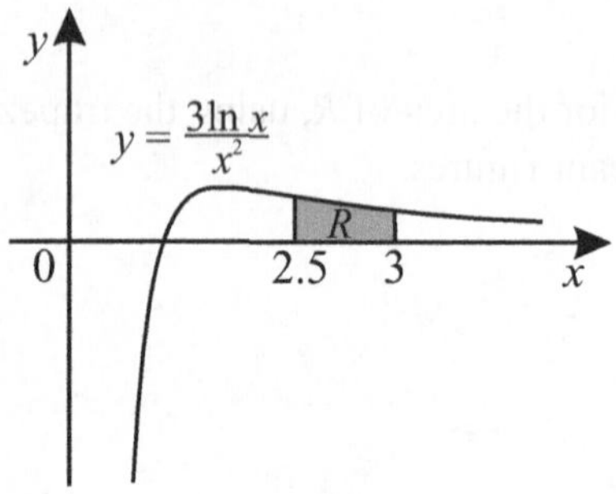

a) Find an approximation for the area of R, using the trapezium rule with 5 intervals.
Give your answer to 4 significant figures.

....

(4 marks)

b) By considering the areas of appropriate rectangles, show that the area of R is 0.2, correct to 1 decimal place.

PROBLEM SOLVING

You need one rectangle that sits above the curve and one that sits below it.

(3 marks)

EXAM TIP

A bit of calculator wizardry can save a lot of time in the exam — especially for iteration questions. Put in your starting value of x and press =, then input the rest of your iteration equation (or Newton-Raphson formula) in terms of ANS. Each time you press =, you'll get the next value of x (without having to type out the full formula each time). What a lifesaver.

Score

59

Vectors

Aaah, good old dependable vectors. They've got a certain magnitude about them, and they always have a clear direction. Much like an inspirational leader. It's kind of how I see myself after I've brought about the revolution.

1 A speedboat is attempting to travel due south-east at a speed of $4\sqrt{2}$ ms^{-1}. At the same time, an ocean current moves the boat north at 7 ms^{-1}.

MODELLING

Find the resultant velocity vector of the boat in terms of **i** and **j**, where **i** and **j** are unit vectors pointing east and north respectively. Circle your answer.

(4**i** + 3**j**) ms^{-1} (4**i** – 3**j**) ms^{-1} (4**i** + 4**j**) ms^{-1} (4**i** – 4**j**) ms^{-1}

(1 mark)

2 Points X and Y have position vectors 5**i** – 2**j** – 6**k** and 2**i** – **j** + 3**k** respectively. Find the exact magnitude of $\overrightarrow{XY}$. Circle your answer.

$\sqrt{27}$ $\sqrt{73}$ $\sqrt{91}$ $\sqrt{99}$

(1 mark)

3 Points A, B and C have position vectors –**i** + 7**j** – 2**k**, 5**i** – 3**j** + 6**k** and 5**i** + 4**j** + 3**k** respectively. M is the midpoint of AB.

Find the exact value of k such that $|\overrightarrow{CM}| = k\,|\overrightarrow{AB}|$.

k = ...

(5 marks)

4 Given that $\overrightarrow{OA} = -2\mathbf{i} + 4\mathbf{j} - 5\mathbf{k}$, $\overrightarrow{OB} = 14\mathbf{i} + 12\mathbf{j} - 9\mathbf{k}$ and $\overrightarrow{OC} = 2\mathbf{i} + \mu\mathbf{j} + \lambda\mathbf{k}$, find the values of μ and λ such that points A, B and C are collinear.

PROBLEM SOLVING

μ = ... λ = ...

(5 marks)

Vectors

5 Points A, B and C have position vectors $\begin{pmatrix} 1 \\ -3 \\ 2 \end{pmatrix}$, $\begin{pmatrix} 4 \\ -12 \\ 8 \end{pmatrix}$ and $\begin{pmatrix} -3 \\ 9 \\ -6 \end{pmatrix}$ respectively.

PROBLEM SOLVING

Point D lies on AB such that $AD:DB = 2:1$.

Point E is positioned such that $\overrightarrow{OD} = -\frac{1}{2}\overrightarrow{CE}$.

Find the position vector of point E.

Don't get overwhelmed by the amount of information in the question — start with a sketch, then see if you can work out any unknown vectors mentioned in the question.

....

(5 marks)

6 Figure 1 shows a sketch of a parallelogram, $PQRS$. Given that $\overrightarrow{PR} = \begin{pmatrix} 2 \\ -9 \\ 3 \end{pmatrix}$ and $\overrightarrow{PQ} = \begin{pmatrix} -14 \\ -6 \\ -7 \end{pmatrix}$, find the angle $\angle RPS$. Give your answer in degrees to 1 decimal place.

PROBLEM SOLVING

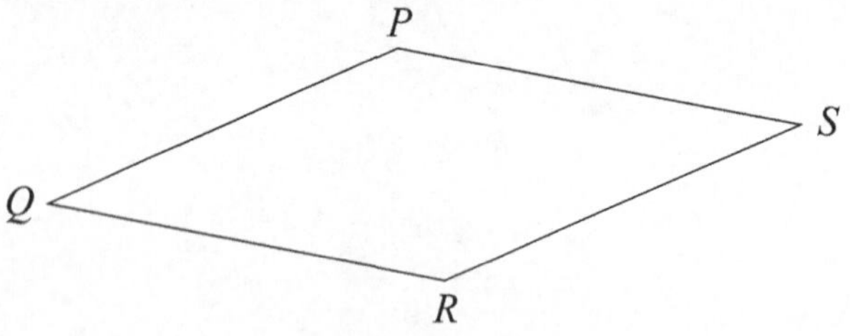

Figure 1

$\angle RPS$ = ... °

(5 marks)

Vectors

7 Two drones, A and B, take off from a launch pad at origin O and follow a series of movements based on the vectors $\mathbf{a} = (4\mathbf{i} + 6\mathbf{j} + 5\mathbf{k})$ metres, $\mathbf{b} = (-\mathbf{i} - 2\mathbf{j} - 2\mathbf{k})$ metres and $\mathbf{c} = (-3\mathbf{j} + \mathbf{k})$ metres, where $\mathbf{i}$ and $\mathbf{j}$ are horizontal unit vectors and $\mathbf{k}$ is a vertical unit vector with the upwards direction being positive.

MODELLING

Drone A follows the vectors $\mathbf{a}$, then $\mathbf{b}$, then $\mathbf{c}$, and then maintains its final position.
Drone B follows the vectors $2\mathbf{a}$, then $\mathbf{b}$, then $-3\mathbf{c}$, and then maintains its final position.

a) Calculate to 3 s.f. the distance between the final positions of drones A and B.

.... m

(4 marks)

b) Drone A now moves in a straight line to a position exactly 2 m directly below drone B. Find the vector that describes this movement of drone A.

....

(2 marks)

c) To maintain contact with the controller on the ground, drone B must always stay within 50 m of the origin O. How far can drone B move in the positive $\mathbf{j}$ direction from its current position before it passes out of range? Give your answer to 3 s.f.

PROBLEM SOLVING

.... m

(5 marks)

EXAM TIP

Fun, fun, fun, vectors are just pure fun, don't you think... ... ... Well anyway, make sure you're comfortable finding their magnitudes and using trig to find angles. Don't be put off by 3D ones — they're generally pretty much the same as their 2D counterparts. Some questions can be quite involved, but always start with a sketch, take it step by step and you'll be OK.

Score

33

Data Presentation and Interpretation

As I am sure you will agree, the only thing more exciting than presenting data is interpreting it. This is exactly the kind of topic where the examiners will test your large data set skills, so take another look at those spreadsheets.

1 Justin is researching the mean carbon dioxide emissions from vehicles registered in the North West. He takes a sample of the vehicles from the large data set and calculates the mean of his sample, $\overline{e}$, to be 135.625 g/km.

MODELLING

Given that $\sum e = 1085$ g/km, work out the number of data values in Justin's sample. Circle your answer.

14 8 9 7

(1 mark)

2 A group of 10 friends play a round of mini-golf and record their scores, x. It is given that $\sum x = 500$ and $\sum x^2 = 25\,622$.

MODELLING

a) Find the mean and the standard deviation for the data.

mean = ..., standard deviation = ...

(3 marks)

b) Another friend wants to incorporate his score of 50. Giving reasons, but without further calculation, explain the effect of adding this score on:
(i) the mean,

....

....

(2 marks)

(ii) the standard deviation.

....

....

(2 marks)

3 Morwenna groups the vehicles in the large data set by both the make of vehicle and the region in which the owner lives to create 15 groups (BMW-London, BMW-South West, BMW-North West, Ford-London, ... etc.). She calculates the mean mass, m kg, of the vehicles in each group. The results are shown in the table below.

Mean mass (m kg)	$1200 \leq m < 1300$	$1300 \leq m < 1350$	$1350 \leq m < 1400$	$1400 \leq m < 1500$	$1500 \leq m < 1700$
Frequency	1	4	4	3	3

Morwenna draws a histogram to represent the data.
The bar for the $1300 \leq m < 1350$ class has a width of 1.25 cm and a height of 8 cm.

MODELLING

Find the width and height, in centimetres, of the bar for the $1500 \leq m < 1700$ class.

width = ... cm, height = ... cm

(3 marks)

Data Presentation and Interpretation

4 The sales figures, x, for a gift shop over a 12-week period are shown below. MODELLING

Week	1	2	3	4	5	6	7	8	9	10	11	12
Sales, x (£'000s)	5.5	4.2	5.8	9.1	3.8	4.6	6.4	6.2	4.9	5.9	6.0	4.1

a) Find the median and quartiles of the sales data.

median = £ ...., lower quartile = £ ...., upper quartile = £ ....

(3 marks)

The shop's manager is considering excluding any outliers from his analysis of the data, to get a more realistic idea of how the shop is performing.

He decides to define outliers as values satisfying either of the following conditions:

- below $Q_1 - 1.5 \times (Q_3 - Q_1)$
- above $Q_3 + 1.5 \times (Q_3 - Q_1)$.

b) Identify any outliers in the data. Show your working.

....

(2 marks)

c) Do you think the manager should include any outliers in his analysis? Explain your answer.

....

....

(1 mark)

d) The mean and standard deviation for this sales data are calculated to be: mean = £5540, standard deviation = £1370 (both to 3 s.f.). Do you think these two measures, or the median and interquartile range, are more useful measures of location and spread for this data? Explain your answer.

....

....

(2 marks)

The manager breaks the sales figures down into 'jewellery' and 'other gifts' and displays his results on the chart on the right.

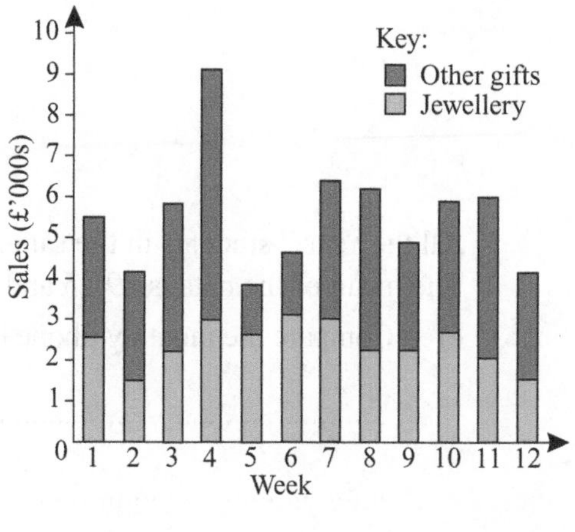

e) There was a two-week special offer on jewellery during the 12-week period. Which two weeks of sales figures correspond to this special-offer period? Explain your answer.

....

....

....

....

(2 marks)

Data Presentation and Interpretation

5 All the Year 12 students in a school were asked how much their monthly phone bill is (in £). The histogram below shows the results.

MODELLING

a) Use the histogram to complete the table below.

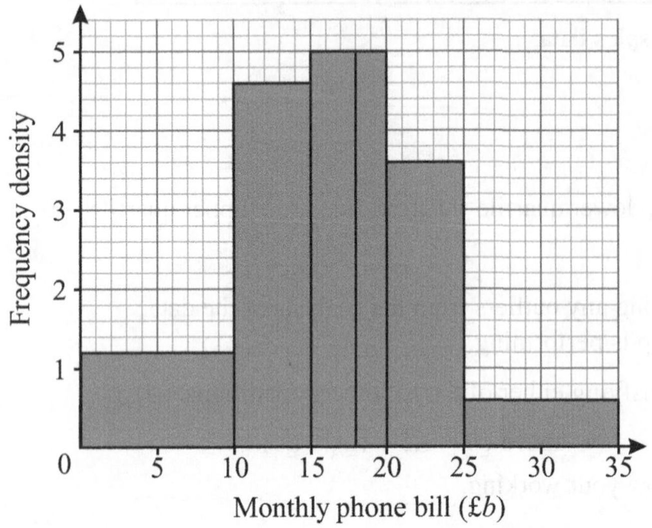

Monthly phone bill, £b	Frequency
$0 \leq b < 10$	12
$10 \leq b < 15$	23
$15 \leq b < 18$	
$18 \leq b < 20$	
$20 \leq b < 25$	18
$25 \leq b < 35$	6

(2 marks)

b) Estimate the number of students that have a monthly phone bill of between £12.50 and £17.50.

....

(2 marks)

c) Estimate the mean monthly phone bill for the Year 12 students.

£ ....

(3 marks)

d) Estimate the standard deviation for the data.

£ ....

(3 marks)

All the Year 7 students in the same school were also asked about their monthly phone bill.
The mean of the data is £9.25 and the standard deviation is £4.13.

e) Compare the monthly phone bills for the Year 12 and Year 7 students, using your answers to parts c) and d).

....

....

(2 marks)

Data Presentation and Interpretation

6 The graph below shows the total number of miles that two satellite television salespeople, Isaac and Niamh, travelled during their work days each year over a period of 14 years.

MODELLING

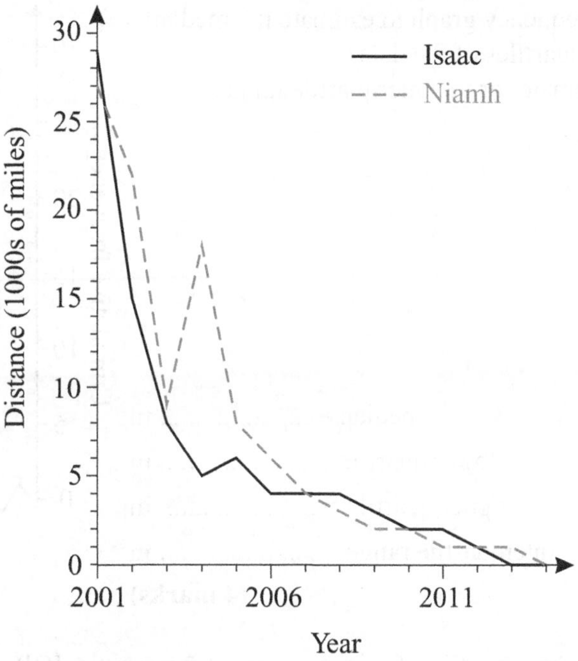

The mean distance travelled each year by Isaac over the 14 years was 5850 miles and the standard deviation was 7360 miles (both to 3 s.f.). For Niamh, the mean was 7480 miles and the standard deviation was 8380 miles (both to 3 s.f.).

a) An outlier is defined as a value that lies more than two standard deviations from the mean. Using the graph and the information given above, identify any outliers for each of Isaac and Niamh and circle them on the graph. You must show your working.

(2 marks)

b) With reference to the data, suggest a reason for any outliers.

....

....

....

(1 mark)

c) Khalid claims that the data shows that Niamh has made more sales than Isaac. Do you agree with Khalid's claim? Explain your answer.

....

....

....

(1 mark)

Data Presentation and Interpretation

7 The heights of giraffes living in a zoo were measured. The results are shown on the cumulative frequency graph on the right.

MODELLING

a) Use the cumulative frequency graph to estimate the median and lower and upper quartiles of the data.
Then calculate an estimate for the interquartile range.

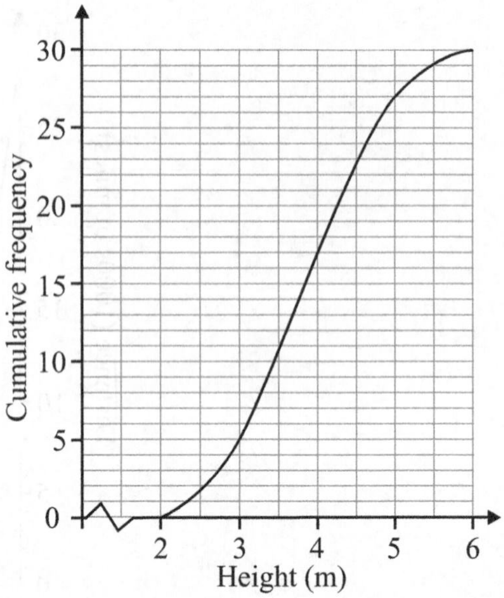

median = ... m

lower quartile = ... m

upper quartile = ... m

interquartile range = ... m

(4 marks)

b) A data value is said to be an outlier if it is more than 1.5 times the IQR above the upper quartile or more than 1.5 times the IQR below the lower quartile. Show that this data set contains no outliers.

(2 marks)

c) Use the cumulative frequency graph to complete the table below.

Height, h (metres)	$0 < h \leq 2$	$2 < h \leq 3$	$3 < h \leq 4$	$4 < h \leq 5$	$5 < h \leq 6$
Frequency	0	5			

(2 marks)

The tallest giraffe in the zoo measures 5.56 m and the shortest giraffe measures 2.7 m.

The heights of giraffes living in a nature reserve were also measured.
The data is summarised in the box plot below.

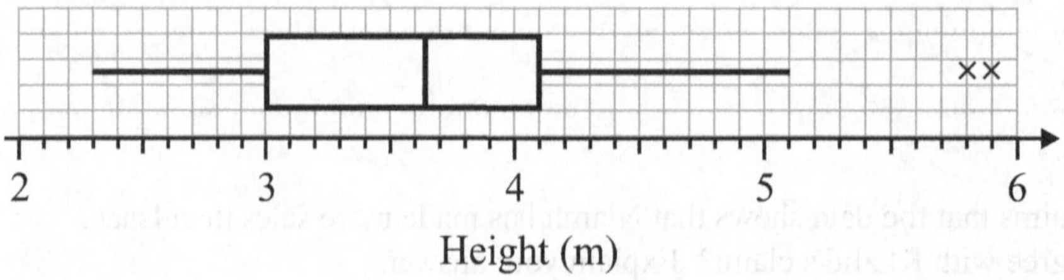

d) Compare the heights of the two groups of giraffes.

....

....

....

(3 marks)

Data Presentation and Interpretation

8 The graph below shows some data about the times taken for runners to finish the Alverston marathon. The graph shows the mean time taken, in minutes, by different age groups of runners, who ran the marathon in 2000, 2005, 2010 and 2015.

MODELLING

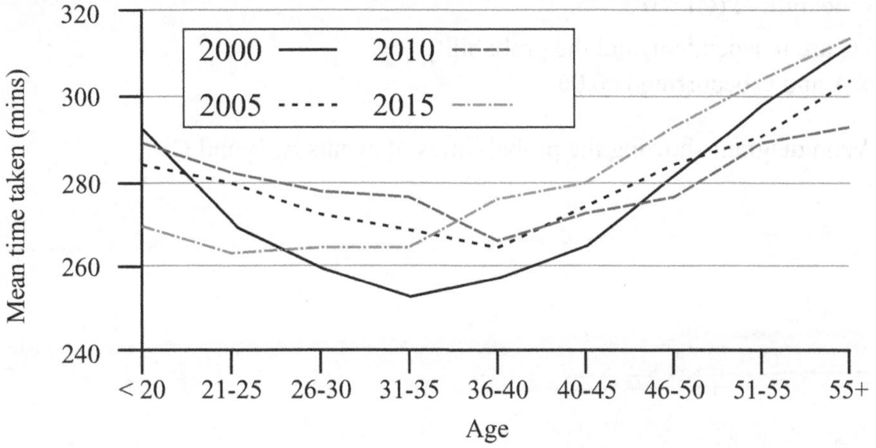

a) State the mean time taken for people aged 40-45 years to finish the marathon in 2015.

.... minutes

(1 mark)

b) A researcher studies a randomly-chosen sample of runners who were in the 21-25 age group in 2000. Does the graph suggest these runners' times improved in 2010? Justify your answer.

PROBLEM SOLVING

....

....

....

(2 marks)

c) Write down one assumption you have made about the runners in your answer to part b).

....

....

(1 mark)

Serj wants to find the overall mean time for the marathon runners in 2015. To calculate this, he intends to add up the mean times for the 9 individual age categories, then divide by 9.

d) Explain why Serj's calculation is unlikely to be accurate, and suggest how he could improve his method.

....

....

....

(2 marks)

EXAM TIP

As well as being able to calculate measures like the mean and the standard deviation, it's important to know what they tell you about a data set. Once you understand what they are and why they're useful, questions asking you to interpret or discuss data become a breeze — which means picking up those extra marks in the exam without needing to do any tricky maths.

Score

54

Probability

Venn diagrams. My question is, Vhat about the Vhere, the Vhich and the Vhy diagrams? I'm sorry, that isn't even remotely funny. In fact, I often find that me making jokes and people laughing are mutually exclusive events...

1 The events A and B are mutually exclusive. P(A) = 0.1 and P(B) = 0.4.
Event C has probability P(C) = 0.3.

Events B and C are independent, and the probability
of both events A and C occurring is 0.06.

a) Draw a Venn diagram showing the probabilities of events A, B and C.

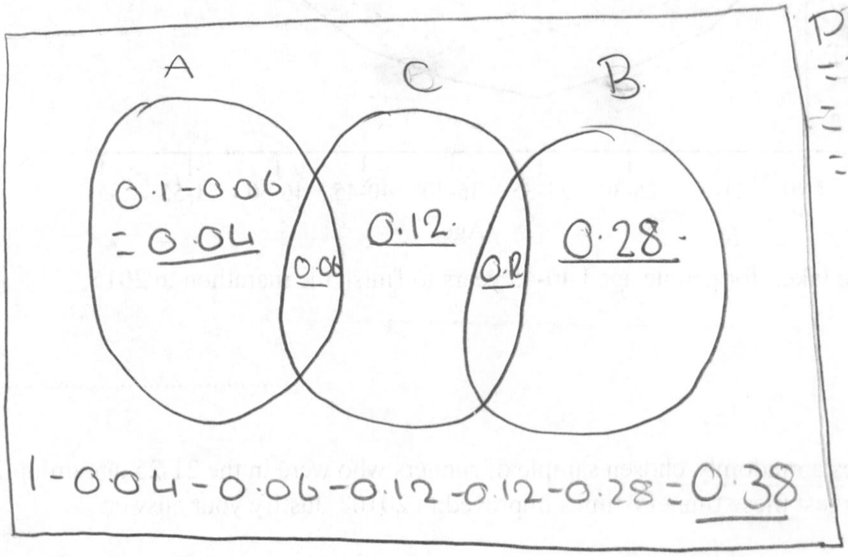

$P(B \cap C)$
$= P(B) \times P(C)$
$= 0.4 \times 0.3$
$= 0.12$

A: $0.1 - 0.06 = 0.04$
C: 0.12
0.06
0.12
B: 0.28

$1 - 0.04 - 0.06 - 0.12 - 0.12 - 0.28 = \underline{0.38}$

(5 marks)

b) Are events A and C independent? Explain your answer.

No. $P(A \cap C) = P(A) \times P(C) = 0.03$
therefore not independent as $(P A \cap C) = 0.06$.

(2 marks)

c) Find P(B ∪ C)

$P(B \cup C) = P(B) + P(C) - P(B \cap C)$
$= 0.4 + 0.3 - 0.12$
$= 0.58$

(1 mark)

d) Find P(A' ∩ B')

$P(A' \cap B') = 0.12 + 0.38$
$= 0.5$

(1 mark)

e) Find P(B'|A'), to 2 decimal places.

$P(B'|A') = \dfrac{P(A' \cap B')}{P(A')}$

$= \dfrac{0.5}{0.12 + 0.12 + 0.28 + 0.38} = \dfrac{0.5}{0.9}$

$= 0.55$ $= 0.56$

Probability

2 This incomplete Venn diagram shows the probabilities of two independent events L and M. Calculate P(L' ∩ M').

PROBLEM SOLVING

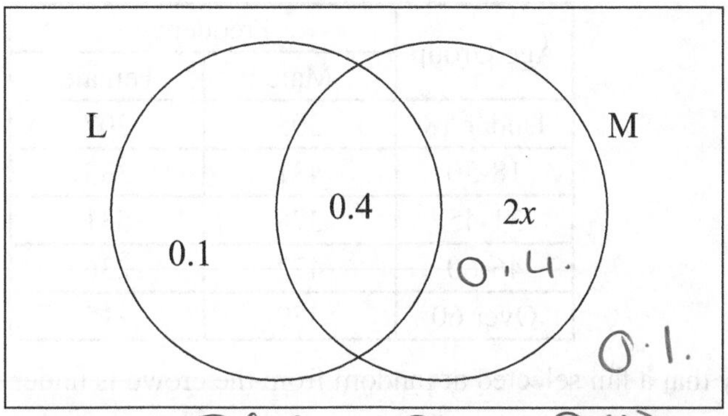

Independent ∴ P(A ∩ B) = P(A) × P(B)

P(L ∩ M) = (0.1 + 0.4) × (0.4 + 2x)

= 0.5 × (0.4 + 2x)

= 0.2 + x

∴ x = 0.2.

P(L' ∩ M')

= 1 − 0.9 = 0.1

....

(4 marks)

3 Of 30 drivers interviewed, 9 have been involved in a car crash in the last year. Of those who have been involved in a crash, 5 wear glasses. The probability of wearing glasses, given that the driver has not been involved in a car crash is $\frac{1}{3}$.

MODELLING

Find the probability that a glasses-wearer interviewed has been involved in a car crash.

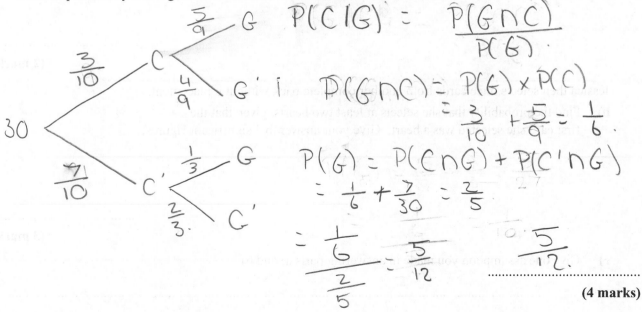

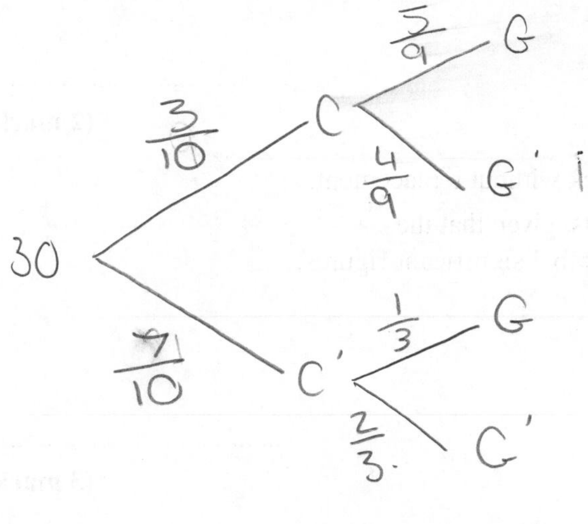

P(C | G) = P(G ∩ C) / P(G)

P(G ∩ C) = P(G) × P(C) = 3/10 + 5/9 = 1/6.

P(G) = P(C ∩ G) + P(C' ∩ G)

= 1/6 + 7/30 = 2/5

= (1/6) / (2/5) = 5/12

5/12.

....

(4 marks)

Probability

4 Alan is studying the age of people attending Ulverston Dynamo's home matches. He surveyed every fan attending the match against Cark Sportif, and recorded their ages and gender in the table shown below.

MODELLING

Age Group	Frequency	
	Male	Female
Under 18	305	207
18-30	431	333
31-45	378	531
46-60	472	236
Over 60	359	115

a) Find the probability that a fan selected at random from the crowd is under 18 given that they are male.

P(U/M) =

....

(2 marks)

b) Alan uses his data to model probabilities for the crowd at Ulverston Dynamo's next home match, which is against AC Flookburgh. He says the probability that a fan selected at random from the crowd is in the 18-30 age group is $\frac{764}{3367}$. Describe one assumption Alan has made in his model, and explain why this assumption may not be valid.

....

....

(2 marks)

5 Jessica has two packs of cards. One pack has some cards missing. The probability of selecting a heart from this pack, P(S), is 0.3. Jessica selects one card from this pack and one card from a complete pack of 52 cards.

MODELLING

a) Find the probability that at least one of the cards is a heart.

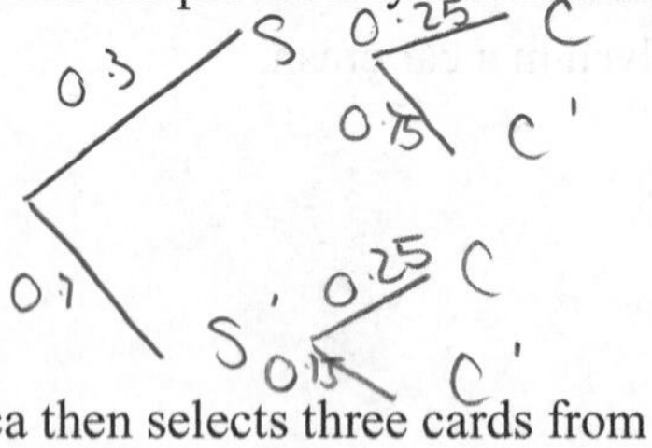

P(C|S)

....

(2 marks)

Jessica then selects three cards from another complete pack without replacement.

b) Find the probability that she selects at least two hearts, given that the first card she selected was a heart. Give your answer to 3 significant figures.

PROBLEM SOLVING

....

(3 marks)

c) Give one assumption you made in answering parts a) and b).

....

....

(1 mark)

Probability

6 P(A | B) = 0.31, P(B | A) = 0.25 and P(B) = 0.4.

a) Which of the following best describes events A and B? Circle your answer.

independent not independent mutually exclusive impossible

(1 mark)

b) Find P(A). Circle your answer.

0.1 0.124 0.496 0.6

(1 mark)

7 At a school cafeteria, every child takes at least one type of fruit with their lunch. The cafeteria has bananas, apples and oranges.

65 children use the cafeteria.
25 take a banana, 28 take an orange, 32 take an apple, 5 take a banana and an orange, 6 take an orange and an apple, and 4 take an orange, an apple and a banana.

a) Find the number of children who take a banana and an apple.

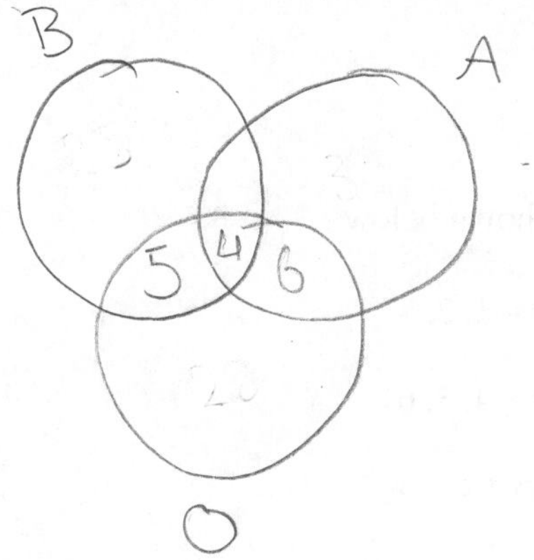

....

(4 marks)

Two children are picked at random, one after the other, without replacement.

b) Given that at least one child takes an apple, find the exact probability that the first child took an apple.

PROBLEM SOLVING

You'll need to use the conditional probability formula here.

....

(4 marks)

EXAM TIP

Even if the question doesn't ask you to draw a Venn or tree diagram, it's often helpful to draw one. They make your life so much easier. Also, make sure you understand all the different bits of set notation — it'd be silly to get a question wrong because you mixed up the union (∪) and intersection (∩) symbols. Just remember, 'u for union and n for intersection'.

Score

39

Statistical Distributions

Another treat for probability fans (like me), and your first glimpse of the binomial and normal distributions. If you don't warm to these distributions here, you'll get another chance with hypothesis testing in the next topic.

1 The number of points awarded to each contestant in a talent competition is modelled by the discrete random variable X with the following probability distribution:

MODELLING

x	0	1	2	3
$\mathrm{P}(X = x)$	0.4	0.3	0.2	a

a) Find the value of a. Circle your answer.

0.1 0.2 0.3 1

(1 mark)

b) Two contestants are chosen at random and their scores added together.
Calculate the probability that their combined score is exactly 1. Circle your answer.

0.12 0.24 0.35 0.7

(1 mark)

2 The discrete random variable X has the probability function shown below.

PROBLEM SOLVING

$$\mathrm{P}(X = x) = \begin{cases} \dfrac{kx}{6} & \text{for } x = 1, 2, 3 \\ \dfrac{k(7-x)}{6} & \text{for } x = 4, 5, 6 \\ 0 & \text{otherwise} \end{cases}$$

a) Find $\mathrm{P}(X = 10)$.

....

(1 mark)

b) Find the value of k.

$k =$ ....

(2 marks)

c) Find $\mathrm{P}(1 < X \leq 4)$.

....

(2 marks)

Statistical Distributions

3 In a game, a player tosses three fair coins. If three heads occur then the player wins 20p. If two heads occur then the player wins 10p. For any other outcome, the player wins nothing.

MODELLING PROBLEM SOLVING

a) If X is the random variable 'amount won in pence', draw a table to show the probability distribution of X.

(3 marks)

b) The player pays 10p to play each game. Find the probability that the player wins 40p in total over two games, given that they make a profit over the two games.

....

(4 marks)

4 5% of chocolate bars made by a particular manufacturer contain a 'golden ticket'. A student buys 5 of the chocolate bars every week for 8 weeks.

MODELLING

The number of golden tickets he finds is represented by the random variable X.

a) State two necessary conditions for X to follow the binomial distribution B(40, 0.05).

....

....

(2 marks)

Assuming that $X \sim \text{B}(40, 0.05)$:

b) Find $\text{P}(X > 1)$.

....

(2 marks)

c) Find the probability that more than 35 of the chocolate bars bought by the student do not contain a golden ticket.

....

(2 marks)

Statistical Distributions

5 A particular model of car, the Dystopia, is prone to developing a rattle in the first year after being made. The probability of any particular Dystopia developing the rattle in its first year is 0.65.

MODELLING

A random sample of 20 one-year-old Dystopias is selected.

a) Find the probability that at least 12 but fewer than 15 of the cars rattle.

....

(3 marks)

b) Find the probability that more than half of the cars rattle.

....

(2 marks)

c) A further five random samples of Dystopias are tested. There are 20 cars in each sample. Find the probability that more than half of the cars in exactly three of these five samples rattle.

Define a new random variable that follows a binomial distribution with n = 5 and p = P(more than half of cars rattle).

....

(3 marks)

6 An ice cream shop owner finds that, on 1st July, 880 out of the 1100 customers chose a sugar cone.

MODELLING

a) A random sample of 20 customers from 2nd July is selected. Use a binomial distribution and the data from the previous day to estimate the probability that exactly 12 of them chose a sugar cone.

Use the info to find p.

....

(4 marks)

The owner claims that 42% of customers buy an ice cream with at least one scoop of chocolate ice cream.

b) Assuming that this claim is correct, and that the next 75 customers form a random sample of customers, find the probability that more than 30 of them choose at least one scoop of chocolate ice cream.

....

(3 marks)

c) Comment on the validity of the binomial model you used in part b).

....

....

(1 mark)

Statistical Distributions

7 The histogram below represents the masses of newborn babies in a particular hospital in 2016. The masses have a mean of 3.55 kg and a standard deviation of 0.5 kg.

MODELLING

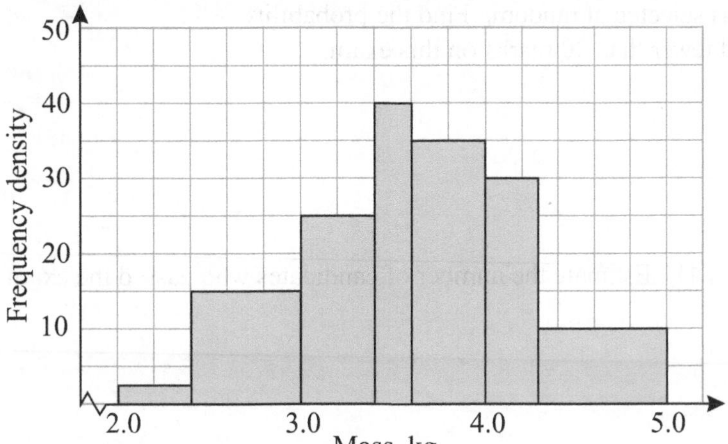

a) A nurse models the data using a normal distribution with mean 3.55 kg and standard deviation 0.5 kg. Based on the histogram, do you think this is an appropriate choice of model? Give two reasons to support your answer.

....

....

(2 marks)

b) Babies who have a mass of less than 2.5 kg at birth are said to have a low birth weight. Using the nurse's model, estimate the probability that a randomly-selected newborn baby at the hospital has a low birth weight.

....

(2 marks)

8 The volumes of water in a certain brand of fire extinguisher approximately follow a normal distribution, as shown in the diagram below. The points of inflection of the graph are labelled.

MODELLING

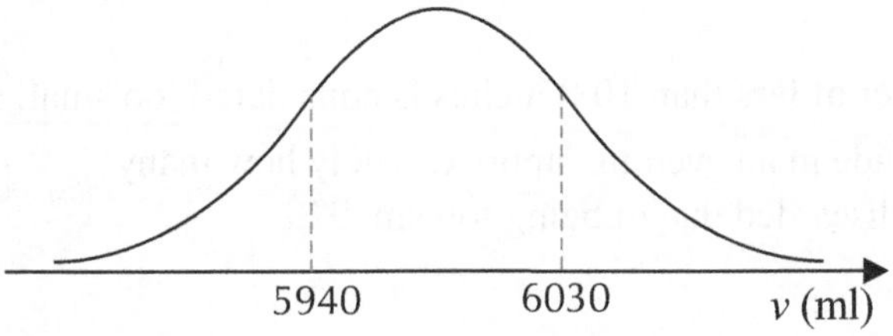

a) Use the diagram to estimate the mean, μ, and standard deviation, σ, for the model.

μ = ... ml, σ = ... ml

(2 marks)

b) Hence use the model to estimate the probability that a randomly-selected fire extinguisher contains between 5900 ml and 6100 ml of water.

....

(2 marks)

Statistical Distributions

9 The exam marks for 1000 candidates can be modelled by a normal distribution with mean 50 marks and standard deviation 15 marks. MODELLING

a) One candidate is selected at random. Find the probability that they scored fewer than 30 marks on this exam.

....

(2 marks)

b) The pass mark is 41. Estimate the number of candidates who passed the exam.

....

(2 marks)

c) Find, to the nearest whole number, the mark needed for a distinction if the top 10% of the candidates achieved a distinction. PROBLEM SOLVING

....

(2 marks)

10 The diameters of the pizza bases made at a restaurant are normally distributed. The mean diameter is 12 inches, and 5% of the bases measure more than 13 inches. MODELLING

a) Find the standard deviation of the diameters of the pizza bases to 3 significant figures.

....

(3 marks)

Any pizza base with a diameter of less than 10.8 inches is considered too small and is discarded.

b) If 100 pizza bases are made in an evening, approximately how many would you expect to be discarded due to being too small? PROBLEM SOLVING

....

(3 marks)

Three pizza bases are selected at random.

c) Find the probability that at least one of these bases is too small. PROBLEM SOLVING

....

(3 marks)

Statistical Distributions

11 The time in minutes, X, that it takes a window cleaner to clean each window of an office block is normally distributed with a mean of 4 minutes and a standard deviation of 1.1 minutes.

MODELLING

a) Find the probability that a randomly-selected window takes less than 3.5 minutes to clean.

....

(2 marks)

b) Find the probability that the time taken to clean a randomly-selected window deviates from the mean by more than 1 minute.

PROBLEM SOLVING

....

(3 marks)

c) Find the time taken t, in minutes to 1 decimal place, such that there is a 1% probability that a randomly-selected window will take longer than t minutes to clean.

PROBLEM SOLVING

.... mins

(2 marks)

12 The mass, M g, of sweets in a packet is normally distributed, with a mean of 93 g. In 20% of packets of these sweets, there are at least 95 g of sweets.

MODELLING PROBLEM SOLVING

a) Packets with less than 88 g of sweets cannot be sold. Calculate the probability that a randomly-selected packet of sweets cannot be sold.

....

(5 marks)

b) 20 packets are selected at random. Find the probability that exactly one of them cannot be sold.

....

(3 marks)

Statistical Distributions

13 One weekend, 48% of customers at Soutergate Cinema went to see the latest superhero film. A random sample of 200 customers was taken.

MODELLING

a) Write down the binomial distribution that could be used to model S, the number of customers in the sample who went to see the superhero film.

....

(1 mark)

b) Explain why the normal distribution could be used to approximate this binomial distribution.

....

....

....

(2 marks)

c) Approximate the mean and standard deviation of the customers who saw the superhero film.

mean = ... standard deviation = ...

(2 marks)

The same weekend, 3% of customers at Vulcan Cinema went to see the latest horror film. The manager takes a random sample of 90 customers.

d) Could a normal distribution be used to accurately approximate probabilities for this sample? Explain your answer.

....

....

....

(2 marks)

e) Find the probability that more than 4 of the sampled customers at Vulcan Cinema went to see the horror film.

....

(3 marks)

EXAM TIP

Make sure you can use the binomial and normal functions on your calculator — you'll need them in the exam. Remember, you can use a normal distribution to approximate a binomial distribution if n is large and p is close to 0.5. You could also be asked to comment on whether a probability model or any assumptions made are appropriate for a given context.

Score

84

Statistical Hypothesis Testing

Here we enter the murky world of hypothesis testing, but we welcome back our friends the binomial and normal distributions. You should remember them from the previous topic... they remember you...

1 Mike works for a farm that produces organic cheese. He needs to carry out a survey to find out people's opinions about cheese. He is told to interview 25 females under 30, 10 males under 30, 35 females over 30 and 20 males over 30. He goes to a supermarket and asks people near the cheese counter to take part.

Name the sampling method used by Mike. Circle your answer.

simple random sampling   cluster sampling   systematic sampling   quota sampling

(1 mark)

2 Josie wants to find out what pupils in her school think about politics. She takes a sample of the pupils.

a) Identify the population that Josie is interested in.

....

(1 mark)

b) Josie plans to select everyone in her A-level politics class as her sample. Name Josie's sampling method and explain whether or not her sample is likely to be representative of the population.

....

....

(2 marks)

3 Jamila is investigating the pay rises given to working adults in her town last year. The table below shows the number of working adults in Jamila's town.

Age (in years)	18-27	28-37	38-47	48-57	Over 57
No. of working adults	1200	2100	3500	3200	1500

Jamila plans to use stratified sampling to select a sample of 50 working adults from her town.

a) Suggest one reason why it might be sensible for Jamila to stratify her sample by age.

....

....

(1 mark)

b) Calculate how many people from each age group should be in the sample.

Remember to round decimals to the nearest whole number, and check your total is 50.

18-27 = ..., 28-37 = ..., 38-47 = ..., 48-57 = ..., Over 57 = ...

(3 marks)

c) Jamila wants to investigate the pay rises given to working adults across the UK last year. Can she use her sample data to draw conclusions about the whole population? Explain your answer.

....

....

(1 mark)

Statistical Hypothesis Testing

4 On a tropical island it is known that it usually rains on 50% of days on average.
Adil wants to carry out a hypothesis test to investigate whether this proportion has changed recently.

MODELLING

a) Adil randomly samples 20 days from the latest year for which he has data. It rained on 4 of the sampled days. Use this information to carry out Adil's test at the 1% level of significance.

You can either work out the p-value or find the critical region.

....

....

(6 marks)

b) Adil carries out a hypothesis test on a different sample of 20 days at the 5% level of significance and rejects his null hypothesis to conclude that the proportion of days on which it rains has changed. Find, to 3 significant figures, the probability that he incorrectly rejected the null hypothesis.

....

(3 marks)

5 Nate teaches judo classes at 'basic' and 'advanced' levels. Last year, 20% of his students had done judo for at least two years. Nate moves to a different judo club and claims that at this club, the percentage of his students who have done judo for at least two years is different.
To test this, he surveys a random sample of 20 of his new students.

MODELLING

a) Given that 7 of the sampled students have done judo for at least two years, use a binomial distribution to carry out a test of Nate's claim at the 5% significance level.

....

....

(6 marks)

b) State two assumptions that are needed for the binomial model you used in part a) to be valid. Comment on whether each assumption is likely to be true for Nate's test.

....

....

....

....

(4 marks)

Statistical Hypothesis Testing

6 2016 records suggest that 45% of the members of a gym use the swimming pool. The gym's manager claims that the popularity of the swimming pool has decreased since then. He surveys a random sample of 50 members to test his claim.

After carrying out his test at the 5% level of significance, the manager concludes that there is evidence to suggest that the popularity of the pool has decreased.

Find the maximum possible number of gym members in the sample of 50 who use the pool.

(4 marks)

7 A bakery makes different flavours of muffins. The masses of their blueberry muffins can be modelled by a normal distribution with mean 110 g and standard deviation 3 g. A customer claims that the bakery's chocolate muffins weigh less than the blueberry muffins. A random sample of 15 chocolate muffins was found to have a mean mass of 108.5 g.

Assuming that the masses of the chocolate muffins can be modelled by a normal distribution with standard deviation 3 g, test the customer's claims at the 10% level of significance.

(5 marks)

8 The mean height of the sunflowers in a particular field is 150 cm. The heights of the sunflowers in a second field are known to follow a normal distribution, with a standard deviation of $\sqrt{20}$ cm. The mean height of a random sample of 6 of these sunflowers is 140 cm.

Test at the 1% level of significance whether the mean height of the sunflowers in the second field is the same as for the sunflowers in the first field.

(5 marks)

Statistical Hypothesis Testing

9 The duration in minutes, X, of a car wash is normally distributed with mean 8 and standard deviation $\sqrt{1.2}$. After some maintenance work is carried out, the manager claims that the mean duration of the car wash has decreased. A hypothesis test is to be carried out to investigate this claim.

MODELLING

a) A random sample of 20 washes are timed and the mean duration is found to be 7.8 minutes. Carry out the test at the 5% significance level. You may assume that the standard deviation of the washes' durations is unchanged.

....

....

(5 marks)

b) Find the least value for the sample mean car wash duration that would have provided insufficient evidence to reject the null hypothesis for the test you carried out in part a). Give your answer to 3 significant figures.

PROBLEM SOLVING

....

(2 marks)

10 The mean time taken by an employee at Sahil's company to get to work has previously been found to be 27 minutes, and the standard deviation of times was found to be 6.1 minutes. The times are assumed to be normally distributed.

MODELLING

Sahil claims that the mean time is now less than 27 minutes. He asks 45 randomly selected employees one day how long it had taken them to get to work that morning, and obtained a sample mean of 24.8 minutes.

a) Assuming that the previous values of the mean and standard deviation of journey times are correct, find the probability that a sample of size 45 will have a mean of 24.8 minutes or less.

(3 marks)

b) Sahil says, "this probability is small, so there is sufficient evidence for a hypothesis test to support my claim." Explain what is wrong with this statement.

....

....

(1 mark)

c) Suggest one criticism of Sahil's sampling method in this situation.

....

....

(1 mark)

EXAM TIP

With hypothesis tests, think carefully about whether it's easier to find the p-value or the critical region — and make sure you know how to use your binomial and normal calculator functions. You should always write a proper conclusion as well. For example, don't just say 'reject H_0', you also need to explain what rejecting H_0 means in the context of the question.

Score

54

Correlation and Regression

Correlation and regression are some of my favourite things. In fact, I even named my two dogs 'Correlation' and 'Regression' because I love these topics so much. My children Cora and Reggie thoroughly approved.

1 Karl is investigating how the price of oil affects the price of bananas. He calculates the product moment correlation coefficient, r, and finds that the two variables are strongly positively correlated.

Which of the following values for r best agrees with Karl's findings? Circle your answer.

–0.851 0.248 0.799 1.73

(1 mark)

2 A construction company measures the length, y metres, of a cable when put under different amounts of tension, T kN (kilonewtons). The results of its tests are shown on the scatter diagram below.

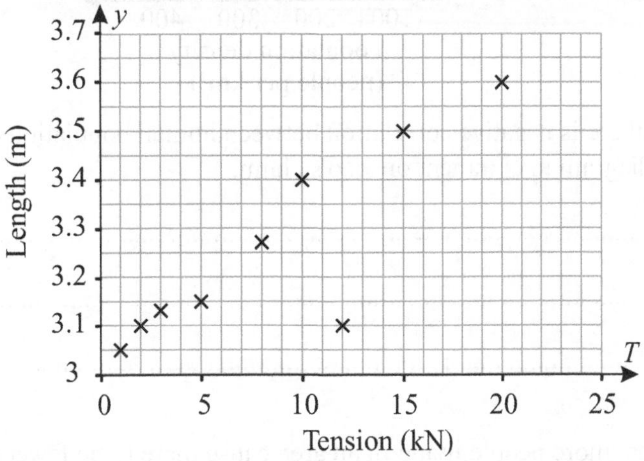

a) One of the readings has been recorded inaccurately. Put a ring around this reading on the graph.

(1 mark)

b) Describe the correlation shown on the scatter diagram.

(1 mark)

An engineer believes a linear regression line of the form $y = a + bT$ could be used to accurately describe the results. She ignores the outlier, and calculates the equation of the regression line to be $y = 3 + 0.03T$.

c) Explain what these values of a and b represent in this context.

(2 marks)

The engineer wants to use the regression line to predict the length of the cable when it is put under a tension of 50 kilonewtons.

d) Comment on the reliability of her estimate.

(1 mark)

Correlation and Regression

3 Some ecologists carry out an investigation into the reindeer populations at different locations. They also record the human population density at the same locations. Their results are displayed in the scatter diagram below.

MODELLING

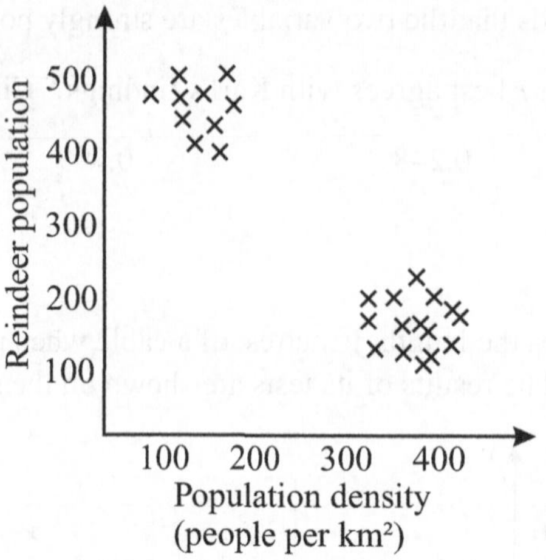

a) Jiao claims that there is negative correlation between human population density and reindeer population. Use the scatter diagram to comment on Jiao's claim.

....

....

....

(2 marks)

b) Killian claims that more people living in an area cause there to be fewer reindeer in that area. Do you agree with Killian's claim? Explain your answer.

....

....

....

(2 marks)

4 A student collects 10 pairs of data values from an estate agent's website. Each pair of values shows the floor area (A) and the advertised price (P) of a randomly-selected house.

MODELLING

Using her 10 pairs of values, the student calculates the PMCC between A and P to be 0.634. The critical value for a 1-tail hypothesis test at a 5% significance level on a sample of size 10 is 0.5494. Carry out a hypothesis test at this significance level of whether the PMCC between A and P for the population of houses advertised on the whole website is positive. State your hypotheses clearly.

....

....

(2 marks)

Correlation and Regression

5 The scatter diagram below uses data from the large data set. It shows the engine size and carbon dioxide emissions of a number of Volkswagen vehicles.

MODELLING

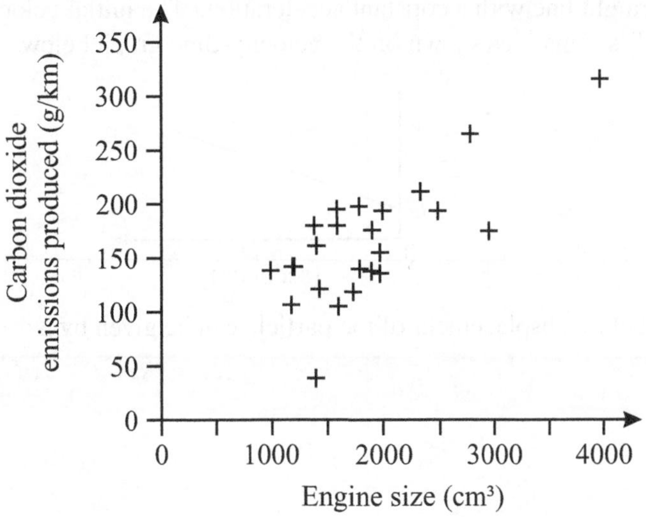

a) Describe the correlation between the engine sizes and the carbon dioxide emissions.

....

(1 mark)

b) Sammi claims that the diagram above shows that, for any make of vehicle, it is generally the case that the greater the engine size, the greater the amount of carbon dioxide emissions produced. Comment on Sammi's claim.

....

....

....

(2 marks)

The hydrocarbon emissions (g/km) are recorded for 17 Volkswagen vehicles, each with different engine sizes. The product moment correlation coefficient between their emissions and engine size is 0.3371 (to 4 d.p.). The critical value for a 2-tail test at a 1% significance level on a sample size of 17 is 0.6055.

c) Carry out a hypothesis test at the 1% significance level of whether the PMCC for this data is non-zero. State your hypotheses clearly.

....

....

(2 marks)

EXAM TIP

Scatter diagrams, regression lines and the PMCC help you to understand relationships between different sets of data — but just because two data sets are correlated, that doesn't necessarily mean that changes in one cause changes in the other. Apparently, ice cream sales and murder rates are correlated... but that doesn't mean the next person you see eating ice cream is a killer.

Score

17

Kinematics — 1

Kinematics is all about the way things move — by the end of this topic your flamboyant dance skills should be most impressive. For these questions, give non-exact answers to 3 significant figures, unless told otherwise.

1 A particle moves in a straight line with a constant acceleration. The initial velocity of the particle is U ms^{-1} and its velocity at time T is V ms^{-1}, as shown on the velocity-time graph below.

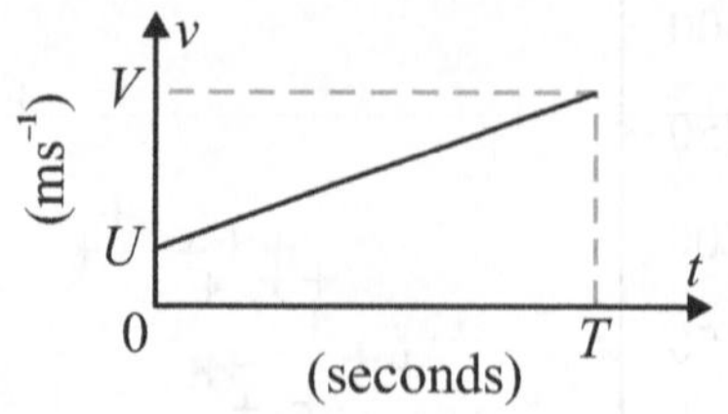

Using the graph, show that the displacement of the particle can be given by $S = \frac{1}{2}(U + V)T$.

(3 marks)

2 **In this question use $g = 9.8$ ms^{-2}.**
A ball is thrown vertically upwards with velocity 5 ms^{-1} from a point 2 m above the ground. The velocity-time graph below models the motion of the ball.

MODELLING

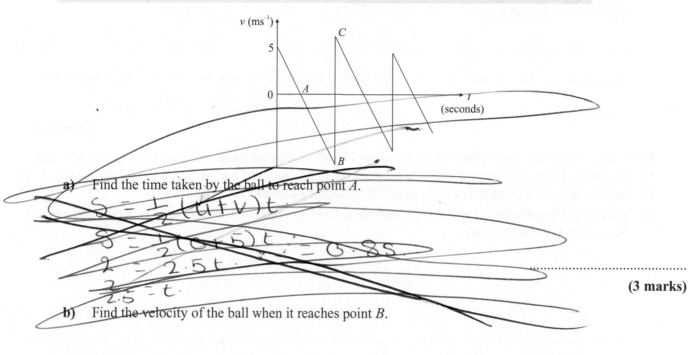

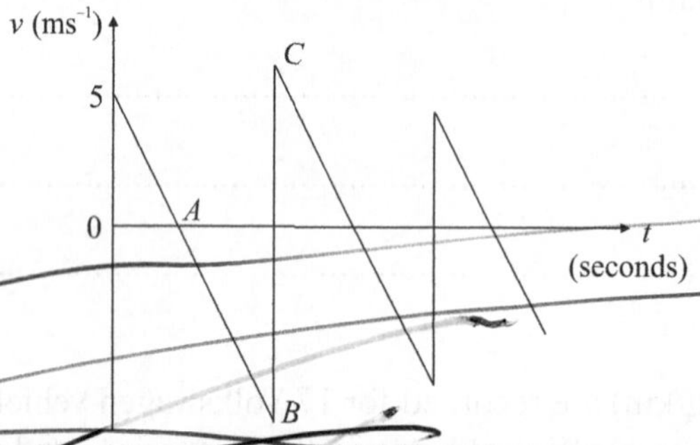

a) Find the time taken by the ball to reach point A.

$S = \frac{1}{2}(u+v)t$

$8 = \frac{1}{2}(0+5)t = 0.8s$

$2 = 2.5t$

$\frac{2}{2.5} = t$

....

(3 marks)

b) Find the velocity of the ball when it reaches point B.

....

(3 marks)

c) Explain why, in reality, this graph may not be an accurate model of the velocity of the ball.

....

(1 mark)

Kinematics — 1

3 A train is moving along a straight horizontal track with constant acceleration.
The train enters a tunnel which is 760 m long and exits 24 seconds later.
8 seconds before entering the tunnel, the train passes a sign.
The sign is 110 m from the tunnel's entrance.

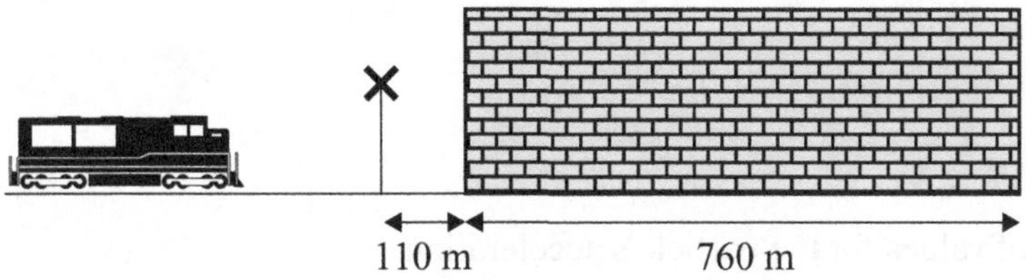

Find the train's acceleration and its speed when it passes the sign.

$a =$ .... $u =$ ....

(6 marks)

4 A particle P has initial velocity $(7\mathbf{i} - 3\mathbf{j})$ ms^{-1}. It accelerates at a constant rate of $(\mathbf{i} + 4\mathbf{j})$ ms^{-2} for 2 seconds. Find the final velocity of P. Circle your answer.

$(8\mathbf{i} + \mathbf{j})$ ms^{-1} $(2\mathbf{i} + 8\mathbf{j})$ ms^{-1} $(9\mathbf{i} + 5\mathbf{j})$ ms^{-1} $(5\mathbf{i} - 11\mathbf{j})$ ms^{-1}

(1 mark)

5 A particle P sets off from the origin at $t = 0$ and starts to move along the x-axis in the direction of increasing x. After t seconds, P has velocity v ms^{-1}, where v is given by:

$$v = \begin{cases} 11t - 2t^2 & 0 \leq t \leq 5 \\ 25 - 4t & t > 5 \end{cases}$$

Find the displacement of P from the origin at $t = 5$, using a suitable algebraic method.

....

(4 marks)

Kinematics — 1

6 A particle moves in a straight line, beginning at the origin at $t = 0$. Its velocity, v ms^{-1}, at time t seconds is given by $v = 2t - 3e^{-2t} + 4$.

a) Find an expression for the particle's acceleration, a ms^{-2}, at time t.

$a =$ ....

(2 marks)

b) Find the range of values for the particle's acceleration. PROBLEM SOLVING

....

(3 marks)

c) Find an expression for the particle's displacement from O, s m, at time t.

$s =$ ....

(3 marks)

7 At time $t = 0$, a particle, P, sets off from rest at the point O and accelerates uniformly. At time $t = 3$ seconds, the particle has position vector $(9\mathbf{i} - 18\mathbf{j})$ m relative to O.

a) Given that the particle continues to move with this constant acceleration, find an expression for the position vector, $\mathbf{p}$, of the particle at time t.

$\mathbf{p} =$ ....

(4 marks)

Also at time $t = 0$, a second particle, Q, moving with constant velocity $(3\mathbf{i} - 5\mathbf{j})$ ms^{-1} has position vector $(a\mathbf{i} + b\mathbf{j})$ m, where a and b are constants.

b) Given that the two particles collide at time $t = 8$ seconds, find the values of a and b.

$a =$ .... $b =$ ....

(3 marks)

Kinematics — 1

8 An object has constant acceleration a and an initial velocity of u.

Given that the object sets off from the origin, use integration to show that the object's displacement at time t is given by the formula $s = ut + \frac{1}{2}at^2$.

(4 marks)

9 A particle P is at position vector $(5t^3 + 7t^2 + 6)\mathbf{i} + (5t^2 + 8)\mathbf{j}$ m, relative to a fixed origin, at time $t \geq 0$. Find the speed of the particle when $\tan \theta = \frac{1}{2}$, where θ is the angle of the direction of motion.

PROBLEM SOLVING

....

(5 marks)

10 A ball's velocity is modelled by the vector $\mathbf{v} = [(2t - 5)\mathbf{i} + (3t - 8)\mathbf{j}]$ ms^{-1}, where $\mathbf{i}$ and $\mathbf{j}$ are unit vectors pointing east and north respectively. At time $t = 2$ s, the ball is at position vector $(-2\mathbf{i} + 10\mathbf{j})$ m.

MODELLING

a) Find the value of t at which the ball is travelling directly eastwards.

$t =$ ....

(2 marks)

b) Calculate the range of t for which the ball is to the west of the origin.

PROBLEM SOLVING

....

(5 marks)

Kinematics — 1

11 At $t = 0$, Robot 1 is at point A moving with a constant velocity of $(\mathbf{i} + 3\mathbf{j})$ ms^{-1}, and Robot 2 accelerates from rest at point B. Robot 2 moves with a constant acceleration of $(0.4\mathbf{i} + 0.2\mathbf{j})$ ms^{-2}. After 6 seconds, the robots collide at point C.

MODELLING

a) Calculate the speed of Robot 2 as it collides with Robot 1.

....

(3 marks)

b) Find the displacement vector $\overrightarrow{AB}$.

PROBLEM SOLVING

....

(4 marks)

c) Give two modelling assumptions you have made in parts **a)** and **b)**.

....

....

(2 marks)

12 A particle is moving in a curved path. Its velocity, $\mathbf{v}$ ms^{-1}, at time t seconds is given by $\mathbf{v} = (2\cos 3t + 5t)\mathbf{i} + (2t - 7)\mathbf{j}$, where the unit vectors $\mathbf{i}$ and $\mathbf{j}$ are in the directions of east and north respectively.

PROBLEM SOLVING

Calculate the magnitude of the particle's maximum acceleration. Give an exact value.

....

(5 marks)

EXAM TIP

Kinematics questions can be tough, because they combine lots of skills — you need to be comfortable with using vectors, differentiating and integrating, as well as all the mechanics-y stuff. Just remember, whenever you see 'constant' or 'uniform' acceleration in an exam question you should think 'suvat'. If acceleration isn't constant, then it's time to whip out the calculus.

Score

66

Kinematics — 2

These questions are all about projectiles. Master the maths of trajectories and you'll be a pro-golfer in no time. Here, you should give your answers to 3 significant figures and take $g = 9.8 \text{ ms}^{-2}$, unless asked otherwise. Fore!

1 **In this question use $g = 9.81 \text{ ms}^{-2}$.**
A stone is thrown upwards from point A on a cliff, 22 m above horizontal ground, with speed 14 ms^{-1} at an angle of 46° to the horizontal. After projection, the stone moves freely under gravity and lands at B on the horizontal ground, as shown below.

MODELLING

a) Find the length of time for which the stone is at least 22 m above the ground.

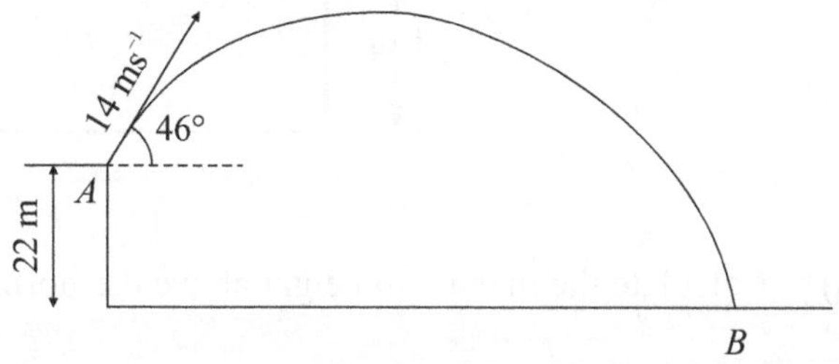

....

(4 marks)

b) Calculate the speed of the stone as it hits the ground.

....

(5 marks)

2 **In this question use $g = 9.8 \text{ ms}^{-2}$.**
A golf ball is at point T, which is partway up a slope. When struck, it moves with initial velocity $(29\mathbf{i} + 24\mathbf{j}) \text{ ms}^{-1}$ in the direction of the line of greatest incline and lands again on the slope. The position vector of T is $(0\mathbf{i} + 0\mathbf{j})$.
The slope is at an angle of 10° to the horizontal, as shown below.

MODELLING PROBLEM SOLVING

a) Show that when the ball lands on the slope, $(X\mathbf{i} + X \tan 10°\mathbf{j}) = 29t\mathbf{i} + (24t - 4.9t^2)\mathbf{j}$, where X is the horizontal displacement of the ball and t is time.

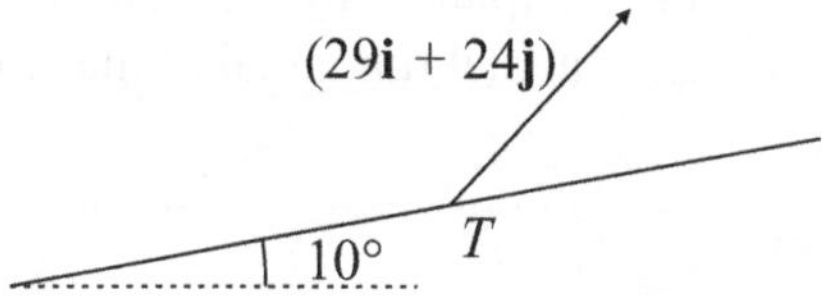

(3 marks)

b) Hence or otherwise, find the position vector of the golf ball when it hits the ground.

....

(5 marks)

Kinematics — 2

3 **In this question use g = 9.8 ms^{-2}.**
A stone is thrown from A, at a height of 1 m above the ground. The stone's initial velocity is 10 ms^{-1} at an angle of 20° above the horizontal. The stone lands on the horizontal ground at B.

MODELLING

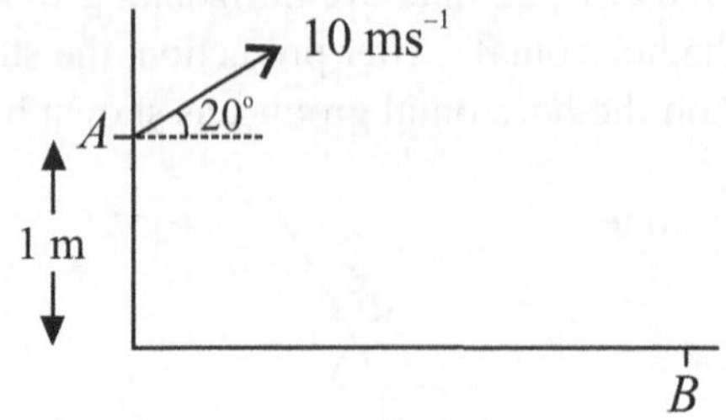

a) Calculate the maximum height above the horizontal ground that the stone reaches during its flight.

(4 marks)

b) Find the time it takes the stone to travel from A to B.

(3 marks)

c) Explain why the answer you found in part b) might not be the actual time it takes the stone to travel from A to B.

(1 mark)

EXAM TIP

Projectiles questions can look really complicated. The trick is: take a deep breath, write out the variables you've been given in the question and then think which suvat equation will let you work out the next bit of the question. Sometimes, you'll have to go through this process a couple of times before you get to the final answer, but so long as you're careful you'll get there.

Score

25

Forces and Newton's Laws

Try as you might, there's no escaping Newton's laws — they pretty much govern the way everything moves. Give any non-exact answers to an appropriate degree of accuracy and use the given value of g when necessary.

1 Three forces act at a point, O, as shown below.

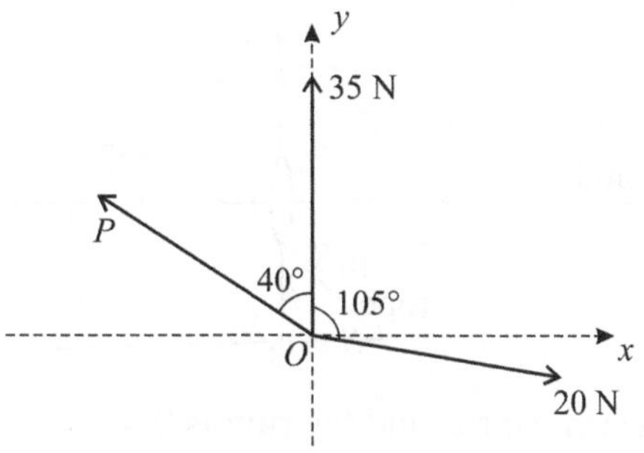

Given that there is no resultant force in the direction of the x-axis, find P to 3 s.f. Circle your answer.

25.2 N   –38.9 N   8.05 N   30.1 N

(1 mark)

2 A bird feeder is hung between two trees using light, inextensible strings. The bird feeder has a weight of 5.2 N and the strings form angles of 47° and 32° with the horizontal, as shown in the diagram below.

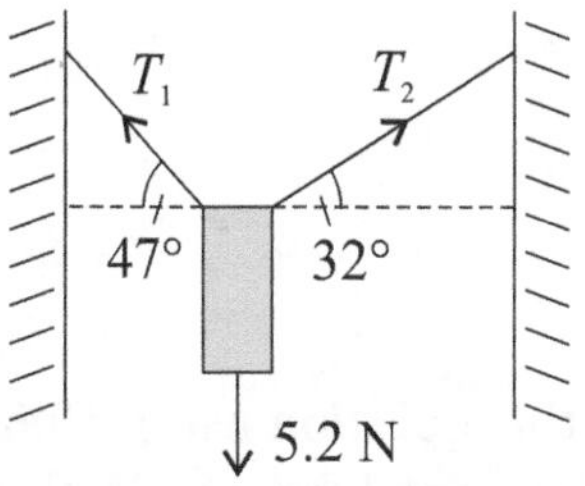

Modelling the bird feeder as a particle, find the tension in each string. Fully justify your answer.

T_1 = ...

T_2 = ...

(5 marks)

3 Two forces, $\mathbf{A} = (2\mathbf{i} - 11\mathbf{j})$ N and $\mathbf{B} = (7\mathbf{i} + 5\mathbf{j})$ N, act on a toy helicopter of mass 500 g.

If the helicopter starts from rest, find the velocity of the helicopter after 4 seconds.

$\mathbf{v}$ = ...

(3 marks)

Forces and Newton's Laws

4 **In this question use $g = 9.81\ \text{ms}^{-2}$.**
A 2 kg ring is threaded on a rough horizontal rod. A rope is attached to the ring, and is held at 40° below the horizontal, as shown. The normal reaction of the rod on the ring is R N, the tension in the rope is S N and the frictional force between the rod and the ring is F N.

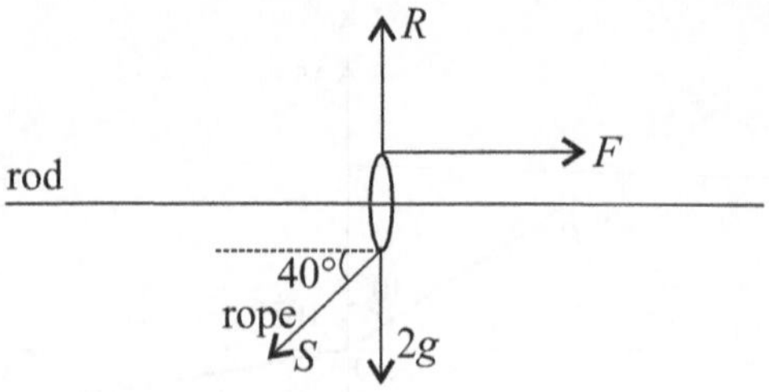

The coefficient of friction between the rod and the ring is 0.3.
Given that the ring is stationary, find the range of possible values that S can take.

....

(5 marks)

5 **In this question use $g = 9.8\ \text{ms}^{-2}$.**
A horizontal force of 25 N causes a particle of mass 7 kg to accelerate up a rough plane inclined at 15° to the horizontal, with acceleration of magnitude $0.2\ \text{ms}^{-2}$, as shown on the diagram to the right.

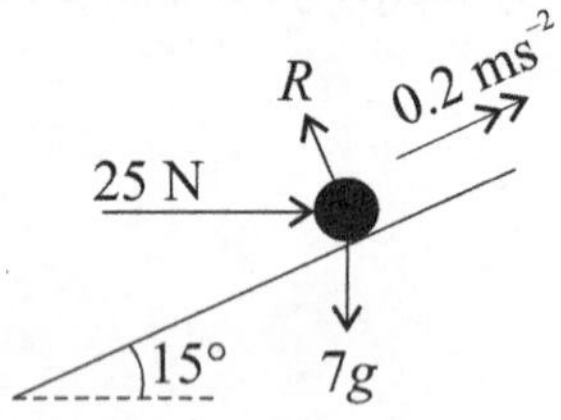

a) Calculate the coefficient of friction between the mass and the plane to 2 decimal places.

μ = ...

(6 marks)

b) The 25 N force is now removed and the particle is released from rest.
Find how long the particle takes to slide a distance of 3 m down the plane.

....

(6 marks)

Forces and Newton's Laws

6 **In this question use $g = 9.8 \text{ ms}^{-2}$.**
A block of mass m kg rests on rough horizontal ground. The block is held in limiting equilibrium by a string under tension T N pulling upwards at an angle of 51.3° to the horizontal. The coefficient of friction between the block and the ground is 0.6 and the magnitude of the frictional force is 1.5 N.

Find the tension in the string, T, and the mass of the block, m.

$T =$ ....

$m =$ ....

(5 marks)

7 A ball of weight W N is attached to a string under tension T N on a rough plane inclined at β to the horizontal. The string is parallel to the plane. The ball is held in limiting equilibrium by friction force F N, acting in the same direction as T.

PROBLEM SOLVING

Assuming that T acts parallel to the plane, show that the coefficient of friction $\mu = \tan\beta - \frac{T}{W}\sec\beta$.

(5 marks)

Forces and Newton's Laws

8 **In this question use $g = 9.81 \text{ ms}^{-2}$.**
A woman is travelling in a lift. The lift is rising vertically and is accelerating at a rate of 0.75 ms^{-2}. The lift is pulled upwards by a light, inextensible cable. The tension in the cable is T N and the lift has mass 500 kg. The floor of the lift exerts a force of 675 N on the woman. Find T.

MODELLING

T = ...

(4 marks)

9 One end of a light inextensible string is attached to a block A, of mass 35 kg. The string passes over a fixed, smooth pulley and is attached at the other end to a block B, of mass M kg.

The system is held at rest by a vertical light inextensible string attached to B at one end and to horizontal ground at the other, as shown. The tension in this second string is K N.

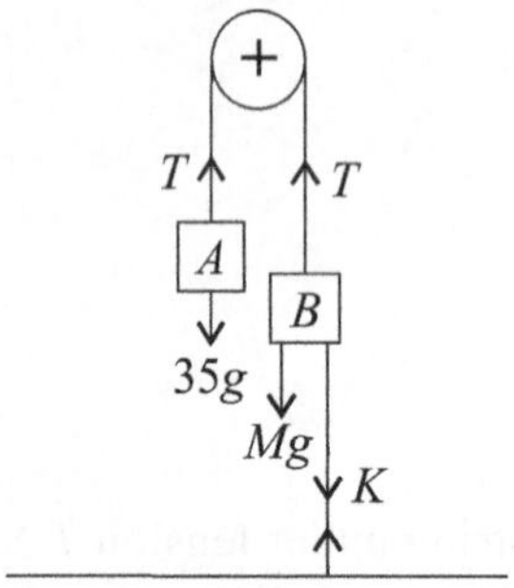

a) Find an expression for K in terms of M and g.

....

(2 marks)

b) (i) In this question use $g = 9.81 \text{ ms}^{-2}$.
The string fixing B to the ground is cut. Three seconds after the string is cut, A is travelling at 1 ms^{-1} towards the ground. Calculate M.

M = ...

(5 marks)

(ii) Give one assumption you have made about the behaviour of the system after the string is cut.

....

(1 mark)

Forces and Newton's Laws

10 **In this question use $g = 9.8$ ms^{-2}.**
A particle, A, is attached to a weight, W, by a light inextensible string which passes over a smooth pulley, P, as shown. When the system is released from rest, with the string taut, A and W experience an acceleration of 4 ms^{-2}. A moves across a rough horizontal plane and W falls vertically. The mass of W is 1.5 times the mass of A.

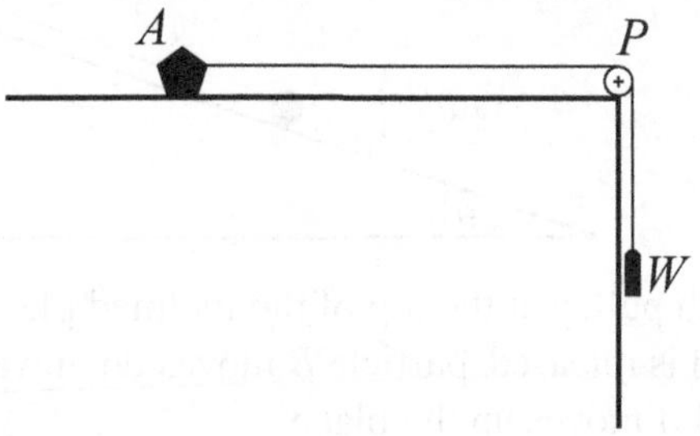

a) Given that the mass of A is 0.2 kg, find the coefficient of friction, μ, between A and the horizontal plane.

μ = ...

(6 marks)

W falls for h m until it impacts the ground and does not rebound. A continues to move until it reaches P with speed 3 ms^{-1}. The initial distance between A and P is $\frac{7}{4}h$.

b) Find the value of h. PROBLEM SOLVING

h = ...

(5 marks)

c) Find the time taken for W to impact the ground.

....

(2 marks)

d) How did you use the information that the string is inextensible?

....

....

(1 mark)

Forces and Newton's Laws

11 **In this question use $g = 9.8$ ms^{-2}.**
A particle A of mass 3 kg is placed on a rough plane inclined at an angle of $\theta = \tan^{-1}\frac{3}{4}$ above the horizontal and is attached by a light inextensible string to a second particle B of mass 4 kg.

PROBLEM SOLVING

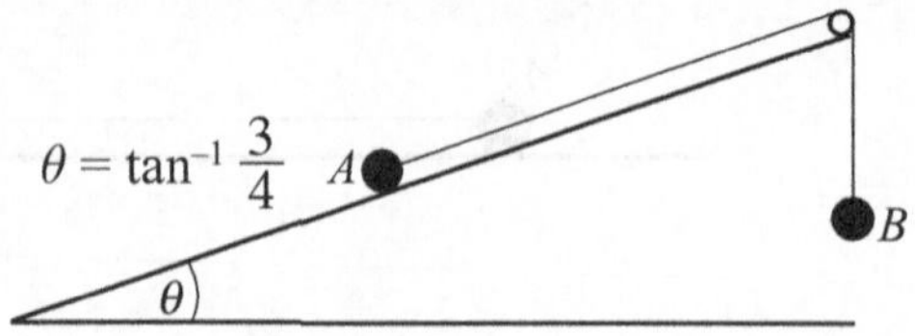

The string passes over a smooth pulley at the top of the inclined plane so that particle B hangs freely. When the system is released, particle B moves downwards vertically with an acceleration of 1.4 ms^{-2} and A moves up the plane.

a) Find the coefficient of friction between particle A and the plane.

μ = ...

(7 marks)

Two seconds after the particles are released, the string breaks. A then continues up the plane until it comes instantaneously to rest. At no point does A reach the pulley.

b) Find how far particle B moves from the start of the motion until the string breaks.

....

(2 marks)

c) Calculate how far particle A moves from the instant the string breaks until it comes to rest.

....

(5 marks)

EXAM TIP

Never in the history of mathematics has drawing a detailed diagram been more important. You don't stand a chance of keeping all the numbers involved in these questions in your head. For connected-particle questions, you might even want to draw more than one diagram — one for each particle. Trust me on this one, a sketch is worth a thousand words.

Score

76

Moments

It had to happen sooner or later, and there's no putting it off any longer — it's your favourite topic... moments. Don't let them get your head in a spin — maintain your equilibrium and your results will be uniformly successful.

1 A non-uniform rod, *PQ*, is supported at its centre of mass, 4 m from *P*, as shown below. A mass of 7 kg is placed 2 m from *P* and a mass of 3 kg is placed 9 m from *P*.

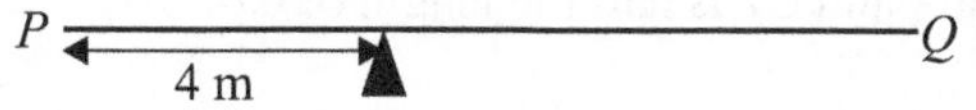

Which of the following statements best describes the system? Circle your answer.

Resultant anticlockwise moment   Static equilibrium   Resultant clockwise moment   Resultant moment in both directions

(1 mark)

2 A uniform rod AB of length 4 m and weight 20 N hangs in equilibrium in a horizontal position supported by two vertical inextensible strings attached at A and B. A bead of weight 16 N rests on the rod at a point C, which is 3 m from A. The bead can be modelled as a particle.

a) Find the tensions in the strings at A (T_1) and at B (T_2).

T_1 = ...

T_2 = ...

(3 marks)

b) The bead is now moved along the rod so that the tension in the string at B is twice the tension in the string at A. Find the distance of the bead from A.

....

(3 marks)

3 A non-uniform rod, *AB*, of length 7 m and mass 5 kg rests on supports at *A* and point *C*, 1 m from *B*, as shown below. The rod's centre of mass is 3 m from *A*. A particle is attached at point *D*, 0.5 m from *B*. The rod is on the point of tilting about *C*.

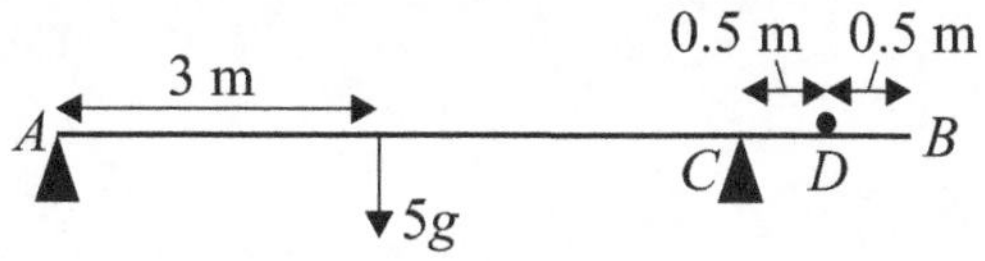

Find the mass of the attached particle. Circle your answer.

7.5 kg   30 kg   5 kg   15 kg

(1 mark)

Moments

4 **In this question use $g = 9.8$ ms^{-2}.**
A skateboarder balances a skateboard on a rail. The skateboard has mass 4 kg and can be modelled as a uniform horizontal rod, AB, 0.8 m in length. The skateboard is in contact with the rail at point C, where $AC = 0.5$ m. The skateboarder has mass 80 kg and places her feet at points X and Y. The skateboard is in equilibrium when the force applied at Y is three times the force applied at X and CY is half the length of CB.

MODELLING PROBLEM SOLVING

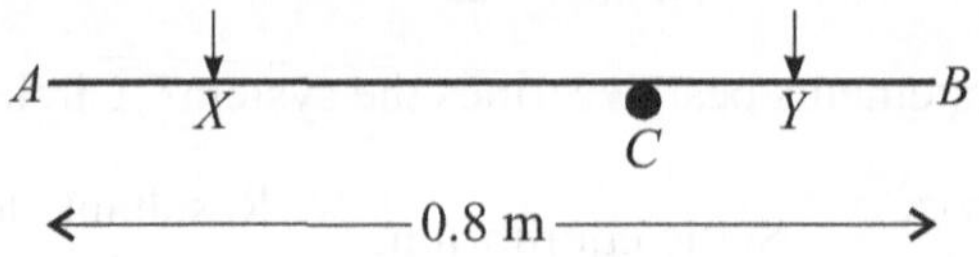

a) Find the distance AX.

....

(5 marks)

b) Find the magnitude of the normal reaction, R, at the rail.

....

(2 marks)

c) An object of mass 3 kg is placed on the skateboard at point A. The skateboarder moves her foot such that AX is increased by 13 cm. The skateboard remains horizontal and in equilibrium. Find the magnitude of the forces applied at X (F_X) and Y (F_Y).

F_X = ...

F_Y = ...

(5 marks)

5 A uniform rectangular lamina, $ABCD$, of weight 70 N, has dimensions x m by 3 m, as shown. The lamina is pivoted at B. It is kept in equilibrium by a horizontal force of 75 N acting at C and a downwards force of 15 N acting at D.

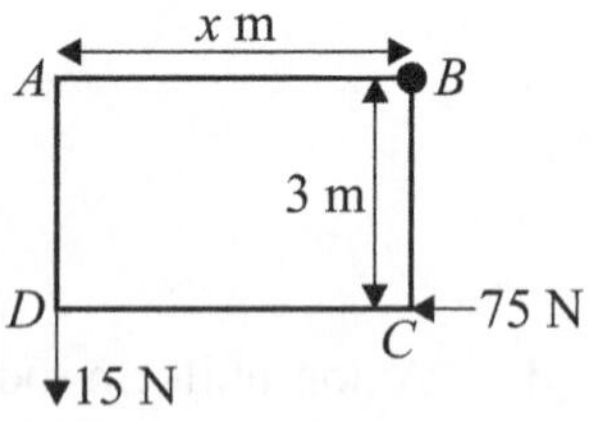

Find the value of x.

....

(2 marks)

EXAM TIP

If I had to sum up this topic in 5 words, I'd say this: "Equate moments and balance forces." Okay, fair enough, you have to be able to actually do the equating of moments and balancing of forces, and if I had about 800 more words to play with, I'd talk you through that. But used wisely I reckon those 5 words will get you around 80% of the marks on these pages.

Score

22

Problem Solving — 1

Sometimes you'll have to do some thinking about how to find the answer to a question — scary, I know...
If your problem is that you need more practice with these tricky questions, then the next few pages are the solution.

1 A small, submersible robot can move anywhere in a 10 × 8 × 7 m cuboid-shaped pool. One corner at the bottom of the pool is chosen to be the origin, O. The corner of the pool furthest from O has position vector $(10\mathbf{i} + 8\mathbf{j} + 7\mathbf{k})$ m.

PROBLEM SOLVING MODELLING

- The robot starts at point A, which has position vector $(p\mathbf{i} + 4\mathbf{j} + (p - 3)\mathbf{k})$ m, where p is a constant.
- The robot then moves to point B, and then to point C.
  $\overrightarrow{AB} = (-2\mathbf{i} - (p - 1)\mathbf{j} + \mathbf{k})$ m and $\overrightarrow{BC} = (\mathbf{i} - \mathbf{j} - \mathbf{k})$ m.
- The distance between point C and the origin is $\sqrt{10}$ m.

Find the value of p, and hence state the position vector of point A.

p = ...

A = ... m

(4 marks)

2 A company is monitoring the amount of CO_2 they emit. The amount of CO_2 emitted per year is forecast to decrease by 12% annually. The amount of CO_2 emitted in 2020 was 56 000 tonnes.

PROBLEM SOLVING MODELLING

a) Write down an equation to model the amount of CO_2, A tonnes, emitted in a given year, y, where $y \geq 2020$.

....

(2 marks)

b) Find the following amounts, giving your answers to 3 significant figures.

(i) The total amount of CO_2 that will be emitted from 2020 up to and including 2040.

.... tonnes

(2 marks)

(ii) The greatest possible total amount of CO_2 that could be emitted.

.... tonnes

(2 marks)

Problem Solving — 1

3 Two curves are defined by the following parametric equations, where M and N are integers.

- Curve C has equations $x = 2t - 3$ and $y = Mt^2 + 34t + N - 8$.
- Curve D has equations $x = u + 2$ and $y = 3u^2 + Nu - M - 11$.

PROBLEM SOLVING

The curves intersect at the point (1, 2).

Use algebra to find the values of M and N.

$M =$ .... $N =$ ....

(5 marks)

4 The function $f(x) = kx^3 - 49x^2 + 70x - k$, where k is a constant. PROBLEM SOLVING

a) Given that $f(2) = 0$, fully factorise $f(x)$ as the product of three distinct linear factors.

....

(5 marks)

b) Hence solve the equation $70 - 8 \operatorname{cosec} x = 49 \sin x - 8 \sin^2 x$, where $0 < x < \pi$.
Give your answers to 3 significant figures.

....

(4 marks)

Problem Solving — 1

5 $f(x) = \dfrac{4x^2 - 2x - 18}{4x^2 - 9}, x \neq \pm\dfrac{3}{2}$ PROBLEM SOLVING

a) Given that $f(x) = A + \dfrac{px + q}{4x^2 - 9}$, find the values of the constants A, p and q.

$A =$ .... $p =$ .... $q =$ ....

(2 marks)

b) Hence show that $\displaystyle\int_3^4 \frac{4x^2 - 2x - 18}{4x^2 - 9}\, dx$ can be written in the form $r + \ln s$, where r and s are constants to be found.

(6 marks)

6 In an experiment, argon gas is being added to a container of oxygen gas. The concentration of argon gas in the container is modelled by the equation $C = \dfrac{3^t + 3^{3t}}{9^t}$, where C is measured in parts per million (ppm) and t is the time in seconds. PROBLEM SOLVING MODELLING

Find the exact time at which the concentration of argon gas is changing at a rate of (5 ln 3) ppm s^{-1}. Give your answer as a single logarithm.

....

(6 marks)

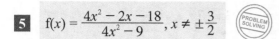

Problem Solving — 1

7 $f(\theta) = \dfrac{\sin\theta}{1 + \sin 2\theta} + \dfrac{1}{\sec\theta + 2\sin\theta}$, where $0 \leq \theta \leq 2\pi$ and $\theta \neq \dfrac{3\pi}{4}, \dfrac{\pi}{2}, \dfrac{3\pi}{2}, \dfrac{7\pi}{4}$.

PROBLEM SOLVING

a) Show that $f(\theta) = \dfrac{1}{\sin\theta + \cos\theta}$.

(4 marks)

In the diagram below, α is an obtuse angle.

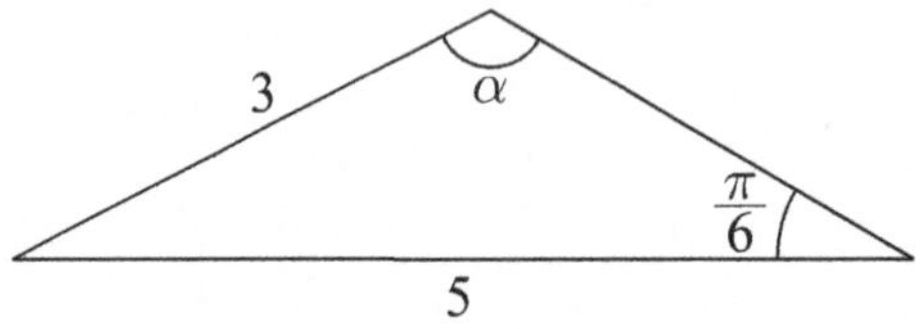

b) Using the result from part a), find the exact value of $f(\alpha)$.
Give your answer in the form $p + q\sqrt{r}$, where p and q are rational numbers and r is an integer.

....

(5 marks)

EXAM TIP

Some questions will involve less problem solving than others. If you get stuck on a tricky one, write down what you can — that way you might still get marks, even without the final answer. Then it might help to try a different question (if you've got any left) — you can come back to the tricky one later with a fresh mind, so long as you've left yourself a bit of time.

Score

47

Problem Solving — 2

Poor old statistics and mechanics, always having to wait for Pure maths to go first. Don't worry, my friends, I still love you. So much so that I've given the next few pages over to you and your best problem solving questions.

1 A random variable X has the cumulative distribution function $F(x) = \frac{x}{m}$, where x and m are integers with $0 \leq x \leq m$.

a) Find an expression for $P(X = x)$ in terms of m.

(2 marks)

A scientist uses X to model the possible outcomes, numbered from 1 to m, of an experiment. The experiment is conducted 20 times and the random variable Y is used to model the number of times that the outcome $X = 7$ is observed.

b) State an assumption that is required for Y to follow a binomial distribution and state the distribution of Y in terms of m.

(2 marks)

c) Given that $P(Y \geq 5) < 0.029$, find the minimum possible value of m.

(3 marks)

2 Three common traits among a population of plants are red flowers (F), broad leaves (L) and thorns (T).

The Venn diagram below shows the probabilities of a randomly selected plant exhibiting these traits. For a randomly selected plant:
$P(F' \cap T \mid L') = 0.2$, $P((F \cup T) \cap L') = 0.56$ and $P(F' \cap L \cap T) : P(F \cap L \cap T) = 2:1$.

a) Showing your working, find the unknown values in the Venn diagram.

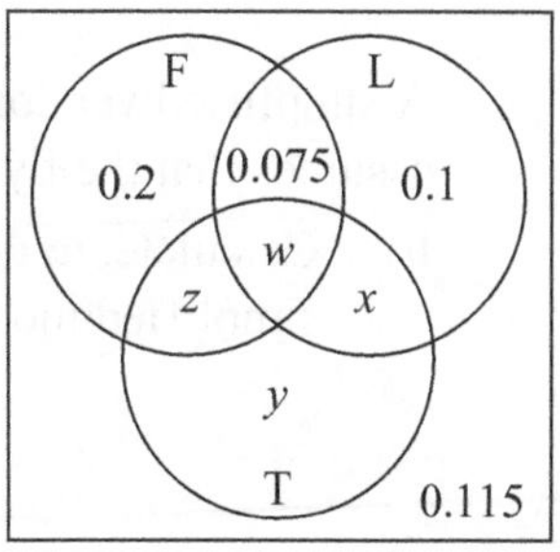

(5 marks)

b) 90 of the plants in the population have at least two of the three traits. Determine how many plants in the population have none of them.

(2 marks)

Problem Solving — 2

3 The velocity of a fly, in ms^{-1}, is modelled by the equation $v = (2t + 1)\ln(t + 1)$, where t is the time in seconds. In its first second of motion, the fly travels from point A to point B.

a) Find the following amounts to 3 significant figures.
Use of a calculator for numerical integration or differentiation is not accepted in this question.

(i) the acceleration of the fly when $t = 0.5$,

(3 marks)

(ii) the distance between points A and B.

(5 marks)

A simplified version of this model uses the same initial velocity but assumes that the fly moves with a constant acceleration of $2\ \text{ms}^{-2}$.

b) Calculate, to one decimal place, the percentage error in using the simplified model to find the distance between points A and B.

(4 marks)

General Certificate of Education
Advanced Level

A-Level Mathematics
Practice Exam Paper 1

Time Allowed: 2 hours

There are 100 marks available for this paper.

Formulas are given on page 174.

1 What are the coordinates of the stationary point of the graph of $y = x^2 - 8x + 7$? Circle your answer.

(2, 16) (–1, 16) (–7, 112) (4, –9)

(1 mark)

2 What is $2\log a^3b - \log ab$ as a single logarithm in its simplest form? Circle your answer.

$\log 2a^2b$ $\log a^2$ $\log a^5b$ $\log a^7b^3$

(1 mark)

3 a) $f(x) = \dfrac{x^3 - 9x^2 + 14x}{x^2 - 4} \times \dfrac{x+2}{x}$. Write f(x) in its simplest form.

(3 marks)

b) Find the coordinates of the points of intersection between $y = |f(x)|$ and the line $y = -\frac{1}{2}x + 5$. Fully justify your answer.

(4 marks)

4 The functions f, g and h are defined below.

$f(x) = \dfrac{2x+7}{3x-5}, x \in \mathbb{R}, x \neq \dfrac{5}{3}$ $g(x) = x^2 - k, x \in \mathbb{R}$ where k is a positive constant $h(x) = \cos x, x \in \mathbb{R}$

a) Find $f^{-1}(x)$.

(2 marks)

b) $gf(2) = 120$. Find the value of k.

(3 marks)

c) Find gh(x) and hg(x), and hence show that the range of gh(x) is not the same as the range of hg(x).

(4 marks)

5 For small values of θ, show that $\frac{1 - \tan 3\theta}{\cos 4\theta - \sin \theta^2} \approx \frac{1}{1 + 3\theta}$.

(3 marks)

6 Prove that $\sqrt{2}$ is an irrational number.

(4 marks)

7 **a)** Show that the graph of $y = xe^x$ only crosses the x-axis once, at (0, 0).

(2 marks)

The graph of $y = xe^x$ for $-1 \leq x \leq 1$ is shown below.

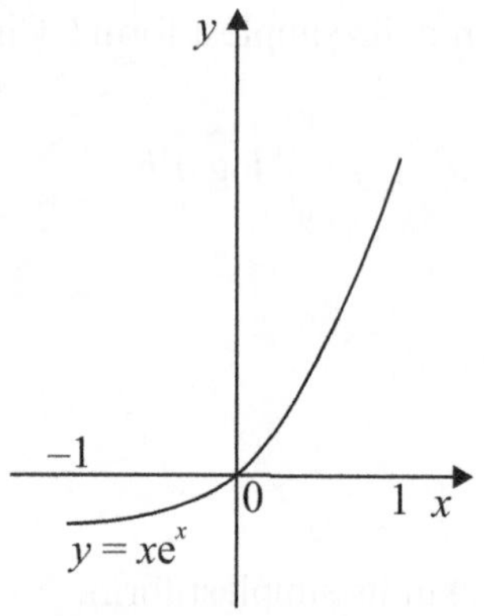

b) Showing the coordinates of any points of intersection with the y-axis, sketch:

(i) $y = xe^x + 0.2, \quad -1 \leq x \leq 1$

(2 marks)

(ii) $y = |xe^x|, \quad -1 \leq x \leq 1$

(2 marks)

8 The curve C has parametric equations:

$$x = t^3 + 2, \; y = t^2 + 2$$

The point P lies on the curve where $t = 1$.

a) Find the coordinates of P.

(1 mark)

The line l is the tangent to C at P.

b) Find the Cartesian equation of the line l in the form $y = mx + c$.

(4 marks)

9 A curve has equation $x^2 - xy = 2y^3$. Find the gradient of the curve at the point (2, 1).

(5 marks)

10 The diagram shows a section of the graph of $y = 2\cos\frac{x}{4}$.
It crosses the x-axis at $x = 2\pi$ and the y-axis at $y = 2$.

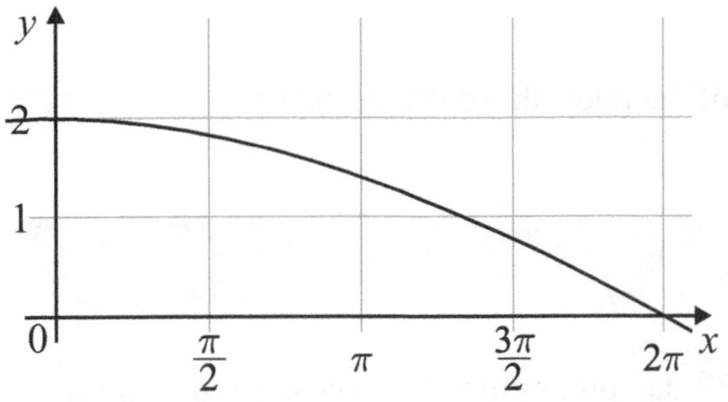

a) Lily works out $\int_0^{2\pi} 2\cos\frac{x}{4}\,dx$ and gets an answer of 4π. Her teacher doesn't do the integration, but tells her that she is wrong, and that her answer is too big. Explain how the teacher knew this by looking at the graph.

(1 mark)

b) Use algebraic integration to find the value of $\int_0^{2\pi} 2\cos\frac{x}{4}\,dx$.

(3 marks)

11 a) Find the coordinates of the stationary point on the curve $y = x\ln x$.
Give your answer in exact form.

(5 marks)

b) Determine the nature of the stationary point. Give a reason for your answer.

(2 marks)

12 The rate of growth of a population of bacteria is proportional to the number of bacteria in the population.

a) Show that the number of bacteria in the population, P, can be modelled by the function $P = Qe^{kt}$, where t is the time in hours after the population was first observed and Q and k are constants.

(3 marks)

b) When the experiment begins, there are 5300 bacteria. After 6 hours, there are 876 bacteria present.
Find k to 1 decimal place.

(3 marks)

c) Use your value of k to describe how the population of bacteria is changing.

(1 mark)

13 A buoy floats on the surface of the sea.
The height, H metres above the sea bed, of the buoy at time t hours is modelled by the equation

$$H = 2\cos\left(\frac{4\pi t}{25}\right) + 4, \quad 0 < t \leq 12$$

a) Find $\frac{dH}{dt}$.

(1 mark)

b) Find the rate of change of the height of the buoy after 7 hours.

(2 marks)

c) Find the minimum height of the buoy above the sea bed.

(2 marks)

14 A group of musicians follow a 30-day programme to practise for a concert.
The length of time for which the pianist practises will increase by 10 minutes every day.
On day 1 the pianist practises for 1 hour.

a) On which day will the pianist practise for exactly 4 hours 40 minutes?

(3 marks)

The length of time for which the violinist practises will increase by 4% each day.
On day 1 the violinist practises for 1 hour 40 minutes.

b) On which day does the violinist first practise for more than 4 hours 40 minutes?

(4 marks)

c) Which of the two musicians practises for the longest time in total over the 30 days?
Give working to show how you came to your conclusion.

(3 marks)

15 In trapezium $ABCD$, the acute angle $BAD = x$ radians. Angles BCD and ABC are $\frac{\pi}{2}$.
$DA = 5$ cm and $AB = 2CD$, as shown in the diagram.

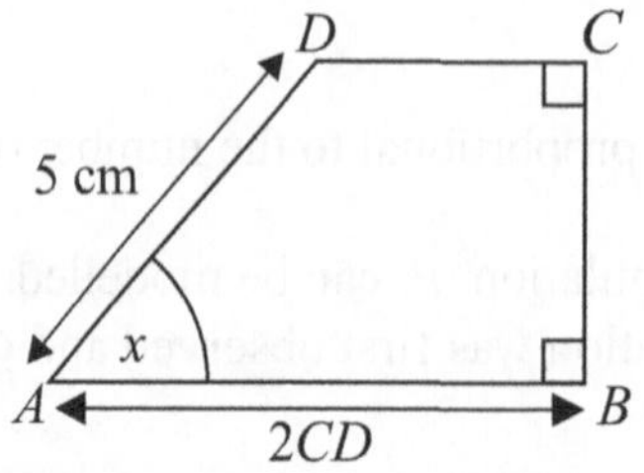

a) Show that an expression for the perimeter, P cm, can be written as $P = R\sin(x + \alpha) + 5$, where R and α are values to be found.

(7 marks)

b) Given that the perimeter of the trapezium is 17 cm, find the value of x to 3 significant figures.

(4 marks)

16 Find $\int \frac{\ln x}{x^5}\,dx$.

(4 marks)

17 Part of a concrete sculpture is modelled as a cube with sides of length x m. Concrete costs £65 per cubic metre. Each face is then covered in gold leaf which costs £150 per square metre.

a) Given that the cost of materials used for the cube is £250, prove that x satisfies the equation

$$x = \sqrt{\frac{250 - 65x^3}{900}}$$

(4 marks)

b) Hence show that the length of the cube is between 0.5 m and 1 m.

(2 marks)

c) Using the iteration formula $x_{n+1} = \sqrt{\frac{250 - 65x_n^3}{900}}$ with $x_1 = 0.75$, find x_2 and x_5. Give your answers correct to 4 decimal places.

(2 marks)

d) Use your value for x_5 to estimate the percentage of the total cost of the cube that was spent on concrete. Give your answer correct to 1 decimal place.

(2 marks)

The graph below shows the curve $y = \sqrt{\frac{250 - 65x^3}{900}}$ and the line $y = x$. The position of x_1 is indicated.

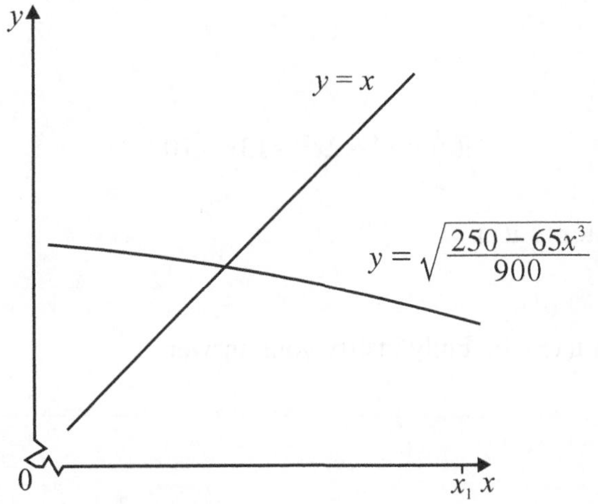

e) Use the graph to show the positions of x_2 and x_3.

(1 mark)

END OF EXAM PAPER

TOTAL FOR PAPER: 100 MARKS

General Certificate of Education
Advanced Level

A-Level Mathematics
Practice Exam Paper 2

Time Allowed: 2 hours

There are 100 marks available for this paper.

Formulas are given on page 174.

Section A

1 Which equation below is a rearrangement of $y = ax^b$? Circle your answer.

$\log y = \log a + x \log b$ $\quad$ $\log y = \log a + b \log x$ $\quad$ $\log y = b \log ax$ $\quad$ $y = \log a + b \log x$

(1 mark)

2 For the continuous function f(x), f(–1) = 1.17 and f(1) = –1.18 (both to 3 s.f.).
Which one of the statements below cannot be true for f(x)? Circle your answer.

There are no roots in the interval (–1, 1). $\quad$ There is an odd number of roots in the interval (–1, 1).

There is exactly 1 root in the interval (–1, 1). $\quad$ There are 2 distinct roots in the interval (–1, 1).

(1 mark)

3

$$f(x) = x^3 - 2x^2 - 13x - 10$$

a) Show that $(x + 1)$ is a factor of f(x).

(2 marks)

b) Hence solve the equation f(x) = 0. Fully justify your answer.

(3 marks)

4 A sequence satisfies the recurrence relation $u_{n+1} = 5u_n - 2$, where $n \geq 1$.

a) Given that $u_3 = 38$, find u_1.

(2 marks)

b) Suppose instead that the sequence is decreasing. Find the range of possible values of u_1.

(2 marks)

c) Find a value of u_1 for which $\sum_{n=1}^{r} u_n = \frac{1}{2}r$ for any value of r.

(1 mark)

5 Find $\int \frac{45x^2 + 12x}{5x^3 + 2x^2 + 6}\,dx$.

(3 marks)

6 Solve the equation $2\text{ cosec}^2 x + 5\cot x = 9$, for $-90° < x < 90°$.
Give your answers to 1 decimal place where appropriate.

(6 marks)

7 **a)** Find $f'(x)$ for $f(x) = 4x^3 + e^{x^2}$.

(2 marks)

b) Show that the graph of $f(x)$ convex when $x > 0$.

(5 marks)

8 The curve C has parametric equations

$$x = 1 + 5\cos t,\ y = 2 + 5\sin t,\quad 0 \le t \le 2\pi$$

a) Show that the Cartesian equation of the curve C is the circle given by the equation

$$(x - 1)^2 + (y - 2)^2 = 25$$

(3 marks)

The line l is the tangent to the circle at the point P (4, 6).

b) Find the equation of the line l. Give your answer in the form $ax + by + c = 0$, where a, b and c are integers to be found.

(4 marks)

9 The parallelogram $ABCD$ has sides of length 5 units and 9 units.

a) The coordinates of A are (2, 4, 1). B has coordinates (9, 8, z).
Find the two possible values of z.

(4 marks)

b) Given that z is a positive integer and that the unit vector in the direction of $\overrightarrow{BC}$ is $0.8\mathbf{j} + 0.6\mathbf{k}$, show that the coordinates of C are (9, 12, 8).

(3 marks)

c) Hence find the exact length of the diagonal $\overrightarrow{AC}$.

(3 marks)

10 The diagram on the right shows the graph of $y = \dfrac{e^{\sin x} + x}{(x+1)^3}$ for $0 \le x \le 2$.

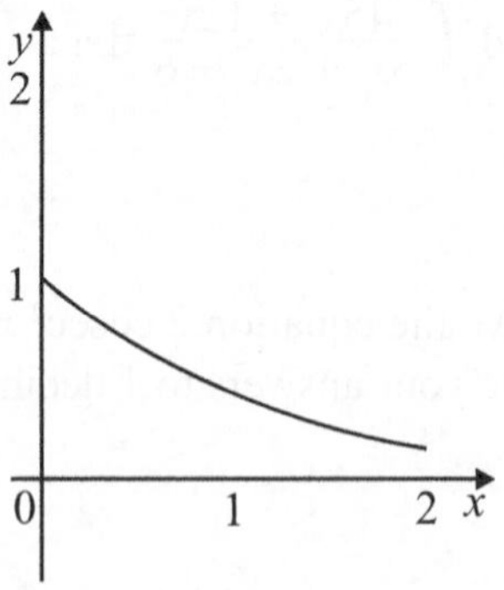

The table below shows values of y for values of x between 0 and 2.
The y-values have been rounded to 3 and 5 decimal places.

x	0	0.5	1	1.5
y (3 d.p.)	1		0.415	0.270
y (5 d.p.)	1		0.41497	0.26953

a) Complete the table.

(1 mark)

b) Using the trapezium rule with 3 strips, and the values of y that have been rounded to 3 decimal places, find an approximation for $\displaystyle\int_0^{1.5} \frac{e^{\sin x} + x}{(x+1)^3}\, dx$.

(3 marks)

c) Sophie calculates that the actual area bounded by the curve, the x-axis, the y-axis and the line $x = 1.5$ is 0.8224, correct to four decimal places. She says that the estimate found using the trapezium rule was larger than this because each rounded value of y was larger than its true value. By considering the graph above, comment on Sophie's claim.

(1 mark)

END OF SECTION A

Section B

11 A particle of mass 120 g is accelerating at a rate of 6 ms^{-2}. Find the resultant force acting on the particle. Circle your answer.

720 N   0.02 N   0.72 N   20 N

(1 mark)

12 A particle P of mass 2.5 kg is moving in a horizontal plane under the action of a single force, $\mathbf{F}$ newtons. At t seconds, the position vector of P is $\mathbf{r}$ m, where $\mathbf{r}$ is given by:

$$\mathbf{r} = (t^3 - 6t^2 + 4t)\mathbf{i} + (7t - 4t^2 + 3)\mathbf{j},$$

where $\mathbf{i}$ and $\mathbf{j}$ are the unit vectors directed due east and due north respectively.

a) Show that when $t = 5$, the velocity of P is $19\mathbf{i} - 33\mathbf{j}$.

(3 marks)

b) Find the value of t when P is moving due south.

(4 marks)

c) Find the magnitude of the resultant force acting on P when $t = 3$.

(5 marks)

13 **In this question use $g = 9.81\ ms^{-2}$.**

A uniform rod, *AB*, of length 6 m and mass 6 kg rests on two supports, *P* and *Q*, as shown.

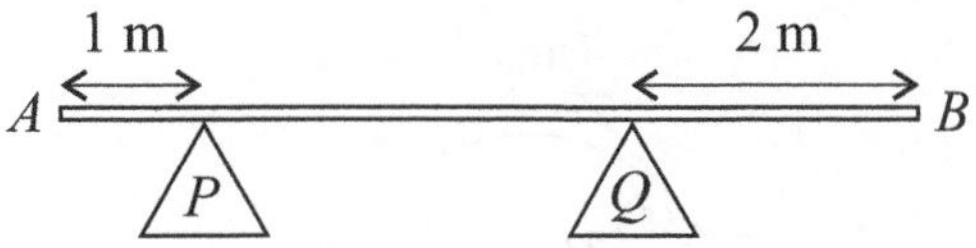

A 4 kg particle is placed on the rod at a distance of *x* m from *A*.

a) Given that the reaction forces on the rod at *P* and *Q* are now equal, and that the rod is in equilibrium, find the value of *x*.

(3 marks)

b) Another particle, of mass *M* kg, is added to the end of the rod, at *B*. Find the maximum value of *M* for which the rod will remain in equilibrium.

(2 marks)

14 A helicopter *E* is modelled as a particle. It sets off from its base *O* on the coast and flies at constant height with initial velocity $(40\mathbf{i} + 108\mathbf{j})\ kmh^{-1}$ and constant acceleration $(4\mathbf{i} + 12\mathbf{j})\ kmh^{-2}$, where **i** and **j** are the unit vectors in the direction of east and north respectively. Thirty minutes after *E* has left the base, the pilot informs the base that he has engine failure and is ditching into the sea.

a) Find the position vector of *E* relative to *O* at the time it experiences engine failure.

(3 marks)

The base immediately informs another helicopter, *F*, that *E* is in need of assistance. *F* is modelled as a particle flying towards *E*'s position at a constant height from position $(2.5\mathbf{i} + 25.5\mathbf{j})$ km, with constant acceleration and initial velocity $(60\mathbf{i} + 120\mathbf{j})\ kmh^{-1}$.

b) Given that *F* takes 15 minutes to reach *E*, find the magnitude of the acceleration of *F*.

(3 marks)

The base sends out a third helicopter, *G*, on another mission. *G* is modelled as a particle, and leaves the base *O* with velocity $(30\mathbf{i} - 40\mathbf{j})\ kmh^{-1}$ and accelerates at a constant $(5\mathbf{i} + 8\mathbf{j})\ kmh^{-2}$ towards its destination.

c) Find the position vector of *G* when it is travelling due east.

(6 marks)

15 A golf ball is hit off a rock of height 0.5 m with initial velocity U ms^{-1} at an angle $\alpha°$ above the horizontal. The golf ball lands on horizontal ground at point X, as shown.

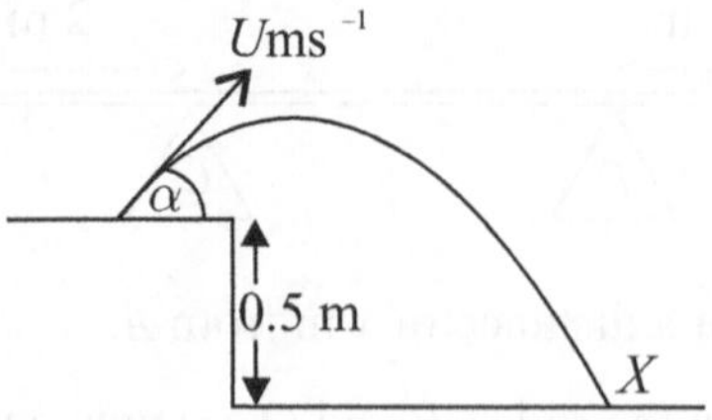

a) Show that the golf ball reaches maximum height $h = \dfrac{g + U^2 \sin^2 \alpha}{2g}$ m above the ground, where g is acceleration due to gravity.

(4 marks)

b) Show that V, the speed of the golf ball when it lands at X, is $V = \sqrt{U^2 + g}$ ms^{-1}.

(5 marks)

A beach ball is projected from the same point as the golf ball, with velocity U ms^{-1} and angle of projection α.

c) Suggest one way in which the model used in parts a) and b) could be adapted for the beach ball.

(1 mark)

16 **In this question use $g = 9.8$ ms^{-2}.**

Two particles, A and B, are connected by a light inextensible string that passes over a smooth pulley. A rests on a smooth plane inclined at an angle of $\theta°$ to the horizontal, where $\theta = \tan^{-1}\left(\frac{3}{4}\right)$, and B rests on a rough plane inclined at 70° to the horizontal, as shown. The coefficient of friction between B and the plane is 0.45. A has mass m kg and B has mass $2m$ kg.

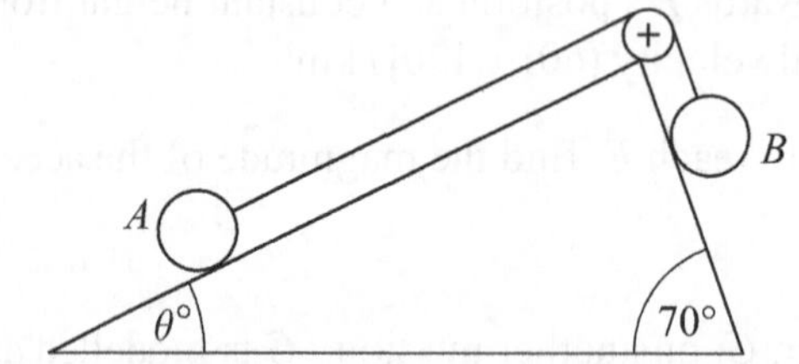

The system is released from rest and B starts to move down the plane.

a) Find the acceleration of particle A towards the pulley.

(6 marks)

b) The mass of A is increased to 10 kg. It is now on the point of sliding down the plane. Find the mass of B.

(4 marks)

END OF EXAM PAPER

TOTAL FOR PAPER: 100 MARKS

General Certificate of Education
Advanced Level

A-Level Mathematics
Practice Exam Paper 3

Time Allowed: 2 hours

There are 100 marks available for this paper.

Formulas are given on page 174.

Section A

1 A curve has parametric equations:

$$x = t - 3,\ y = (t + k)^2 \text{, where } k \text{ is a constant.}$$

Given that the curve passes through the point (–7, 0), find the value of k. Circle your answer.

4 7 –4 3

(1 mark)

2 Point $P(a, b)$ lies on the curve $y = f(x)$, where f is some function of x. At P, $\frac{dy}{dx} = 1$ and $\frac{d^2y}{dx^2} = 0$. When $x < a$, $\frac{d^2y}{dx^2} > 0$ and when $x > a$, $\frac{d^2y}{dx^2} < 0$. What type of point is P? Circle your answer.

maximum point minimum point point of inflection stationary point of inflection

(1 mark)

3 Prove that

$$\sec 2\theta \equiv \frac{\sec^2\theta}{2 - \sec^2\theta}$$

(3 marks)

4 Sketch the graph of $y = \frac{2}{x^2 - 1}$, giving the equations of any asymptotes and coordinates of any points of intersection with the axes.

(4 marks)

5 **a)** Express $\frac{11x - 7}{(2x - 4)(x + 1)}$ in partial fractions.

(4 marks)

b) Hence find the binomial expansion of $\frac{11x - 7}{(2x - 4)(x + 1)}$, in ascending powers of x, up to and including the term in x^2.

(6 marks)

6 The diagram below shows a rectangular field 20 m long and 8 m wide enclosed by fences. Inside the field is a rabbit pen, which is a regular hexagon with sides of length 2 m. The pen is positioned with one of its sides up against one of the 20 m fences.

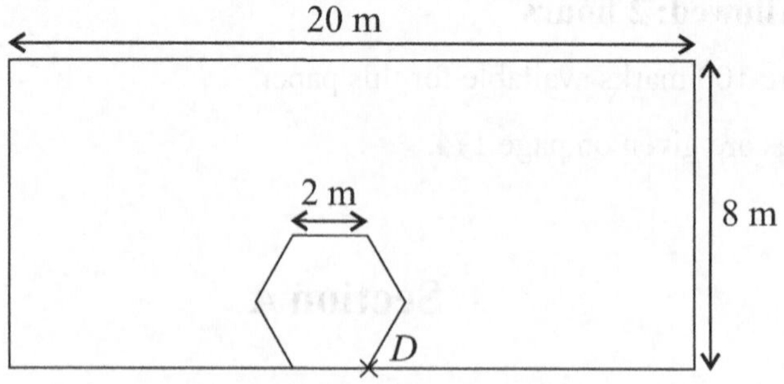

A dog is tied to the point labelled D on the diagram. The dog's lead is 2 m long. It is not able to enter the pen.

a) Calculate the exact area of the field the dog can reach.

(3 marks)

b) A cat now enters the field. It stays out of the area that the dog can get to and it is not able to enter the rabbit pen. Find the area of the field that the cat might go in. Give your answer correct to 3 significant figures.

(4 marks)

7 Find $f'(x)$ for $f(x) = \dfrac{3 + \sin x}{(2x+1)^4}$.

(4 marks)

8 Use the substitution $u = \sqrt{x-1}$ to find the exact value of $\int_5^{10} \dfrac{2x}{\sqrt{x-1}}\,dx$. Fully justify your answer.

(5 marks)

9 **a)** Show that the x-coordinate of the point of intersection of the curves $y = \dfrac{1}{x^3}$ and $y = x + 3$ satisfies the equation $x^4 + 3x^3 - 1 = 0$.

(1 mark)

$x^4 + 3x^3 - 1 = 0$ has a root α in the interval $[0.5, 1]$

b) Apply the Newton-Raphson method to obtain a second and third approximation for α, using 0.6 as the first approximation for α. Give your answers to 4 decimal places.

(5 marks)

10 A pan containing soup at a temperature of 95°C is removed from a stove and the soup is left to cool in a kitchen. t minutes after being removed from the stove, the temperature of the soup is T °C.

The rate of heat loss of the soup over time is modelled as being directly proportional to the difference in temperature between the soup and the kitchen.
The temperature of the kitchen is 15°C.

a) Explain why $\frac{dT}{dt} = -k(T - 15)$, for some positive constant k.

(1 mark)

b) Find an expression for T in terms of t and k.

(3 marks)

After 10 minutes, the temperature of the soup is 55°C.

c) Find the exact value of k, and hence show that $T = 80(0.5)^{pt} + 15$ where p is a positive constant to be found.

(4 marks)

d) State one assumption that has been made for this model.

(1 mark)

END OF SECTION A

Section B

11 Chloe wants to survey some of the residents of her town to ask their opinion about the local supermarket. She obtains a copy of the electoral roll and selects one person at random from the first 20 people listed. She then surveys every 20th person on the electoral roll.

a) What type of sampling has Chloe used to collect her data? Circle your answer.

Opportunity sampling Stratified sampling Systematic sampling Quota sampling

(1 mark)

Chloe visits the supermarket each weekday. The probability that she has to queue for longer than 2 minutes on any visit is 0.4.

b) She records how long she has to wait on a random sample of 50 visits to the supermarket. She uses a normal approximation to the binomial distribution to represent the number of times she has to queue for longer than 2 minutes. What is the normal approximation she should use? Circle your answer.

N(50, 0.4) N(20, 12) N(100, 40) N(25, 30)

(1 mark)

12 The graph below shows the average carbon monoxide emissions (to 2 decimal places) of the vehicles in the large data set registered in London in 2016 with different body types. The graph includes these body types: 4-door saloons (A), convertibles (B), coupes (C), estates (D), 3-door hatchbacks (E), 5-door hatchbacks (F), and multi-purpose vehicles (G).

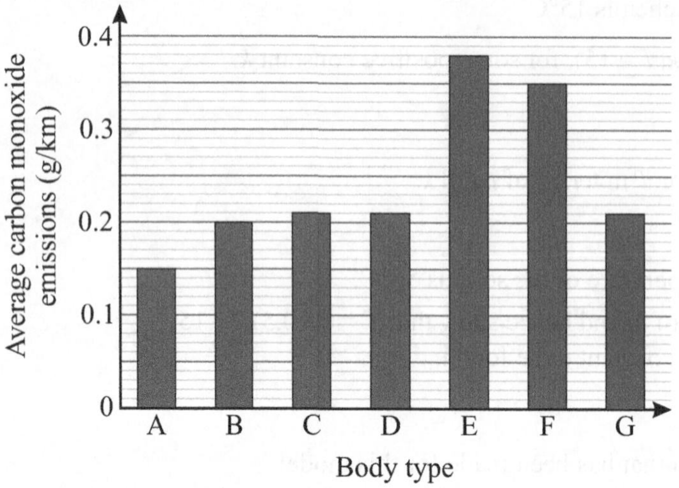

a) An outlier is defined as a value that is less than $Q_1 - 1.5 \times \text{IQR}$ or greater than $Q_3 + 1.5 \times \text{IQR}$. By working out any necessary statistics, determine if any of the body types are outliers.

(4 marks)

b) 3-door hatchbacks and 5-door hatchbacks are combined to create a single hatchback body type (H) and the average carbon monoxide emissions of the vehicles in this group, h g/km, calculated. Show that body type H is an outlier, and decide whether the data values for this body type should be excluded from any analysis. Explain your answer.

(3 marks)

c) Mason wants to know about the carbon monoxide emissions of vehicles in the South West. Do you think he can use the information in the graph above for this purpose? Use your knowledge of the large data set to explain your answer.

(1 mark)

13 Aliyah usually goes to the gym on Saturdays. When she does, she uses only the swimming pool or the rowing machines. On any given Saturday:

R represents the event that she uses the rowing machines.

S represents the event that she uses the swimming pool.

$$P(R \cup S) = \frac{8}{10} \quad P(R|S) = \frac{4}{9} \quad P(S|R) = \frac{4}{11}$$

a) Calculate P(R) and P(S).

(5 marks)

b) Explain whether the events R and S are independent.

(2 marks)

T represents the event that Aliyah has a takeaway on any given Saturday.

The events S and T are independent.

$$P(T) = 0.15 \quad P(R \cap T) = 0.08 \quad P(R \cap S \cap T) = 0.05$$

c) Draw a Venn diagram to show events R, S and T, giving the probabilities for each region.

(4 marks)

14 Hashim wants to investigate the mass of vehicles registered in 2002 in London.
He collects data on 400 vehicles from the large data set and represents the results on a histogram, shown below.

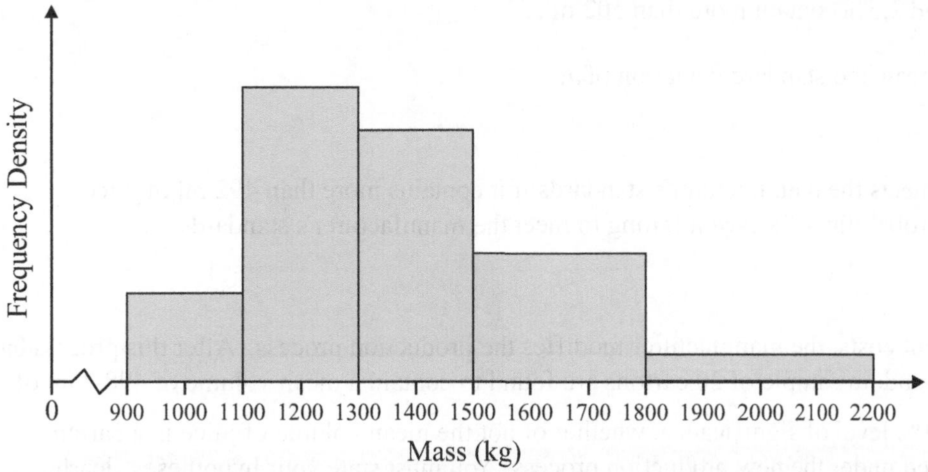

a) Hashim calculates the following summary statistics: $\sum fx = 557\,250$, $\sum fx^2 = 804\,302\,500$.
Use these values to find the mean and standard deviation of x.

(3 marks)

b) Hashim suggests modelling the data using a normal distribution with the mean and standard deviation calculated in part a). With reference to the histogram, explain why this would not be an appropriate model.

(1 mark)

c) Leanne collects her own data from her town in the North West.
For her data, she calculates the mean and standard deviation to be 1597 kg and 278 kg respectively.
The values for the upper and lower quartiles are $Q_3 = 1786$ kg and $Q_1 = 1399$ kg.
Based on these statistics, explain whether the normal distribution $N(1597, 278^2)$ could be a suitable model for Leanne's data. Use calculations to support your answer.

(3 marks)

15 Lara is investigating particulate emissions from diesel vehicles in the South West. Lara finds particulate emission data for 131 diesel vehicles in this region from the large data set, and she records that 105 of these vehicles have emissions of less than 0.04 g/km. One Saturday afternoon in August 2018, she takes a sample of 15 diesel vehicles parked at a service station on the M5 motorway in Somerset. She models the number of vehicles in this sample with particulate emissions of less than 0.04 g/km using a binomial distribution. In her model, she uses the data from the large data set to give $p = 105 \div 131 = 0.80$ (2 d.p.).

a) According to Lara's model, find the probability that at least five but fewer than 10 vehicles in her sample have particulate emissions of less than 0.04 g/km.

(3 marks)

b) Explain why Lara's value of p may not represent the true probability of a diesel vehicle at the service station having particulate emissions of less than 0.04 g/km.

(1 mark)

c) State an assumption that Lara has made in order to use a binomial model.

(1 mark)

16 A juice manufacturer produces orange juice in cartons. The volume of juice in a carton, J ml, is assumed to be normally distributed. Based on previous data, the quality control officer finds that 5% of cartons contain less than 493 ml, and 2.5% contain more than 502 ml.

a) Find the mean and standard deviation of J.

(5 marks)

b) A carton meets the manufacturer's standards if it contains more than 492 ml of juice. Find the probability of a carton failing to meet the manufacturer's standards.

(2 marks)

In an effort to cut costs, the manufacturer modifies the production process. After this process has been in place for a month, a random sample of 20 cartons are found to contain a mean volume of 498.7 ml of juice.

c) Test, at a 1% level of significance, whether or not the mean volume of juice in a carton has changed under the new production process. You must state your hypotheses clearly.

(5 marks)

17 Amira and Ben are studying the approximate number of a particular bacteria, y, in ponds of different maximum depths, x m. They collect data from 8 ponds, with maximum depths varying from 0.5 m to 12 m, and calculate the product moment correlation coefficient between x and y for their data. Amira obtains a value of $r_A = 0.71$, and Ben calculates his value to be $r_B = 1.09$.

a) Interpret, in context, the value of Amira's correlation coefficient, and explain how you can tell that Ben must have made a mistake in his calculation.

(2 marks)

b) Amira claims that her results show that deeper ponds result in higher numbers of bacteria. Comment on this claim.

(1 mark)

c) The critical value for a 1-tail test at a 5% significance level on a sample size of 8 is 0.6215. Stating your hypotheses clearly, test at the 5% significance level whether Amira's results are statistically significant evidence of positive correlation between the number of this type of bacteria and pond depth in the population of ponds.

(2 marks)

END OF EXAM PAPER

TOTAL FOR PAPER: 100 MARKS

Answers

Section One — Pure Maths

Pages 3-4: Proof

1 A $\Leftrightarrow$ B ***[1 mark]***
You can show A $\Rightarrow$ B by simplifying A. Conversely, to show B $\Rightarrow$ A you can cube both sides of B, then add 1. So A $\Leftrightarrow$ B is the best description.

2 Proof by exhaustion: $n^3 - 16n = n(n^2 - 16) = n(n+4)(n-4)$ ***[1 mark]***
If n is a multiple of 3, then the first factor is a multiple of 3.
If n is 1 more than a multiple of 3, then $n = 3k + 1$ for some integer k.
Then $n - 4 = 3k + 1 - 4 = 3k - 3 = 3(k-1)$, which is a multiple of 3.
If n is 2 more than a multiple of 3, then $n = 3k + 2$ for some integer k.
Then $n + 4 = 3k + 2 + 4 = 3k + 6 = 3(k+2)$, which is a multiple of 3.
[1 mark for substituting in all three possible values]
So by exhaustion, either n, $(n-4)$ or $(n+4)$ is a multiple of 3, meaning $n^3 - 16n$ is a multiple of 3 for any integer n ***[1 mark]***.

3 Take two prime numbers, p and q ($p \neq q$ and $p, q > 1$). As p is prime, its only factors are 1 and p ***[1 mark]***, and as q is prime, its only factors are 1 and q ***[1 mark]***. So the product pq has factors 1, p, q, and pq ***[1 mark]*** (these factors are found by multiplying the factors of each number together in every possible combination). $pq \neq 1$ as $p, q > 1$. Hence the product of any two distinct prime numbers has exactly four factors.

4 As n is even, write n as $2k$ for some integer k ***[1 mark]***.
So $n^3 + 2n^2 + 12n = (2k)^3 + 2(2k)^2 + 12(2k)$
$= 8k^3 + 8k^2 + 24k$ ***[1 mark]***
This can be written as $8x$, where $x = k^3 + k^2 + 3k$, so is always a multiple of 8 when n is even ***[1 mark]***.

5 a) E.g. Let both x and y be $\sqrt{2}$. $\sqrt{2}$ is irrational, but $\frac{\sqrt{2}}{\sqrt{2}} = 1$ which is rational, hence Riyad's claim is false.
[1 mark for any valid counter-example]

b) Let x be a rational number, where $x \neq 0$.
Let z be an irrational number.
Assume that the product zx is rational, so $zx = \frac{a}{b}$ where a and b are integers ($a, b \neq 0$) ***[1 mark]***.
x is rational, so $x = \frac{l}{m}$ where l and m are integers ($l, m \neq 0$).
So, the product $zx = \frac{zl}{m} = \frac{a}{b} \Rightarrow z = \frac{ma}{lb}$ ***[1 mark]***.
ma and lb are the products of non-zero integers, so are non-zero integers themselves. So, z is rational. This is a contradiction, as z is irrational by definition, ***[1 mark]*** therefore, zx must be irrational.

6 Proof by contradiction: Assume that $\sqrt[4]{x}$ is rational ***[1 mark]***.
Then $\sqrt[4]{x} = \frac{a}{b}$ where a and b are non-zero integers ***[1 mark]***.
This gives $x = \left(\frac{a}{b}\right)^4 = \frac{a^4}{b^4}$. Since a and b are non-zero integers, a^4 and b^4 are also non-zero integers. This means that x is rational. This is a contradiction, since x is irrational by definition ***[1 mark]***.
So $\sqrt[4]{x}$ is irrational.

7 a) E.g. The student's proof shows that if x is even, then x^3 is even. This is not the same as showing if x^3 is even, then x is even.
[1 mark for any sensible explanation of why the proof is not valid]

b) Proof by contradiction:
Assume that the statement is false. So, that means for some value of x, x^3 is even but x is odd ***[1 mark]***.
x is odd so $x = 2n + 1$, where n is an integer ***[1 mark]***.
So, $x^3 = (2n+1)^3 = (4n^2 + 4n + 1)(2n + 1)$
$= 8n^3 + 12n^2 + 6n + 1$
$= 2(4n^3 + 6n^2 + 3n) + 1$ ***[1 mark]***
$4n^3 + 6n^2 + 3n$ is an integer, call it m, so $x^3 = 2m + 1$ is odd.
This contradicts the assumption that x^3 is even but x is odd, ***[1 mark]*** hence if x^3 is even, then x is even.

8 A four-digit number can be written as $1000a + 100b + 10c + d$, where a, b, c and d are the integer digits of the number ***[1 mark]***.
If the number is a multiple of 3, then for some integer k:
$1000a + 100b + 10c + d = 3k$ ***[1 mark]***
$\Rightarrow 999a + a + 99b + b + 9c + c + d = 3k$
$\Rightarrow a + b + c + d = 3k - 999a - 99b - 9c$
$\Rightarrow a + b + c + d = 3(k - 333a - 33b - 3c)$ ***[1 mark]***
$k - 333a - 33b - 3c$ is an integer,
so the sum of the digits is a multiple of 3 ***[1 mark]***.

Pages 5-7: Algebra and Functions — 1

1 $\sqrt[m]{a^n} = a^{\frac{n}{m}}$ so $\sqrt{a^4} = a^2$ and $a^6 \times a^3 = a^{6+3} = a^9$

So $\frac{a^6 \times a^3}{\sqrt{a^4}} \div a^{\frac{1}{2}} = \frac{a^9}{a^2} \div a^{\frac{1}{2}}$ ***[1 mark]***

$= a^{7-\frac{1}{2}} = a^{\frac{13}{2}}$ ***[1 mark]***

2 a) $3 = \sqrt[3]{27} = 27^{\frac{1}{3}}$, so $x = \frac{1}{3}$ ***[1 mark]***

b) $81 = 3^4 = (\sqrt[3]{27})^4 = 27^{\frac{4}{3}}$, so $x = \frac{4}{3}$ ***[1 mark]***

3 $\frac{(3ab^3)^2 \times 2a^6}{6a^4b} = \frac{3^2 \times a^2 \times (b^3)^2 \times 2a^6}{6a^4b} = \frac{18a^8b^6}{6a^4b} = 3a^4b^5$ ***[1 mark]***

4 $\frac{(5+4\sqrt{x})^2}{2x} = \frac{25 + 40\sqrt{x} + 16x}{2x}$ ***[1 mark]***

$= \frac{1}{2}x^{-1}(25 + 40x^{\frac{1}{2}} + 16x)$ ***[1 mark]***

$= \frac{25}{2}x^{-1} + 20x^{-\frac{1}{2}} + 8$ ***[1 mark]***

So P = 20 and Q = 8.

5 $(5\sqrt{5} + 2\sqrt{3})^2 = (5\sqrt{5} + 2\sqrt{3})(5\sqrt{5} + 2\sqrt{3})$
$= (5\sqrt{5})^2 + 2(5\sqrt{5} \times 2\sqrt{3}) + (2\sqrt{3})^2$

First term: $(5\sqrt{5})^2 = 5\sqrt{5} \times 5\sqrt{5}$
$= 5 \times 5 \times \sqrt{5} \times \sqrt{5} = 5 \times 5 \times 5 = 125$ ***[1 mark]***

Second term: $2(5\sqrt{5} \times 2\sqrt{3}) = 2 \times 5 \times 2 \times \sqrt{5} \times \sqrt{3}$
$= 20\sqrt{15}$ ***[1 mark]***

Third term: $(2\sqrt{3})^2 = 2\sqrt{3} \times 2\sqrt{3} = 2 \times 2 \times \sqrt{3} \times \sqrt{3}$
$= 2 \times 2 \times 3 = 12$ ***[1 mark]***

So $(5\sqrt{5})^2 + 2(5\sqrt{5} \times 2\sqrt{3}) + (2\sqrt{3})^2$
$= 125 + 20\sqrt{15} + 12 = 137 + 20\sqrt{15}$ ***[1 mark]***

So a = 137, b = 20 and c = 15.

6 $\frac{1}{(4\sqrt{7} - \sqrt{2})^2} = \frac{1}{112 - 8\sqrt{14} + 2}$
$= \frac{1}{114 - 8\sqrt{14}}$

Multiply top and bottom by $114 + 8\sqrt{14}$:

$\frac{114 + 8\sqrt{14}}{(114 - 8\sqrt{14})(114 + 8\sqrt{14})}$ ***[1 mark]*** $= \frac{114 + 8\sqrt{14}}{12\,996 - 896}$ ***[1 mark]***

$= \frac{114 + 8\sqrt{14}}{12\,100}$

$= \frac{57 + 4\sqrt{14}}{6050}$ ***[1 mark]***

So a = 57, b = 14 and c = 6050.

7 Multiply top and bottom by $1 - \sqrt{8}$:

$\frac{14(1-\sqrt{2})(1-\sqrt{8})}{(1+\sqrt{8})(1-\sqrt{8})} = \frac{14(1 - \sqrt{8} - \sqrt{2} + \sqrt{16})}{1 - 8}$
$= -2(1 + 4 - \sqrt{8} - \sqrt{2})$
$= 2\sqrt{8} + 2\sqrt{2} - 10$

$2\sqrt{8}$ can be written as $\sqrt{4 \times 8} = \sqrt{32} = \sqrt{2 \times 16} = 4\sqrt{2}$
$\Rightarrow 2\sqrt{8} + 2\sqrt{2} - 10 = 4\sqrt{2} + 2\sqrt{2} - 10$
$= 6\sqrt{2} - 10$

[4 marks available — 1 mark for a correct method to rationalise the denominator, 1 mark for correctly simplifying the numerator, 1 mark for correctly simplifying the denominator, 1 mark for obtaining the given result]

8 $\dfrac{(x^2-9)(3x^2-10x-8)}{(6x+4)(x^2-7x+12)} = \dfrac{(x+3)(x-3)(3x+2)(x-4)}{2(3x+2)(x-3)(x-4)}$

$= \dfrac{x+3}{2}$

[3 marks available — 1 mark for factorising the numerator, 1 mark for factorising the denominator, 1 mark for the correct answer]

9 a) $\dfrac{x^2+5x-14}{2x^2-4x} = \dfrac{(x+7)(x-2)}{2x(x-2)} = \dfrac{x+7}{2x}$

[2 marks available — 1 mark for factorising the numerator and the denominator, 1 mark for cancelling to obtain the correct answer]

b) $\dfrac{x^2+5x-14}{2x^2-4x} + \dfrac{14}{x(x-4)} = \dfrac{x+7}{2x} + \dfrac{14}{x(x-4)}$

$= \dfrac{(x+7)(x-4)}{2x(x-4)} + \dfrac{2\times 14}{2x(x-4)}$

$= \dfrac{x^2+3x-28+28}{2x(x-4)} = \dfrac{x^2+3x}{2x(x-4)}$

$= \dfrac{x(x+3)}{2x(x-4)} = \dfrac{x+3}{2(x-4)}$

[3 marks available — 1 mark for putting fractions over a common denominator, 1 mark for multiplying out and simplifying the numerator, 1 mark for cancelling to obtain the correct answer]

10 $\dfrac{1}{x(2x-3)} \equiv \dfrac{A}{x} + \dfrac{B}{2x-3} \Rightarrow 1 \equiv A(2x-3) + Bx$

Equating constants gives $1 = -3A \Rightarrow A = -\dfrac{1}{3}$

Equating coefficients of x gives $0 = 2A + B \Rightarrow B = \dfrac{2}{3}$

So $\dfrac{1}{x(2x-3)} \equiv \dfrac{2}{3(2x-3)} - \dfrac{1}{3x}$ ***[1 mark]***

11 $\dfrac{6x-1}{x^2+4x+4} \equiv \dfrac{6x-1}{(x+2)^2}$ ***[1 mark]*** $\equiv \dfrac{A}{(x+2)} + \dfrac{B}{(x+2)^2}$

$\Rightarrow 6x-1 \equiv A(x+2) + B$ ***[1 mark]***

Equating coefficients of x gives $6 = A$

Equating constant terms gives $-1 = 2A + B \Rightarrow B = -13$

[1 mark for A or B]

So $\dfrac{6x-1}{x^2+4x+4} \equiv \dfrac{6}{(x+2)} - \dfrac{13}{(x+2)^2}$ ***[1 mark]***

Pages 8-11: Algebra and Functions — 2

1 When $ax^2 + bx + c = 0$ has no real roots, you know that $b^2 - 4ac < 0$ ***[1 mark]***. Here, $a = -j$, $b = 3j$ and $c = 1$.

Therefore $(3j)^2 - (4 \times -j \times 1) < 0 \Rightarrow 9j^2 + 4j < 0$ ***[1 mark]***

To find the values where $9j^2 + 4j < 0$, you need to start by solving $9j^2 + 4j = 0$: $j(9j + 4) = 0$, so $j = 0$ or $9j = -4 \Rightarrow j = -\dfrac{4}{9}$

Now sketch the graph:

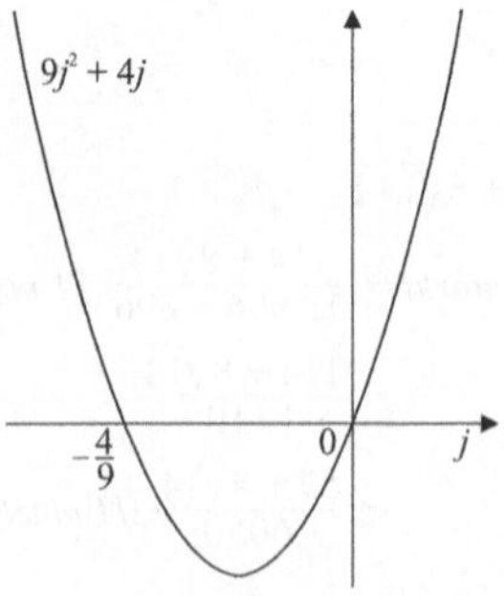

From the graph, you can see that $9j^2 + 4j < 0$ when $-\dfrac{4}{9} < j < 0$ ***[1 mark]***.

2 a) Complete the square by halving the coefficient of x to find the number in the brackets (m):

$x^2 - 7x + 17 = \left(x - \dfrac{7}{2}\right)^2 + n$

$\left(x - \dfrac{7}{2}\right)^2 = x^2 - 7x + \dfrac{49}{4}$, so $n = 17 - \dfrac{49}{4} = \dfrac{19}{4}$

So $x^2 - 7x + 17 = \left(x - \dfrac{7}{2}\right)^2 + \dfrac{19}{4}$

[3 marks available — 1 mark for the correct brackets, 1 mark for finding the right correcting number, 1 mark for the correct final answer]

b) The maximum value of $f(x)$ will be when the denominator is as small as possible — so you want the minimum value of $x^2 - 7x + 17$. Using the completed square from part a), you can see that the minimum value is $\dfrac{19}{4}$ ***[1 mark]*** because the squared part can equal but never be below 0.

So the maximum value of $f(x)$ is $\dfrac{1}{\left(\frac{19}{4}\right)} = \dfrac{4}{19}$ ***[1 mark]***.

3 If the equation has two real roots, then $b^2 - 4ac > 0$ ***[1 mark]***.

For this equation, $a = 3k$, $b = k$ and $c = 2$.

Use the discriminant formula to find k:

$k^2 - (4 \times 3k \times 2) > 0$ ***[1 mark]***

$k^2 - 24k > 0$

$k(k - 24) > 0$

$k < 0$ or $k > 24$ ***[1 mark]***

If you're struggling to solve this inequality, you could always sketch a graph like in the answer to question 1.

As the curve crosses $y = kx + 27$:

$3kx^2 + kx + 2 = kx + 27$ ***[1 mark]***

$x^2 = \dfrac{25}{3k}$

This only has solutions if $\dfrac{25}{3k} > 0$, so k must be greater than 0.

So $k > 24$ ***[1 mark]***

4 Let $y = x^3$. Then $x^6 = 7x^3 + 8$ becomes $y^2 = 7y + 8$ ***[1 mark]***, so solve the quadratic in y:

$y^2 = 7y + 8 \Rightarrow y^2 - 7y - 8 = 0$

$(y - 8)(y + 1) = 0$, so $y = 8$ or $y = -1$ ***[1 mark]***.

Now replace y with x^3. So $x^3 = 8 \Rightarrow x = 2$ ***[1 mark]***

or $x^3 = -1 \Rightarrow x = -1$ ***[1 mark]***.

Here, you had to spot that the original equation was a quadratic of the form $x^2 + bx + c$, just in terms of x^3 not x.

5 a) (i) First, rewrite the quadratic as: $-h^2 + 10h - 27$ and complete the square ($a = -1$):

$-(h - 5)^2 + 25 - 27 = -(h - 5)^2 - 2$

Rewrite the square in the form given in the question:

$T = -(-(5 - h))^2 - 2 \Rightarrow T = -(5 - h)^2 - 2$

[3 marks available — 1 mark for $(5 - h)^2$ or $(h - 5)^2$, 1 mark for 25 – 27, 1 mark for the correct final answer]

The last couple of steps are using the fact that $(-a)^2 = a^2$ to show that $(m - n)^2 = (n - m)^2$...

(ii) $(5 - h)^2 \geq 0$ for all values of h, so $-(5 - h)^2 \leq 0$.

Therefore $-(5 - h)^2 - 2 < 0$ for all h, so T is always negative ***[1 mark]***.

b) (i) The maximum temperature is the maximum value of T, which is –2 (from part a) ***[1 mark]***, and this occurs when the expression in the brackets = 0. The h-value that makes the expression in the brackets 0 is 5 ***[1 mark]***, so maximum temperature occurs 5 hours after sunrise.

(ii) At sunrise, $h = 0$, so $T = 10(0) - 0^2 - 27 = -27$ °C, so the graph looks like this:

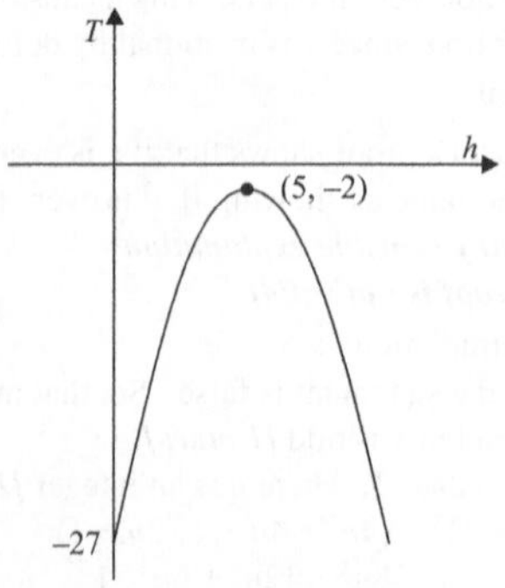

[2 marks available — 1 mark for drawing n-shaped curve that sits below the x-axis with the maximum roughly where shown (even if its position is not labelled), 1 mark for correct T-axis intercept (0, –27)]

6 Rearrange the first equation to get y on its own:
$y + x = 7 \Rightarrow y = 7 - x$ ***[1 mark]***
Substitute the expression for y into the quadratic to get:
$7 - x = x^2 + 3x - 5$ ***[1 mark]***
Rearrange again to get everything on one side of the equation, and then factorise it:
$0 = x^2 + 4x - 12 \Rightarrow (x + 6)(x - 2) = 0$
So $x = -6$ and $x = 2$ ***[1 mark]***
Use these values to find the corresponding values of y:
When $x = -6$, $y = 7 - -6 = 13$
and when $x = 2$, $y = 7 - 2 = 5$ ***[1 mark for both y-values]***
So the solutions are $x = -6$, $y = 13$ or $x = 2$, $y = 5$.

7 a) At the point of intersection, $-dx + 4 = -x^2 + 3$ ***[1 mark]***
$x^2 - dx - 3 + 4 = 0$
$x^2 - dx + 1 = 0$. As l is a tangent to C, this equation must have only one solution, or one real root.
$b^2 - 4ac = 0$ for one real root. ***[1 mark]***
$(-d)^2 - (4 \times 1 \times 1) = 0$
$d^2 = 4$
$d = 2$ (as d is positive) ***[1 mark]***
Substitute back in to quadratic and solve:
$x^2 - 2x + 1 = 0 \Rightarrow x = 1$ ***[1 mark]***.
When $x = 1$, $y = -2x + 4 = 2$,
so point of intersection is $(1, 2)$ ***[1 mark]***.

b)

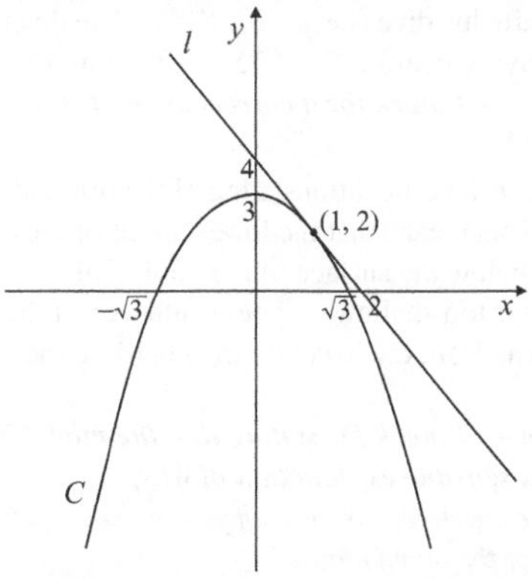

[5 marks available — 1 mark for drawing n-shaped curve, 1 mark for x-axis intercepts at $\pm\sqrt{3}$, 1 mark for maximum point of curve and y-axis intercept at (0, 3). 1 mark for line crossing the y-axis at (0, 4) and the x-axis at (2, 0). 1 mark for line and curve touching in one place at (1, 2).]

8 $y \geq x + 2$ and $y < 4 - x^2$ ***[1 mark]***
A solid line represents ≤ or ≥, and the shaded area is above the line $y = x + 2$, so this inequality is $y \geq x + 2$. A dashed line represents < or >, and the shaded area is below $y = 4 - x^2$, so the other inequality is $y < 4 - x^2$.

9 $x^2 - 8x + 15 > 0 \Rightarrow (x - 5)(x - 3) > 0$
Sketch a graph to see where the quadratic is greater than 0 — it'll be a u-shaped curve that crosses the x-axis at $x = 3$ and $x = 5$.

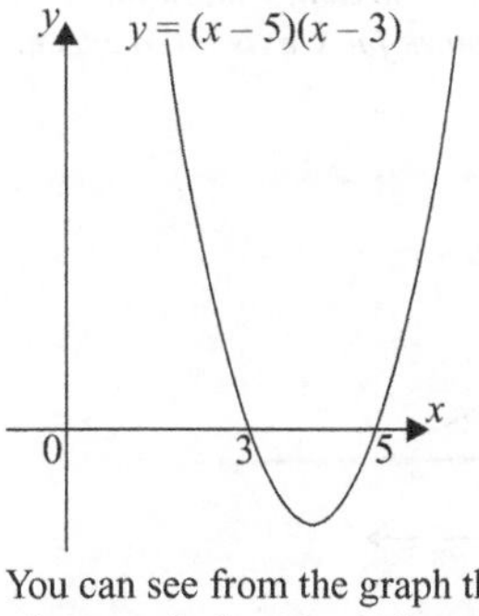

You can see from the graph that the function is positive when $x < 3$ and when $x > 5$. In set notation, this is $\{x : x < 3\} \cup \{x : x > 5\}$.
[4 marks available — 1 mark for factorising the quadratic, 1 mark for finding the roots, 1 mark for x < 3 and x > 5, 1 mark for the correct answer in set notation]

10 a) Multiply out the brackets and rearrange to get 0 on one side:
$(x - 1)(x^2 + x + 1) = 2x^2 - 17$
$x^3 + x^2 + x - x^2 - x - 1 = 2x^2 - 17$ ***[1 mark]***
$x^3 - 2x^2 + 16 = 0$ ***[1 mark]***

b) By the factor theorem, if $f(-2) = 0$, then $(x + 2)$ is a factor of $f(x)$.
$f(x) = x^3 - 2x^2 + 16$
$f(-2) = (-2)^3 - 2(-2)^2 + 16 = -8 - 8 + 16 = 0$ ***[1 mark]***
$f(-2) = 0$, therefore $(x + 2)$ is a factor of $f(x)$ ***[1 mark]***.

c) From part b) you know that $(x + 2)$ is a factor of $f(x)$.
Dividing $f(x)$ by $(x + 2)$ gives:
$x^3 - 2x^2 + 16 = (x + 2)(x^2 + ?x + 8) = (x + 2)(x^2 - 4x + 8)$
If you find it easier, you can use algebraic long division here.
[2 marks available — 2 marks for all three correct terms in the quadratic, otherwise 1 mark for two terms correct]

d) From b) you know that $x = -2$ is a root. From c),
$f(x) = (x + 2)(x^2 - 4x + 8)$. So for $f(x)$ to equal zero,
either $(x + 2) = 0$ (so $x = -2$) or $(x^2 - 4x + 8) = 0$ ***[1 mark]***.
Completing the square of $(x^2 - 4x + 8)$ gives
$x^2 - 4x + 8 = (x - 2)^2 + 4$, which is always positive so has no real roots. So $f(x) = 0$ has no solutions other than $x = -2$, which means it only has one root ***[1 mark]***.
You could also have shown that $x^2 - 4x + 8$ has no real roots by showing that the discriminant is < 0.

11 If $(x - 1)$ is a factor of $f(x)$, then $f(1) = 0$ by the factor theorem ***[1 mark]***.
$f(1) = 1^3 - 4(1)^2 - a(1) + 10$, so $0 = 7 - a \Rightarrow a = 7$ ***[1 mark]***.
So $f(x) = x^3 - 4x^2 - 7x + 10$.
To solve $f(x) = 0$, first factorise $x^3 - 4x^2 - 7x + 10$.
You know one factor, $(x - 1)$, so find the quadratic that multiplies with that factor to give the original equation:
$x^3 - 4x^2 - 7x + 10 = (x - 1)(x^2 + ?x - 10)$
$= (x - 1)(x^2 - 3x - 10)$ ***[1 mark]***
Again, you could use algebraic long division to do this.
Then factorise the quadratic: $= (x - 1)(x - 5)(x + 2)$ ***[1 mark]***
Finally, solve $f(x) = 0$:
$x^3 - 4x^2 - 7x + 10 = 0 \Rightarrow (x - 1)(x - 5)(x + 2) = 0$, so $x = 1$, $x = 5$ or $x = -2$ ***[2 marks for all three x-values, otherwise 1 mark for either x = 5 or x = −2]***.

Pages 12-17: Algebra and Functions — 3

1 a)

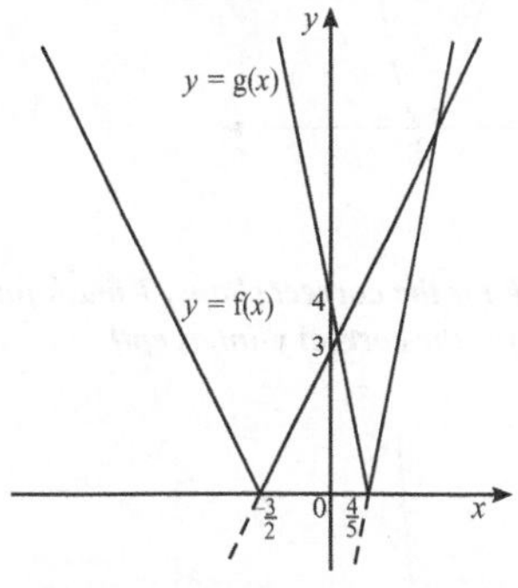

[2 marks available — 1 mark for y = |2x + 3| (with correct x- and y-intercepts), 1 mark for y = |5x − 4| (with correct x- and y-intercepts)]

b) From the graph, it is clear that there are two points where the graphs intersect. One is in the range $-\frac{3}{2} < x < \frac{4}{5}$, where $(2x + 3) > 0$ but $(5x - 4) < 0$.
This gives $2x + 3 = -(5x - 4)$ ***[1 mark]***.
The other one is in the range $x > \frac{4}{5}$, where $(2x + 3) > 0$ and $(5x - 4) > 0$, so $2x + 3 = 5x - 4$ ***[1 mark]***. Solving the first equation gives: $2x + 3 = -5x + 4 \Rightarrow 7x = 1$, so $x = \frac{1}{7}$ ***[1 mark]***.
Solving the second equation gives:
$2x + 3 = 5x - 4 \Rightarrow 7 = 3x$, so $x = \frac{7}{3}$ ***[1 mark]***.

2 a) If $|x| = 2$, then either $x = 2$ or $x = -2$
When $x = 2$, $|4x + 5| = |8 + 5| = |13| = 13$ ***[1 mark]***
When $x = -2$, $|4x + 5| = |-8 + 5|$ ***[1 mark]*** $= |-3| = 3$ ***[1 mark]***

b) First, sketch a quick graph:

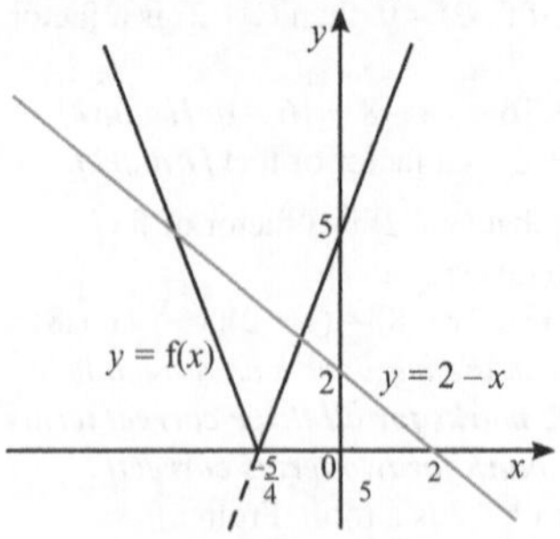

You can see that the lines cross twice, so you need to solve two inequalities:

$4x + 5 \le 2 - x \Rightarrow 5x \le -3 \Rightarrow x \le -\frac{3}{5}$

and $-(4x + 5) \le 2 - x \Rightarrow -7 \le 3x \Rightarrow x \ge -\frac{7}{3}$

So $f(x) \le 2 - x$ when $-\frac{7}{3} \le x \le -\frac{3}{5}$

[3 marks available — 1 mark for each correct value in the inequality, 1 mark for the correct inequality signs]

c) Two distinct roots means that the graphs of $y = f(x) + 2$ and $y = A$ cross twice ***[1 mark]***. From the graph in part b), the graph of $y = f(x) + 2$ is the black line translated up by 2. A horizontal line will intersect this in two places as long as it lies above the point where the graph is reflected, i.e. above $y = 2$.
So the possible values of A are $A > 2$ ***[1 mark]***.

3 The quartic has already been factorised — there are two double roots, one at (2, 0) and the other at (–3, 0). When $x = 0$, $y = (-2)^2(3^2) = 36$, so the y-intercept is (0, 36). The coefficient of the x^4 term is positive, and as the graph only touches the x-axis but doesn't cross it, it is always above the x-axis.
The graph looks like this:

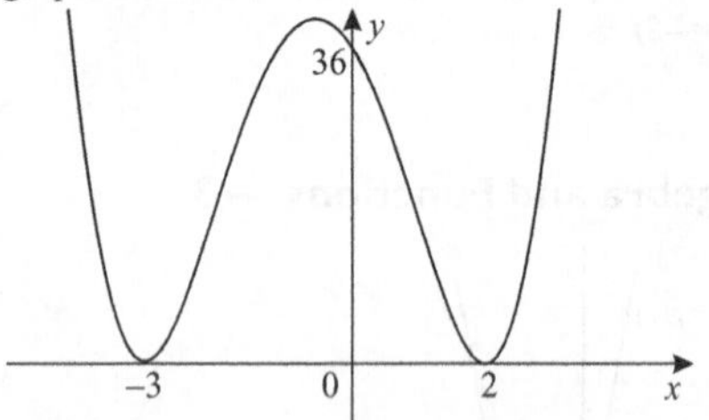

[3 marks available — 1 mark for the correct shape, 1 mark for the correct x-intercepts, 1 mark for the correct y-intercept]

4 a)

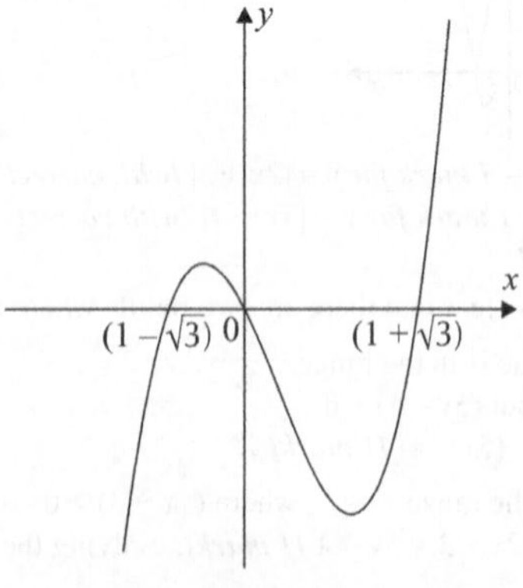

[2 marks available — 1 mark for the correct positive cubic shape with the two turning points the correct side of the y-axis, 1 mark for the x-intercepts correctly labelled.]

b) $x^3 - 2x^2 + px$ can be factorised to give $x(x^2 - 2x + p)$, so the roots of the quadratic factor must be $x = 1 + \sqrt{3}$ and $x = 1 - \sqrt{3}$.
The quadratic factor can be factorised to give $(x - (1 + \sqrt{3}))(x - (1 - \sqrt{3}))$, so the constant term is given by $p = (1 + \sqrt{3})(1 - \sqrt{3}) = 1 - 3 = -2$

[2 marks available — 1 mark for a correct method to find p, 1 mark for the correct answer]

5 a) Expand the brackets to show the two functions are the same:

$$\begin{aligned}(2t + 1)(t - 2)(t - 3.5) &= (2t + 1)(t^2 - 5.5t + 7)\\ &= 2t^3 - 11t^2 + 14t + t^2 - 5.5t + 7\\ &= 2t^3 - 10t^2 + 8.5t + 7 \text{ as required}\end{aligned}$$

[2 marks available — 1 mark for expanding the brackets, 1 mark for rearranging to get the required answer]

b)

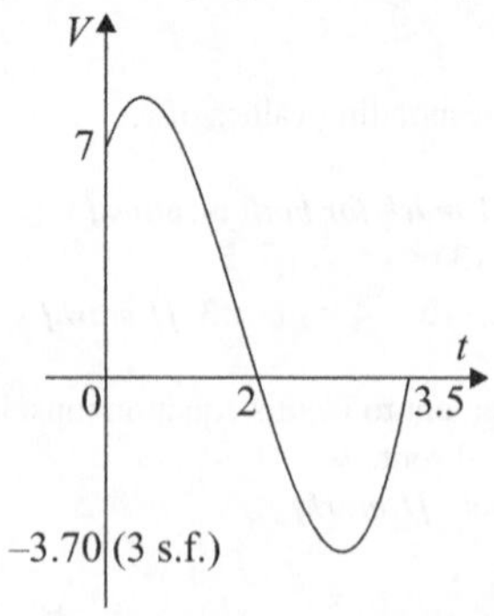

[3 marks available — 1 mark for the correct shape drawn between t = 0 and t = 3.5, 1 mark for the correct t-intercepts, 1 mark for the correct V-intercept]

c) 2 s ***[1 mark]***
This is the first point on the graph at which V = 0.

d) When the diver starts his dive (i.e. $t = 0$), $V = 7$. The diver's height is 1.75 m, so the diving board is 7 – 1.75 = 5.25 m high.
[2 marks available — 1 mark for a correct method, 1 mark for the correct answer]

e) The adapted model is a vertical translation of the original graph by 3 m upwards. This means that the lowest point of the dive is 3.70 – 3 = 0.70 m below the surface of the pool. This is obviously unrealistic as it is far too shallow — you would expect the diver to go at least as deep as from the lower diving board, so the adapted model is not valid.
[2 marks available — 1 mark for stating that the model is not valid, 1 mark for a sensible explanation of why]
This model is a lot easier to comment on if you realise it's just a vertical translation of the original model.

6

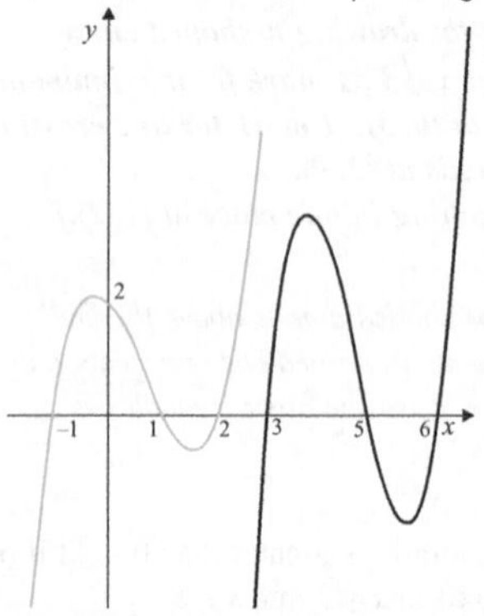

[3 marks available — 1 mark for vertical stretch, 1 mark for horizontal translation to the right, 1 mark for x-axis intercepts at 3, 5 and 6]

7

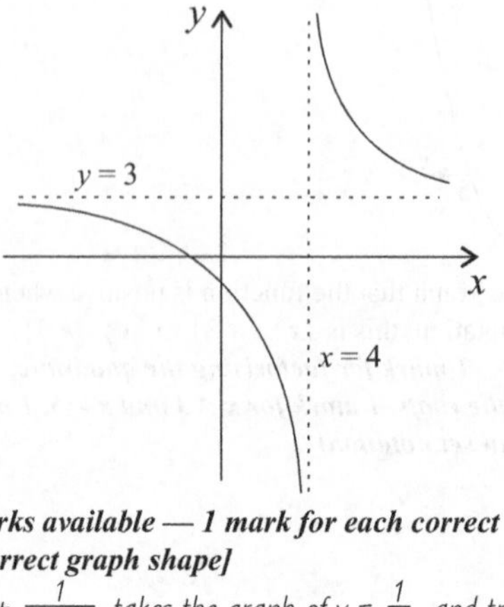

[3 marks available — 1 mark for each correct asymptote, 1 mark for the correct graph shape]

$y = 3 + \frac{1}{x - 4}$ takes the graph of $y = \frac{1}{x}$, and translates it by 3 units up and 4 units right.

8 a) 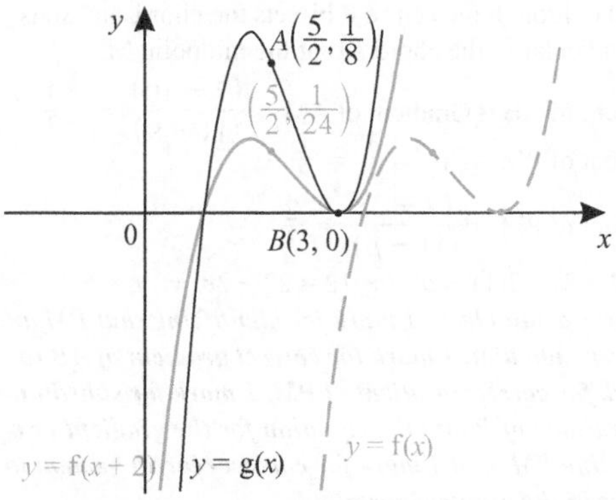

[3 marks available — 1 mark for the correct shape (stretched and translated), 1 mark each for coordinates of transformations of A and B]

The solid grey line shows the graph of y = f(x + 2) — it's easier to do the transformation in two stages, instead of doing it all at once.

b) g(x) has a double root at $x = 3$, so $g(x) = (x - 3)^2(px + q)$, where p and q are constants. ***[1 mark]***
g(x) passes through (0, –18), so:
$(0 - 3)^2(p(0) + q) = -18$
$9q = -18$
$q = -2$ ***[1 mark]***
g(x) passes through $\left(\frac{5}{2}, \frac{1}{8}\right)$, so:
$\left(\frac{5}{2} - 3\right)^2\left(p\left(\frac{5}{2}\right) - 2\right) = \frac{1}{8}$
$\frac{1}{4}\left(\frac{5p}{2} - 2\right) = \frac{1}{8}$
$\frac{5p}{2} - 2 = \frac{1}{2}$
$p = 1$ ***[1 mark]***
$\Rightarrow g(x) = (x - 3)^2(x - 2)$ or $g(x) = x^3 - 8x^2 + 21x - 18$ ***[1 mark]***

9 a) A translation of 3 up is a translation of the form f(x) + 3, then a translation of 2 right is f(x – 2) + 3.
Finally, a reflection in the y-axis gives f(–(x – 2)) + 3. So g(x) = f(2 – x) + 3 ***[1 mark]***.

b) P' = (–3, 5), Q' = (–5, 19) ***[1 mark]***
Do a quick sketch of the graph if you need to.

10 a) (i) $gf(x) = g(2^x) = \sqrt{3(2^x) + 1}$ ***[1 mark]***
(ii) $gf(x) = 5 \Rightarrow \sqrt{3(2^x) + 1} = 5 \Rightarrow 3(2^x) + 1 = 25$
$\Rightarrow 3(2^x) = 24 \Rightarrow 2^x = 8 \Rightarrow x = 3$
[2 marks available — 1 mark for a correct method, 1 mark for the correct answer]

b) First write $y = g(x)$ and rearrange to make x the subject:
$y = \sqrt{3x + 1} \Rightarrow y^2 = 3x + 1 \Rightarrow y^2 - 1 = 3x$
$\Rightarrow \frac{y^2 - 1}{3} = x$
Then replace x with $g^{-1}(x)$ and y with x:
$g^{-1}(x) = \frac{x^2 - 1}{3}$ ***[1 mark]***
g(x) has domain $x \geq -\frac{1}{3}$ and range $g(x) \geq 0$, so $g^{-1}(x)$ has domain $x \geq 0$ ***[1 mark]*** and range $g^{-1}(x) \geq -\frac{1}{3}$ ***[1 mark]***.

11 a) g has range $g(x) \geq -k$ ***[1 mark]***, as the minimum value of g is $-k$.

b) Neither f nor g are one-to-one functions, so they don't have inverses ***[1 mark]***.

c) (i) $gf(1) = g\left(\frac{1}{1^2}\right) = g(1) = 1^2 - k$ ***[1 mark]***
So $1 - k = -8 \Rightarrow k = 9$ ***[1 mark]***
$fg(x) = f(x^2 - 9)$ ***[1 mark]*** $= \frac{1}{(x^2 - 9)^2}$ ***[1 mark]***.
The domain of fg is $x \in \mathbb{R}, x \neq \pm 3$ ***[1 mark]***, as the denominator of the function can't be 0.

(ii) From part (i), you know that $fg(x) = \frac{1}{(x^2 - 9)^2}$, so
$\frac{1}{(x^2 - 9)^2} = \frac{1}{256} \Rightarrow (x^2 - 9)^2 = 256$ ***[1 mark]***
$x^2 - 9 = \pm\sqrt{256} = \pm 16$ ***[1 mark]***
$x^2 = 9 \pm 16 = 25, -7$ ***[1 mark]***
$x = \sqrt{25} = \pm 5$ ***[1 mark]***
You can ignore $x^2 = -7$, as this has no solutions in $x \in \mathbb{R}$.

Pages 18-22: Coordinate Geometry

1 a) $-\frac{1}{3}$ ***[1 mark]***

b) $y = 3x - 7$ ***[1 mark]***

2 a) To find the coordinates of A, solve the equations of the lines simultaneously:
$l_1: x - y + 1 = 0$
$l_2: 2x + y - 8 = 0$
Add the equations to get rid of y:
$3x - 7 = 0$ ***[1 mark]*** $\Rightarrow x = \frac{7}{3}$ ***[1 mark]***
Now put $x = \frac{7}{3}$ back into l_1 to find y:
$\frac{7}{3} - y + 1 = 0 \Rightarrow y = \frac{7}{3} + 1 = \frac{10}{3}$
So A is $\left(\frac{7}{3}, \frac{10}{3}\right)$ ***[1 mark]***

b) There's a lot of information here, so draw a quick sketch to make things a bit clearer:

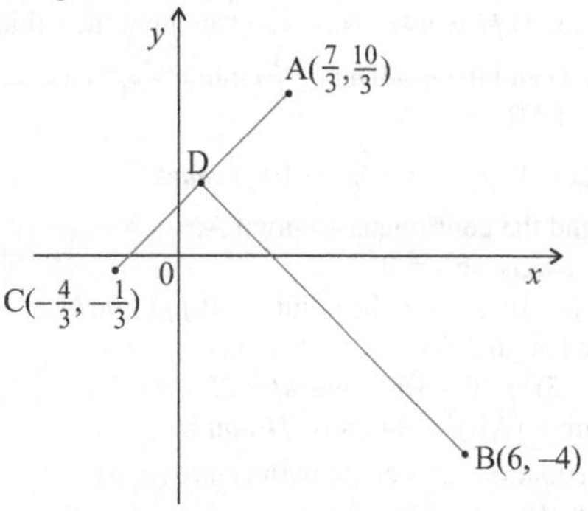

To find the equation of the line through B and D, you need its gradient. But before you can find the gradient, you need to find the coordinates of point D — the midpoint of AC. To find the midpoint of two points, find the average of the x-values and the average of the y-values:

$D = \left(\frac{x_A + x_C}{2}, \frac{y_A + y_C}{2}\right) = \left(\frac{\frac{7}{3} + \frac{-4}{3}}{2}, \frac{\frac{10}{3} + \frac{-1}{3}}{2}\right)$ ***[1 mark]***

$D = \left(\frac{1}{2}, \frac{3}{2}\right)$ ***[1 mark]***

To find the gradient (m) of the line through B and D, use this rule: $m_{BD} = \frac{y_D - y_B}{x_D - x_B}$

$m = \frac{\frac{3}{2} - -4}{\frac{1}{2} - 6} = \frac{\frac{3}{2} + \frac{8}{2}}{\frac{1}{2} - \frac{12}{2}} = \frac{3 + 8}{1 - 12} = -1$ ***[1 mark]***

Now you can find the equation of the line. Input the known values of x and y at B(6, –4) and the gradient (–1) into $y - y_1 = m(x - x_1)$, which gives:
$y - (-4) = -1(x - 6)$ ***[1 mark]***
$\Rightarrow y + 4 = -x + 6 \Rightarrow x + y - 2 = 0$ ***[1 mark]***
You could also have used the point D you found earlier in the question in the formula $y - y_1 = m(x - x_1)$.

c) Look at the sketch in part b). To prove triangle ABD is a right-angled triangle, you need to prove that lines AD and BD are perpendicular — in other words, prove the product of their gradients equals –1.
You already know the gradient of BD = –1.
Use the same rule to find the gradient of AD:
$m_{AD} = \frac{y_D - y_A}{x_D - x_A}$

$m = \frac{\frac{3}{2} - \frac{10}{3}}{\frac{1}{2} - \frac{7}{3}} = \frac{\frac{9}{6} - \frac{20}{6}}{\frac{3}{6} - \frac{14}{6}} = \frac{9 - 20}{3 - 14} = 1$ ***[1 mark]***

$m_{BD} \times m_{AD} = -1 \times 1 = -1$ ***[1 mark]***, so triangle ABD is a right-angled triangle ***[1 mark]***.

3 a) The gradient of the line through B and C equals the coefficient of x when the equation of the line is in the form $y = mx + c$.

$-3x + 5y = 16 \Rightarrow 5y = 3x + 16 \Rightarrow y = \frac{3}{5}x + \frac{16}{5}$,

so gradient $= \frac{3}{5}$.

AB and BC are perpendicular, so the gradient of the line through A and B equals $-1 \div \frac{3}{5} = -\frac{5}{3}$ ***[1 mark]***.

Two lines are parallel if they have the same gradient.

$5x + 3y - 6 = 0 \Rightarrow 3y = -5x + 6 \Rightarrow y = -\frac{5}{3}x + 2$,

so the gradient is $-\frac{5}{3}$ ***[1 mark]***.

The line with equation $5x + 3y - 6 = 0$ has the same gradient as the line through points A and B, so the lines are parallel ***[1 mark]***.

b) To calculate the area, find the length of one side — say AB.

Point B has coordinates $(3, k)$, so you can find k by substituting $x = 3$ and $y = k$ into the equation of the line through B and C:

$-3x + 5y = 16 \Rightarrow (-3 \times 3) + 5k = 16 \Rightarrow 5k = 25 \Rightarrow k = 5$,

so point B = (3, 5) ***[1 mark]***. Now you can input the values of x and y at B(3, 5) and the gradient ($-\frac{5}{3}$) into $y - y_1 = m(x - x_1)$ to find the equation of AB:

$y - 5 = -\frac{5}{3}(x - 3) \Rightarrow y = -\frac{5}{3}x + 10$ ***[1 mark]***

Use this to find the coordinates of point A:

A lies on the y-axis, so $x = 0$.

When $x = 0$, $y = 10$, so A is the point (0, 10) ***[1 mark]***.

Now find the length AB using Pythagoras' theorem:

$(AB)^2 = (10 - 5)^2 + (0 - 3)^2$ ***[1 mark]*** $= 25 + 9 = 34$,

Area of square $= (AB)^2 = 34$ units^2 ***[1 mark]***

4 a) The general equation for a circle with centre (a, b) and radius r is: $(x - a)^2 + (y - b)^2 = r^2$.

The centre of the circle must be the midpoint of AB, since AB is a diameter. Midpoint of AB is:

$\left(\frac{2+0}{2}, \frac{1+-5}{2}\right) = (1, -2)$ ***[1 mark]***

The radius is the distance from the centre (1, –2) to point A:

radius $= \sqrt{(2-1)^2 + (1-(-2))^2}$ ***[1 mark]*** $= \sqrt{10}$ ***[1 mark]***

For a circle with centre (1, –2) and radius $\sqrt{10}$, the equation is $(x - 1)^2 + (y + 2)^2 = 10$ ***[1 mark]***.

To show that the point (4, –1) lies on the ant's route, show that it satisfies the equation of the circle:

$(4 - 1)^2 + (-1 + 2)^2 = 9 + 1 = 10$,

so (4, –1) lies on the ant's route ***[1 mark]***.

b) Start with your equation from part a) and multiply out to get the form given in the question:

$(x - 1)^2 + (y + 2)^2 = 10$

$x^2 - 2x + 1 + y^2 + 4y + 4 = 10$

$x^2 + y^2 - 2x + 4y - 5 = 0$

[2 marks available — 1 mark for correct expansion of the equation of the circle, 1 mark for correct rearrangement to give the answer in the required form]

c) The radius at A has the same gradient as the diameter AB,

so gradient of radius $= \frac{1 - -5}{2 - 0} = 3$ ***[1 mark]***.

The tangent at point A is perpendicular to the radius at point A, so the tangent has gradient $-1 \div 3 = -\frac{1}{3}$ ***[1 mark]***.

Put the gradient $-\frac{1}{3}$ and point A(2, 1) into the formula for the equation of a straight line and rearrange:

$y - y_1 = m(x - x_1) \Rightarrow y - 1 = -\frac{1}{3}(x - 2)$

$\Rightarrow y - 1 = -\frac{1}{3}x + \frac{2}{3} \Rightarrow y = -\frac{1}{3}x + \frac{5}{3}$ ***[1 mark]***

If you've already come across implicit differentiation, you could also use that here to find the gradient of the circle at point A.

5 a) The line through the centre P bisects the chord, and so is perpendicular to the chord AB at the midpoint M.

Gradient of AB = Gradient of AM $= \frac{(7-10)}{(11-9)} = -\frac{3}{2}$.

Gradient of PM $= -1 \div -\frac{3}{2} = \frac{2}{3}$

Gradient of PM $= \frac{(7-3)}{(11-p)} = \frac{2}{3}$

$\Rightarrow 3(7 - 3) = 2(11 - p) \Rightarrow 12 = 22 - 2p \Rightarrow p = 5$.

[5 marks available — 1 mark for identifying that PM and AB are perpendicular, 1 mark for correct gradient of AB (or AM), 1 mark for correct gradient of PM, 1 mark for substitution of the y-coordinate of P into the equation for the gradient or equation of the line PM, and 1 mark for correct rearrangement to give the answer in the required form]

b) The equation of a circle is $(x - a)^2 + (y - b)^2 = r^2$.

The centre of the circle is P(5, 3), so $a = 5$ and $b = 3$. ***[1 mark]***

r^2 is the square of the radius. The radius equals the length of AP, so you can find r^2 using Pythagoras' theorem:

$r^2 = (AP)^2 = (9 - 5)^2 + (10 - 3)^2$ ***[1 mark]*** $= 65$

So the equation of the circle is:

$(x - 5)^2 + (y - 3)^2 = 65$ ***[1 mark]***

6 a) A is on the y-axis, so the x-coordinate is 0.

Just put $x = 0$ into the equation and solve:

$0^2 - (6 \times 0) + y^2 - 4y = 0$ ***[1 mark]***

$\Rightarrow y^2 - 4y = 0 \Rightarrow y = 0$ or $y = 4$

$y = 0$ is the origin, so A is at (0, 4) ***[1 mark]***

b) Complete the square for the terms involving x and y separately:

Completing the square for $x^2 - 6x$ means you have to start with $(x - 3)^2$, but $(x - 3)^2 = x^2 - 6x + 9$, so you need to subtract 9:

$(x - 3)^2 - 9$ ***[1 mark]***

Now do the same for $y^2 - 4y$: $(y - 2)^2 = y^2 - 4y + 4$,

so subtract 4 which gives: $(y - 2)^2 - 4$ ***[1 mark]***

Put these new expressions back into the original equation:

$(x - 3)^2 - 9 + (y - 2)^2 - 4 = 0$

$\Rightarrow (x - 3)^2 + (y - 2)^2 = 13$ ***[1 mark]***

c) In the general equation for a circle $(x - a)^2 + (y - b)^2 = r^2$, the centre is (a, b) and the radius is r.

So for the equation in part b), $a = 3$, $b = 2$, $r = \sqrt{13}$.

Hence, the centre of the forest is (3, 2) ***[1 mark]***

and the radius is $\sqrt{13}$ km ***[1 mark]***.

d) The tangent at point A is perpendicular to the radius at A.

The radius between A(0, 4) and the centre(3, 2) has gradient:

$\frac{y_2 - y_1}{x_2 - x_1} = \frac{2-4}{3-0} = -\frac{2}{3}$ ***[1 mark]***

So the gradient of the tangent at A $= -1 \div -\frac{2}{3} = \frac{3}{2}$ ***[1 mark]***

Put $m = \frac{3}{2}$ and A = (0, 4) into $y - y_1 = m(x - x_1)$ to find the equation of the tangent to the circle at point A:

$y - 4 = \frac{3}{2}(x - 0) \Rightarrow y - 4 = \frac{3}{2}x \Rightarrow y = \frac{3}{2}x + 4$ ***[1 mark]***

Point B lies on the line with equation $y = \frac{3}{2}x + 4$.

B also lies on the x-axis, so substitute $y = 0$ into the equation of the line to find the x-coordinate of B:

$0 = \frac{3}{2}x + 4 \Rightarrow x = -\frac{8}{3}$, so B is the point $\left(-\frac{8}{3}, 0\right)$ ***[1 mark]***

Now find AB using Pythagoras' theorem:

$(AB)^2 = \left(0 - -\frac{8}{3}\right)^2 + (4 - 0)^2$ ***[1 mark]*** $= \frac{64}{9} + 16$,

so AB $= \sqrt{\frac{64}{9} + 16} = \sqrt{\frac{208}{9}} = \frac{4\sqrt{13}}{3}$ km ***[1 mark]***

If the question asks for an exact answer, leave it in surd form.

7 $x = 5 \sin \theta + 2 \Rightarrow 5 \sin \theta = x - 2$

$y = 5 \cos \theta - 3 \Rightarrow 5 \cos \theta = y + 3$

$\cos^2 \theta + \sin^2 \theta = 1 \Rightarrow 5^2 \cos^2 \theta + 5^2 \sin^2 \theta = 5^2$

So $(x - 2)^2 + (y + 3)^2 = 5^2$

a) So the centre of the circle is at (2, –3) ***[1 mark]***.

b) $r = 5$ ***[1 mark]***

8 a) At A, $y = 4$, so $4 \cos \theta = 4 \Rightarrow \cos \theta = 1$

$\Rightarrow \theta = 0$, as $0 \le \theta \le \frac{\pi}{2}$.

At B, $x = 3$, so $3 \sin \theta = 3 \Rightarrow \sin \theta = 1$

$\Rightarrow \theta = \frac{\pi}{2}$, as $0 \le \theta \le \frac{\pi}{2}$.

[2 marks available — 1 mark for each value of θ]

b) $y^2 = 16\cos^2\theta$. Use the identity $\cos^2\theta \equiv 1 - \sin^2\theta$:
$y^2 = 16(1 - \sin^2\theta)$ ***[1 mark]***.
Now, $x^2 = 9\sin^2\theta$, so $\frac{x^2}{9} = \sin^2\theta$. ***[1 mark]***
Substitute this into the equation for y^2:
$y^2 = 16(1 - \frac{x^2}{9}) = 16 - \frac{16x^2}{9} = \left(4 + \frac{4x}{3}\right)\left(4 - \frac{4x}{3}\right)$ ***[1 mark]***
The last step is a difference of squares.

9 For the boat to be further west than the tip of the island, this means $x < 12$, so:
$t^2 - 7t + 12 < 12$ ***[1 mark]*** $\Rightarrow t^2 - 7t < 0 \Rightarrow t(t-7) < 0$
$\Rightarrow 0 < t < 7$ ***[1 mark]***
This means that the boat starts level with the tip of the island (at $t = 0$), and is then level again when $t = 7$. So the boat is west of the tip of the island for 7 hours ***[1 mark]***.

10 a) Substitute the given value of θ into the parametric equations:
$\theta = \frac{\pi}{3} \Rightarrow x = 1 - \tan\frac{\pi}{3} = 1 - \sqrt{3}$
$y = \frac{1}{2}\sin\left(\frac{2\pi}{3}\right) = \frac{1}{2}\left(\frac{\sqrt{3}}{2}\right) = \frac{\sqrt{3}}{4}$
So $P = \left(1 - \sqrt{3}, \frac{\sqrt{3}}{4}\right)$
[2 marks available — 1 mark for substituting $\theta = \frac{\pi}{3}$ into the parametric equations, 1 mark for both coordinates of P correct]

b) Use $y = -\frac{1}{2}$ to find the value of θ:
$-\frac{1}{2} = \frac{1}{2}\sin 2\theta \Rightarrow \sin 2\theta = -1$
$\Rightarrow 2\theta = -\frac{\pi}{2} \Rightarrow \theta = -\frac{\pi}{4}$
[2 marks available — 1 mark for substituting given x- or y-value into the correct parametric equation, 1 mark for finding the correct value of θ]
You can also find θ using the parametric equation for x, with x = 2.

c) $x = 1 - \tan\theta \Rightarrow \tan\theta = 1 - x$
$y = \frac{1}{2}\sin 2\theta = \frac{1}{2}\left(\frac{2\tan\theta}{1 + \tan^2\theta}\right) = \frac{\tan\theta}{1 + \tan^2\theta}$
$= \frac{(1-x)}{1 + (1-x)^2} = \frac{1-x}{1 + 1 - 2x + x^2} = \frac{1-x}{x^2 - 2x + 2}$
[3 marks available — 1 mark for using the given identity to rearrange one of the parametric equations, 1 mark for eliminating θ from the parametric equation for y, 1 mark for correctly expanding to obtain the Cartesian equation given in the question]

11 a) C crosses the y-axis when $x = 0$,
so when $4t - 2 = 0 \Rightarrow 4t = 2 \Rightarrow t = \frac{1}{2}$ ***[1 mark]***
Substitute this into the equation for y:
$y = \left(\frac{1}{2}\right)^3 + \frac{1}{2} = \frac{5}{8}$, so the coordinates are $\left(0, \frac{5}{8}\right)$ ***[1 mark]***

b) Substitute $x = 4t - 2$ into $y = \frac{1}{2}x + 1$:
$y = \frac{1}{2}(4t - 2) + 1 = 2t$. Now solve for t when $y = t^3 + t$:
$2t = t^3 + t \Rightarrow t^3 - t = 0 \Rightarrow t(t^2 - 1) = 0 \Rightarrow t(t-1)(t+1) = 0$.
So $t = 0$, 1 and -1.
When $t = 0$, $x = -2$ and $y = 0$ so the point has coordinates $(-2, 0)$
When $t = 1$, $x = 2$ and $y = 2$ so the point has coordinates $(2, 2)$
When $t = -1$, $x = -6$ and $y = -2$ so the point has coordinates $(-6, -2)$
[4 marks available — 1 mark for a correct method to find t at points of intersection, 1 mark for all values of t correct, 2 marks for all coordinates correct, otherwise 1 mark for two coordinates correct]

c) $x = 4t - 2 \Rightarrow t = \frac{x+2}{4}$ ***[1 mark]***
Substitute this into the equation for y:
$y = \left(\frac{x+2}{4}\right)^3 + \frac{x+2}{4} = \frac{x^3 + 6x^2 + 12x + 8}{64} + \frac{x+2}{4}$ ***[1 mark]***
$= \frac{x^3 + 6x^2 + 28x + 40}{64} = \frac{1}{64}x^3 + \frac{3}{32}x^2 + \frac{7}{16}x + \frac{5}{8}$ ***[1 mark]***
(so $a = \frac{1}{64}$, $b = \frac{3}{32}$, $c = \frac{7}{16}$ and $d = \frac{5}{8}$)

Pages 23-26: Sequences and Series — 1

1 a) In an arithmetic sequence, the nth term is defined by the formula $a + (n-1)d$. The 12th term is 79, so the equation is $79 = a + 11d$, and the 16th term is 103, so the other equation is $103 = a + 15d$ ***[1 mark for both equations]***. Solving these simultaneously (by taking the first equation away from the second) gives $24 = 4d$, so $d = 6$ ***[1 mark]***.
Putting this value of d into the first equation gives
$79 = a + (11 \times 6)$, so $a = 13$. ***[1 mark]***

b) $u_n = 13 + 6(n-1)$
$u_{k+6} = 2u_k - 1$
$\Rightarrow 13 + 6(k + 6 - 1) = 2(13 + 6(k-1)) - 1$ ***[1 mark]***
$\Rightarrow 13 + 6k + 30 = 26 + 12k - 12 - 1$
$\Rightarrow 30 = 6k$
$\Rightarrow k = 5$ ***[1 mark]***

2 a) $h_2 = 2h_1 + 2 = 2 \times 5 + 2 = 12$
$h_3 = 2h_2 + 2 = 2 \times 12 + 2 = 26$
$h_4 = 2h_3 + 2 = 2 \times 26 + 2 = 54$
[2 marks available — 1 mark for a correct method, 1 mark for all three correct answers]

b) $\sum_{r=3}^{6} h_r = h_3 + h_4 + h_5 + h_6$
$h_5 = 2h_4 + 2 = 2 \times 54 + 2 = 110$ and
$h_6 = 2h_5 + 2 = 2 \times 110 + 2 = 222$ ***[1 mark for both correct]***
So $\sum_{r=3}^{6} h_r = 26 + 54 + 110 + 222$ ***[1 mark]*** $= 412$ ***[1 mark]***

3 To find the value of m, sum the series up to the mth term:
$S_n = \frac{1}{2}n(a + l)$
$1935 = \frac{1}{2}m(21 + 108) \Rightarrow 3870 = 129m \Rightarrow m = 30$ ***[1 mark]***
So 108 is the 30th term. Use this to find the common difference, d:
$u_{30} = a + (n-1)d$
$108 = 21 + (30 - 1)d \Rightarrow 29d = 87 \Rightarrow d = 3$ ***[1 mark]***
So $u_{23} = 21 + (23 - 1) \times 3 = 21 + 66 = 87$ ***[1 mark]***

4 a) $H_n = \frac{n}{2}(2a + (n-1)d)$
$H_{60} = H_5 \times H_6$
$\frac{60}{2}(2a + (60-1)d) = \frac{5}{2}(2a + (5-1)d) \times \frac{6}{2}(2a + (6-1)d)$
$30(2a + 59d) = \frac{30}{4}(2a + 4d)(2a + 5d)$
$4(2a + 59d) = (2a + 4d)(2a + 5d)$
$8a + 236d = 4a^2 + 18ad + 20d^2$
$4a + 118d = 2a^2 + 9ad + 10d^2$
$2a^2 - 4a + 9ad - 118d + 10d^2 = 0$
[3 marks available — 1 mark for correct use of H_n formula, 1 mark for correct method, 1 mark for correctly deriving the given result]

b) Substitute a into the expression from part a), and solve for d:
$2 \times 2^2 - 4 \times 2 + (9 \times 2)d - 118d + 10d^2 = 0$ ***[1 mark]***
$8 - 8 + 18d - 118d + 10d^2 = 0$
$10d^2 - 100d = 0$
$10d(d - 10) = 0$
$10d = 0 \Rightarrow d = 0$, but you know that $d \neq 0$, so you can ignore this solution.
$d - 10 = 0 \Rightarrow d = 10$ ***[1 mark]***
So the base block has a height of $a = 2$ cm and the remaining blocks have heights of $d = 10$ cm. The maximum height of a stable tower is $h = 224$ cm, so the 10 cm blocks can be no taller than $224 - 2 = 222$ cm in total. $222 \div 10 = 22.2$, so there can be at most $1 + 22 = 23$ blocks in a stable tower. ***[1 mark]***

5 $u_1 = 18$
$u_2 = 18 \times -1 = -18$
$u_3 = -18 \times -1 = 18$ (which is equal to u_1)
So it's a periodic sequence ***[1 mark]***.

6 a) First put the two known terms into the formula for the nth term of a geometric series, $u_n = ar^{n-1}$:
$u_3 = ar^2 = \frac{5}{2}$ and $u_6 = ar^5 = \frac{5}{16}$ ***[1 mark for both]***
Divide the expression for u_6 by the expression for u_3 to get an expression just containing r and solve it:
$\frac{ar^5}{ar^2} = \frac{5}{16} \div \frac{5}{2} \Rightarrow r^3 = \frac{5}{16} \times \frac{2}{5} = \frac{10}{80}$
$r^3 = \frac{1}{8} \Rightarrow r = \sqrt[3]{\frac{1}{8}} \Rightarrow r = \frac{1}{2}$ ***[1 mark]***
Put this value back into the expression for u_3 to find a:
$a\left(\frac{1}{2}\right)^2 = \frac{5}{2} \Rightarrow \frac{a}{4} = \frac{5}{2} \Rightarrow a = 10$ ***[1 mark]***
The nth term is $u_n = ar^{n-1}$, where $r = \frac{1}{2}$ and $a = 10$
$u_n = 10 \times \left(\frac{1}{2}\right)^{n-1} = 10 \times \frac{1}{2^{n-1}} = \frac{10}{2^{n-1}}$ ***[1 mark]***

b) $S_n = \frac{a(1-r^n)}{1-r}$,
$S_{10} = \frac{10\left(1-\left(\frac{1}{2}\right)^{10}\right)}{1-\left(\frac{1}{2}\right)}$ ***[1 mark]*** $= 10 \times 2 \times \left(1 - \frac{1}{2^{10}}\right)$
$= 20\left(1 - \frac{1}{1024}\right) = \frac{5115}{256}$ ***[1 mark]***

c) Substitute $a = 10$ and $r = \frac{1}{2}$ into the sum to infinity formula:
$S_\infty = \frac{a}{1-r} = \frac{10}{1-\left(\frac{1}{2}\right)} = 10 \div \frac{1}{2} = 10 \times 2 = 20$
[2 marks available — 1 mark for a correct method and 1 mark for showing the sum to infinity is 20]

7 a) The series is defined by $u_{n+1} = 5 \times 1.7^n$ so $r = 1.7$.
r is greater than 1, so the sequence is divergent, which means the sum to infinity cannot be found ***[1 mark]***.

b) $u_3 = 5 \times 1.7^2 = 14.45$ ***[1 mark]***
$u_8 = 5 \times 1.7^7 = 205.17$ (2 d.p.) ***[1 mark]***

8 a) $S_\infty = \frac{a}{1-r} = \frac{20}{1-\frac{3}{4}} = \frac{20}{\frac{1}{4}} = 80$
[2 marks available — 1 mark for substituting into the correct formula, 1 mark for correct answer]

b) Use the formula for the sum of a geometric series to write an expression for S_n:
$S_n = \frac{a(1-r^n)}{1-r} = \frac{20\left(1-\left(\frac{3}{4}\right)^n\right)}{1-\frac{3}{4}}$ ***[1 mark]***
so $\frac{20\left(1-\left(\frac{3}{4}\right)^n\right)}{1-\frac{3}{4}} > 79.76$
Now rearrange and use logs to get n on its own:
$\frac{20\left(1-\left(\frac{3}{4}\right)^n\right)}{1-\frac{3}{4}} > 79.76 \Rightarrow 20\left(1-\left(\frac{3}{4}\right)^n\right) > 19.94$
$\Rightarrow 1-\left(\frac{3}{4}\right)^n > 0.997 \Rightarrow 0.003 > 0.75^n$ ***[1 mark]***
$\Rightarrow \log 0.003 > n \log 0.75$ ***[1 mark]***
$\Rightarrow \frac{\log 0.003}{\log 0.75} < n$ ***[1 mark]***
Remember — if x < 1, then log x has a negative value and dividing by a negative means flipping the inequality.
$\frac{\log 0.003}{\log 0.75} = 20.1929....$
so $n > 20.1929....$
But n must be an integer, so $n = 21$ ***[1 mark]***

9 a) Use $u_n = ar^{n-1}$ with $a = 1$ and $r = 1.5$:
$u_5 = 1 \times (1.5)^4$ ***[1 mark]***
$= 5.06$ km (to the nearest 10 m) ***[1 mark]***

b) Use $u_n = ar^{n-1}$ with $a = 2$ and $r = 1.2$:
$u_9 = 2 \times (1.2)^8 = 8.60$ km (3 s.f.) ***[1 mark]***
$u_{10} = 2 \times (1.2)^9 = 10.3$ km (3 s.f.) ***[1 mark]***
$u_9 < 10$ km and $u_{10} > 10$ km, so day 10 is the first day that Chris runs further than 10 km. ***[1 mark]***
You could've used logs to solve $2(1.2)^{n-1} > 10$ here instead.

c) Alex: 3 × 10 = 30 km ***[1 mark]***
Use the formula for the sum of first n terms: $S_n = \frac{a(1-r^n)}{1-r}$
Chris: $\frac{2(1-1.2^{10})}{1-1.2} = 51.917...$ km ***[1 mark]***
Heather: $\frac{1(1-1.5^{10})}{1-1.5} = 113.330...$ km ***[1 mark]***
Total raised = 30 + 51.917... + 113.330...
= £195.25 (to the nearest penny) ***[1 mark]***

10 a) $S_\infty = \frac{a}{1-r} = -9 \Rightarrow a = -9(1-r)$
and $ar = -2 \Rightarrow a = \frac{-2}{r}$
$\Rightarrow \frac{-2}{r} = -9(1-r)$
$\Rightarrow -2 = -9r + 9r^2 \Rightarrow 9r^2 - 9r + 2 = 0$
[3 marks available — 1 mark for finding two expressions in a and r, 1 mark for setting these expressions equal to each other, 1 mark for rearranging to give answer in required form]

b) By using a calculator or an algebraic method:
$9r^2 - 9r + 2 = 0 \Rightarrow r = \frac{1}{3}$ or $r = \frac{2}{3}$ ***[1 mark for both]***
$ar = -2 \Rightarrow a = \frac{-2}{r}$
$r = \frac{1}{3} \Rightarrow a = \frac{-2}{\frac{1}{3}} = -6$ ***[1 mark]***
$r = \frac{2}{3} \Rightarrow a = \frac{-2}{\frac{2}{3}} = -3$ ***[1 mark]***

11 a) $u_1 = x$ and $u_2 = x^2$.
As it's a geometric sequence, $u_n = x^n$. ***[1 mark]***
$u_3 = 9x = x^3 \Rightarrow x(x^2 - 9) = 0 \Rightarrow x = 3$ (as $x > 0$) ***[1 mark]***
Hence $u_n = 3^n$ ***[1 mark]***

b) $u_1 = x$, $u_2 = x^2$, $u_3 = 9x$
Let d be the common difference, then:
$u_2 = u_1 + d = x + d \Rightarrow x^2 = x + d$
$u_3 = u_2 + d = x + 2d \Rightarrow 9x = x + 2d \Rightarrow d = 4x$
Substitute $d = 4x$ into the equation for u_2:
$x^2 = x + 4x \Rightarrow x^2 - 5x = 0 \Rightarrow x(x-5) = 0 \Rightarrow x = 5$ (as $x \neq 0$)
So $u_n = a + (n-1)d = x + 4x(n-1)$
$= 5 + 20(n-1) = 20n - 15$
[4 marks available — 1 mark for setting up correct simultaneous equations, 1 mark for a correct method to solve simultaneously, 1 mark for the correct value of x, 1 mark for the correct answer]

Pages 27-29: Sequences and Series — 2

1 a) c represents the coefficient of x^3, so find an expression for the coefficient of x^3 using the binomial expansion formula:
$(j + kx)^6 = j^6\left(1 + \frac{k}{j}x\right)^6$
Coefficient of $x^3 = j^6 \times \frac{6 \times 5 \times 4}{1 \times 2 \times 3} \times \left(\frac{k}{j}\right)^3$ ***[1 mark]***
so $j^6 \times \frac{6 \times 5 \times 4}{1 \times 2 \times 3} \times \left(\frac{k}{j}\right)^3 = 20\,000$ ***[1 mark]***
$j^6 \times 20 \times \left(\frac{1}{j^3}\right) \times k^3 = 20\,000$
$j^6 \times j^{-3} \times k^3 = 1000 \Rightarrow j^3 \times k^3 = 1000 \Rightarrow (jk)^3 = 1000$,
so $jk = \sqrt[3]{1000} = 10$ ***[1 mark for correct rearrangement]***

b) Write an expression for the coefficient of x and then solve simultaneously with the equation $jk = 10$.
coefficient of x: $j^6 \times \frac{6}{1} \times \frac{k}{j} = 37\,500$ ***[1 mark]***
$j^6 \times j^{-1} \times k \times 6 = 37\,500 \Rightarrow kj^5 = 6250$
From a), $jk = 10$, so $k = \frac{10}{j}$
$kj^5 = \frac{10}{j} \times j^5 = 6250$ ***[1 mark for using jk = 10]***
$\Rightarrow 10 \times j^{-1} \times j^5 = 6250 \Rightarrow j^4 = 625 \Rightarrow j = \pm 5$
But j and k are positive so $j = 5$ ***[1 mark]***
Now input $j = 5$ into $jk = 10$ to find: $k = 2$ ***[1 mark]***

c) Coefficient of x^2: $b = 5^6 \times \frac{6 \times 5}{1 \times 2} \times \left(\frac{2}{5}\right)^2 = 37\,500$
[2 marks available — 1 mark for formula, 1 mark for correct answer]

2 The x^5 term is $\frac{(-8)(-9)(-10)(-11)(-12)}{1\times2\times3\times4\times5}\times(-3x)^5$

$= -792 \times -243x^5 = 192\,456\,x^5$

So the coefficient is 192 456 ***[1 mark]***.

3 a) $f(x) \approx 1 + n + \frac{n(n-1)}{2!}x^2 + \frac{n(n-1)(n-2)}{3!}x^3$

$f(x) = (2+4x)^{-4} = (2^{-4})(1+2x)^{-4} = \frac{1}{16}(1+2x)^{-4}$ ***[1 mark]***

$\approx \frac{1}{16}\left(1 + (-4)(2x) + \frac{-4\times-5}{2!}(2x)^2 + \frac{-4\times-5\times-6}{3!}(2x)^3\right)$

$= \frac{1}{16}(1 + (-4\times2x) + (10\times4x^2) + (-20\times8x^3))$ ***[1 mark]***

$= \frac{1}{16}(1 - 8x + 40x^2 - 160x^3)$ ***[1 mark]***

$= \frac{1}{16} - \frac{1}{2}x + \frac{5}{2}x^2 - 10x^3$ ***[1 mark]***

b) The coefficient of x^2 in the expansion of g(x) is:

$\frac{-5(-5-1)}{2!}a^2 = 15a^2$ ***[1 mark]***

The coefficients of x^2 for f(x) and g(x) are equal so:

$15a^2 = \frac{5}{2} \Rightarrow a^2 = \frac{1}{6} \Rightarrow a = \pm\frac{\sqrt{6}}{6}$ ***[1 mark]***

$a > 0$, so $a = \frac{\sqrt{6}}{6}$ ***[1 mark]***

4 a) $(27+4x)^{\frac{1}{3}} = 27^{\frac{1}{3}}\left(1+\frac{4}{27}x\right)^{\frac{1}{3}} = 3\left(1+\frac{4}{27}x\right)^{\frac{1}{3}}$ ***[1 mark]***

$\approx 3\left[1 + \left(\frac{1}{3}\right)\left(\frac{4}{27}x\right) + \frac{\frac{1}{3}\times-\frac{2}{3}}{1\times2}\left(\frac{4}{27}x\right)^2\right]$ ***[1 mark]***

$= 3\left[1 + \left(\frac{1}{3}\right)\left(\frac{4}{27}x\right) + \left(-\frac{1}{9}\right)\left(\frac{16}{729}x^2\right)\right]$

$= 3\left(1 + \frac{4}{81}x - \frac{16}{6561}x^2\right)$ ***[1 mark]***

$= 3 + \frac{4}{27}x - \frac{16}{2187}x^2$ ***[1 mark]***

$27 + 4x = 26.2 \Rightarrow x = -0.2$

This lies within $|x| < \frac{27}{4}$, so the expansion is valid, and x is small, so the higher powers can be ignored and it is a valid approximation.

$\sqrt[3]{26.2} = (26.2)^{\frac{1}{3}} \approx 3 + \frac{4}{27}(-0.2) - \frac{16}{2187}(-0.2)^2$ ***[1 mark]***

$= 3 - 0.0296296... - 0.0002926...$

$= 2.9700777... = 2.970078$ (6 d.p.) ***[1 mark]***

b) Percentage error

$= \left|\frac{\text{real value} - \text{estimate}}{\text{real value}}\right| \times 100$

$= \left|\frac{\sqrt[3]{26.2} - 2.970078}{\sqrt[3]{26.2}}\right| \times 100$ ***[1 mark]***

$= 0.0001744...$

$= 0.000174\%$ (3 s.f.) ***[1 mark]***

5 a) (i) $\sqrt{\frac{1+3x}{1-5x}} = \frac{\sqrt{1+3x}}{\sqrt{1-5x}}$

$= (1+3x)^{\frac{1}{2}}(1-5x)^{-\frac{1}{2}}$ ***[1 mark]***

$(1+3x)^{\frac{1}{2}} = 1 + \frac{1}{2}(3x) + \frac{\frac{1}{2}\times-\frac{1}{2}}{1\times2}(3x)^2 + ...$

$\approx 1 + \frac{3}{2}x - \frac{9}{8}x^2$ ***[1 mark]***

$(1-5x)^{-\frac{1}{2}} = 1 + \left(-\frac{1}{2}\right)(-5x) + \frac{-\frac{1}{2}\times-\frac{3}{2}}{1\times2}(-5x)^2 + ...$

$\approx 1 + \frac{5}{2}x + \frac{75}{8}x^2$ ***[1 mark]***

$\sqrt{\frac{1+3x}{1-5x}} \approx \left(1 + \frac{3}{2}x - \frac{9}{8}x^2\right)\left(1 + \frac{5}{2}x + \frac{75}{8}x^2\right)$ ***[1 mark]***

$\approx 1 + \frac{5}{2}x + \frac{75}{8}x^2 + \frac{3}{2}x + \frac{15}{4}x^2 - \frac{9}{8}x^2$

(ignoring any terms in x^3 or above)

$= 1 + 4x + 12x^2$ ***[1 mark for correct simplification]***

(ii) Expansion of $(1+3x)^{\frac{1}{2}}$ is valid for: $|3x| < 1 \Rightarrow |x| < \frac{1}{3}$.

Expansion of $(1-5x)^{-\frac{1}{2}}$ is valid for:

$|-5x| < 1 \Rightarrow |-5||x| < 1 \Rightarrow |x| < \frac{1}{5}$.

The combined expansion is valid for the narrower of these two ranges, so the expansion of $\sqrt{\frac{1+3x}{1-5x}}$ is valid for: $|x| < \frac{1}{5}$.

[2 marks available — 1 mark for identifying the valid range of the expansion as being the narrower of the two valid ranges shown, 1 mark for correct answer]

b) $x = \frac{1}{15} \Rightarrow \sqrt{\frac{1+3x}{1-5x}} = \sqrt{\frac{1+\frac{3}{15}}{1-\frac{5}{15}}} = \sqrt{\frac{\left(\frac{18}{15}\right)}{\left(\frac{10}{15}\right)}} = \sqrt{\frac{18}{10}} = \sqrt{1.8}$

$\sqrt{1.8} \approx 1 + 4\left(\frac{1}{15}\right) + 12\left(\frac{1}{15}\right)^2 = 1 + \frac{4}{15} + \frac{4}{75} = \frac{33}{25}$

[2 marks available — 1 mark for substituting $x = \frac{1}{15}$ into the expansion from part a), 1 mark for correct simplification]

6 a) $2 - 18x \equiv A(1-2x)^2 + B(5+4x)(1-2x) + C(5+4x)$ ***[1 mark]***

Let $x = \frac{1}{2}$, then:

$2 - 9 = 7C \Rightarrow -7 = 7C \Rightarrow C = -1$ ***[1 mark]***

Let $x = -\frac{5}{4}$, then:

$2 - -\frac{45}{2} = \frac{49}{4}A \Rightarrow \frac{49}{2} = \frac{49}{4}A \Rightarrow A = 2$ ***[1 mark]***

Equating the coefficients of the x^2 terms:

$0 = 4A - 8B = 8 - 8B \Rightarrow 8B = 8 \Rightarrow B = 1$ ***[1 mark]***

b) $f(x) = \frac{2}{(5+4x)} + \frac{1}{(1-2x)} - \frac{1}{(1-2x)^2}$

$= 2(5+4x)^{-1} + (1-2x)^{-1} - (1-2x)^{-2}$

Expand each bracket separately:

$(5+4x)^{-1} = 5^{-1}\left(1+\frac{4}{5}x\right)^{-1} = \frac{1}{5}\left(1+\frac{4}{5}x\right)^{-1}$

$= \frac{1}{5}\left(1 + (-1)\left(\frac{4}{5}x\right) + \frac{-1\times-2}{1\times2}\left(\frac{4}{5}x\right)^2 + ...\right)$

$= \frac{1}{5}\left(1 - \frac{4}{5}x + \frac{16}{25}x^2 + ...\right) = \frac{1}{5} - \frac{4}{25}x + \frac{16}{125}x^2 + ...$

$(1-2x)^{-1} = 1 + (-1)(-2x) + \frac{-1\times-2}{1\times2}(-2x)^2 + ...$

$= 1 + 2x + 4x^2 + ...$

$(1-2x)^{-2} = 1 + (-2)(-2x) + \frac{-2\times-3}{1\times2}(-2x)^2 + ...$

$= 1 + 4x + 12x^2 + ...$

Putting it all together gives (ignoring any terms in x^3 or above):

$f(x) \approx 2\left(\frac{1}{5} - \frac{4}{25}x + \frac{16}{125}x^2\right) + (1 + 2x + 4x^2) - (1 + 4x + 12x^2)$

$= \frac{2}{5} - \frac{8}{25}x + \frac{32}{125}x^2 + 1 + 2x + 4x^2 - 1 - 4x - 12x^2$

$= \frac{2}{5} - \frac{58}{25}x - \frac{968}{125}x^2$

[6 marks available — 1 mark for taking out a factor of 5 from $(5+4x)^{-1}$, 1 mark for correct expansion of $(5+4x)^{-1}$, 1 mark for correct expansion of $(1-2x)^{-1}$, 1 mark for correct expansion of $(1-2x)^{-2}$, 1 mark for correct constant and x-terms in final answer, 1 mark for correct x^2-term in final answer]

c) Expansion of $(5+4x)^{-1}$ is valid for

$\left|\frac{4x}{5}\right| < 1 \Rightarrow \frac{4|x|}{5} < 1 \Rightarrow |x| < \frac{5}{4}$

Expansions of $(1-2x)^{-1}$ and $(1-2x)^{-2}$ are valid for

$\left|\frac{-2x}{1}\right| < 1 \Rightarrow \frac{2|x|}{1} < 1 \Rightarrow |x| < \frac{1}{2}$

The combined expansion is valid for the narrower of these two ranges. So the expansion of f(x) is valid for $|x| < \frac{1}{2}$.

Claire had the wrong inequality sign in the second inequality OR she incorrectly combined the two inequalities instead of using the narrower of the two of the ranges. ***[2 marks available — 1 mark for explaining the error Claire had made, 1 mark for correct range]***

Pages 30-36: Trigonometry

1 To find the area of the sector, you need the angle in radians:
$(120° \div 180°) \times \pi = \frac{2\pi}{3}$ radians ***[1 mark]***
Now use the arc length to find r:
Arc length $S = r\theta$, so
$40 = \frac{2\pi}{3} \times r$ ***[1 mark]***
$r = 40 \div \frac{2\pi}{3} = \frac{60}{\pi}$ ***[1 mark]***
Finally, use this value of r to find the area:
$A = \frac{1}{2}r^2\theta = \frac{1}{2} \times (\frac{60}{\pi})^2 \times \frac{2\pi}{3}$ ***[1 mark]***
$= \frac{1200}{\pi} = 381.9718... = 382 \text{ cm}^2$ (to the nearest cm²) ***[1 mark]***

2 a) The total length of the bottom and straight sides is $q + q + 2r$.
The top length is $2x$, so using the right-angled triangle formed by r, x and y:
$\cos\theta = \frac{\text{adjacent}}{\text{hypotenuse}} = \frac{x}{r} \Rightarrow x = r\cos\theta \Rightarrow 2x = 2r\cos\theta$
For the curved lengths, the shaded areas are sectors of circles, and the formula for the length of one arc is given by $r\theta$.
Now add them all up to get the total perimeter:
$P = q + q + 2r + 2r\cos\theta + r\theta + r\theta = 2[q + r(1 + \theta + \cos\theta)]$.
Break the area down into a rectangle, a triangle and two sectors:
Area of rectangle = width × height = $2qr$
Area of triangle $= \frac{1}{2}(2r\cos\theta)(r\sin\theta) = r^2\cos\theta\sin\theta$
Area of one shaded sector $= \frac{1}{2}r^2\theta$
So the total area $A = 2qr + r^2\cos\theta\sin\theta + r^2\theta$
$= 2qr + r^2(\cos\theta\sin\theta + \theta)$.
[4 marks available — 1 mark for all individual lengths correct, 1 mark for all individual areas correct, 1 mark for each correct expression]
You could've used $\frac{1}{2}AB\sin C$ to find the area of the triangle, but then you'd need to use an expressions for x or y to get the final answer.

b) Substitute the given values of P and θ into the expression for the perimeter: $P = 2[q + r(1 + \theta + \cos\theta)]$
$\Rightarrow 40 = 2\left[q + r\left(1 + \frac{\pi}{3} + \cos\frac{\pi}{3}\right)\right]$
$\Rightarrow 20 = q + r\left(\frac{3}{2} + \frac{\pi}{3}\right)$ ***[1 mark]***
And then into the expression for the area:
$A = 2qr + r^2(\cos\theta\sin\theta + \theta)$
$\Rightarrow A = 2qr + r^2\left(\cos\frac{\pi}{3}\sin\frac{\pi}{3} + \frac{\pi}{3}\right)$
$= 2qr + r^2\left(\frac{\sqrt{3}}{4} + \frac{\pi}{3}\right)$ ***[1 mark]***
To rearrange this formula for area into the form shown in the question, you need to get rid of q. Rearrange the perimeter formula to get an expression for q in terms of r, then substitute that into the area expression:
$q = 20 - r\left(\frac{3}{2} + \frac{\pi}{3}\right)$
$A = 2qr + r^2\left(\frac{\sqrt{3}}{4} + \frac{\pi}{3}\right)$
$= 2r\left[20 - r\left(\frac{3}{2} + \frac{\pi}{3}\right)\right] + r^2\left(\frac{\sqrt{3}}{4} + \frac{\pi}{3}\right)$ ***[1 mark]***
$= 40r - 2r^2\left(\frac{3}{2} + \frac{\pi}{3}\right) + r^2\left(\frac{\sqrt{3}}{4} + \frac{\pi}{3}\right)$
$= 40r - r^2\left[\left(3 + \frac{2\pi}{3}\right) - \left(\frac{\sqrt{3}}{4} + \frac{\pi}{3}\right)\right]$
$= 40 - r^2\left(3 - \frac{\sqrt{3}}{4} + \frac{\pi}{3}\right)$
So $A = 40r - kr^2$, where $k = 3 - \frac{\sqrt{3}}{4} + \frac{\pi}{3}$, as required ***[1 mark]***

3 The graph of $y = \sin x$ is mapped onto the graph of $y = \sin\frac{x}{2}$ via a stretch parallel to the x-axis of scale factor 2.
The graph should appear as follows:

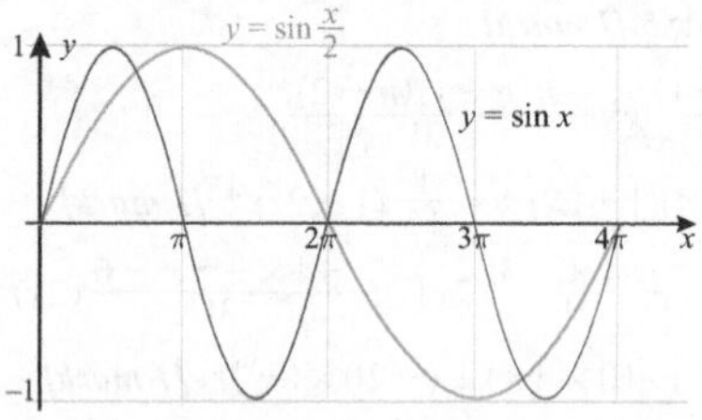

[3 marks available — 1 mark for sin x correct, 1 mark for sin $\frac{x}{2}$ correct, 1 mark for correct axis labelling]

4 a) Use the cosine rule:
e.g. $\cos A = \frac{50^2 + 70^2 - 90^2}{2 \times 50 \times 70}$ ***[1 mark]***
$\cos A = -0.1$ ***[1 mark]***
$A = 95.739...°$ ***[1 mark]***
Now use this value of A to find the area:
Area $= \frac{1}{2} \times 50 \times 70 \times \sin 95.739...°$ ***[1 mark]***
$= 1741.228... = 1741 \text{ m}^2$ (nearest m²) ***[1 mark]***
If you've allocated your values of a, b, c etc. differently, or found a different angle, then the numbers in your working will be different.

b) E.g. the model is unlikely to give an area accurate to the nearest square metre as the given side lengths are most likely rounded, at least to the nearest metre, possibly to the nearest 5 m or 10 m. This means that there is a large range of possible areas. / The sides are unlikely to be perfectly straight, so the model will not be accurate ***[1 mark for a sensible comment]***.

5 $\sin x = -\frac{\sqrt{2}}{2} \Rightarrow x = -\frac{\pi}{4}$. So $\pi - \left(-\frac{\pi}{4}\right) = \frac{5\pi}{4}$ is also a solution.
So $x = \frac{5\pi}{4}$ is a solution in the range ***[1 mark]***.
You could sketch the graph of y = sin x, or use a CAST diagram, to help you find the answer.

6 $7 - 3\cos x = 9\sin^2 x$, and $\sin^2 x \equiv 1 - \cos^2 x$
$\Rightarrow 7 - 3\cos x = 9(1 - \cos^2 x)$
$\Rightarrow 7 - 3\cos x = 9 - 9\cos^2 x$
$\Rightarrow 9\cos^2 x - 3\cos x - 2 = 0$
Substitute y for $\cos x$ and solve $9y^2 - 3y - 2 = 0$ by factorising:
$(3y - 2)(3y + 1) = 0 \Rightarrow y = \frac{2}{3}$ or $y = -\frac{1}{3}$
So $\cos x = \frac{2}{3}$ or $\cos x = -\frac{1}{3}$
For $\cos x = \frac{2}{3}$, $x = 48.189...° = 48.2°$ (1 d.p.).
For $\cos x = -\frac{1}{3}$, $x = 109.471...° = 109.5°$ (1 d.p).
[5 marks available — 1 mark for correct substitution using trig identity, 1 mark for forming a quadratic in cos x, 1 mark for finding correct values of cos x, 1 mark for each of the 2 correct solutions]

7 a) Substituting $t = 35.26...°$ into both sides of the equation gives:
LHS: $\sin(2 \times 35.26...°) = 0.94$ (2 s.f)
RHS: $\sqrt{2}\cos(2 \times 35.26...°) = 0.47$ (2 s.f.)
$0.94 \neq 0.47$, so Adam's solution is incorrect ***[1 mark]***.

b) Adam has incorrectly divided by 2:
$\tan 2t = \sqrt{2} \nRightarrow \tan t = \frac{\sqrt{2}}{2}$ ***[1 mark]***

c) $t = -27.36...°$ is not a solution of the original equation ***[1 mark]***. The error appeared because Bethan has squared the equation and then taken roots ***[1 mark]***.

8 a) Use the trig identity $\tan\theta \equiv \frac{\sin\theta}{\cos\theta}$:

$\tan^2\theta + \frac{\tan\theta}{\cos\theta} = 1 \Rightarrow \frac{\sin^2\theta}{\cos^2\theta} + \frac{\sin\theta}{\cos^2\theta} = 1$ ***[1 mark]***

Put over a common denominator: $\frac{\sin^2\theta + \sin\theta}{\cos^2\theta} = 1$

$\Rightarrow \sin^2\theta + \sin\theta = \cos^2\theta$

Now use the identity $\cos^2\theta \equiv 1 - \sin^2\theta$ to give:

$\sin^2\theta + \sin\theta = 1 - \sin^2\theta$ ***[1 mark]***

$\Rightarrow 2\sin^2\theta + \sin\theta - 1 = 0$ ***[1 mark for rearrangement]***.

b) Factorising the quadratic from a) gives:

$(2\sin\theta - 1)(\sin\theta + 1) = 0$ ***[1 mark]***

$\Rightarrow \sin\theta = \frac{1}{2}$ or $\sin\theta = -1$ ***[1 mark]***

$\sin\theta = \frac{1}{2} \Rightarrow \theta = \frac{\pi}{6}$ and $\theta = (\pi - \frac{\pi}{6}) = \frac{5\pi}{6}$ ***[1 mark for both]***

$\sin\theta = -1 \Rightarrow \theta = \frac{3\pi}{2}$, but $f(\theta)$ is not defined for $\theta = \frac{3\pi}{2}$, so ignore this solution. So the solutions are $\theta = \frac{\pi}{6}$ and $\frac{5\pi}{6}$ ***[1 mark]***

9 a) The start and end points of the cos curve (with restricted domain) are $(0, 1)$ and $(\pi, -1)$, so the coordinates of the start point of arccos (point A) are $(-1, \pi)$ ***[1 mark]*** and the coordinates of the end point (point B) are $(1, 0)$ ***[1 mark]***.

b) $y = \arccos x \Rightarrow y = \cos^{-1} x \Rightarrow x = \cos y$ ***[1 mark]***

c) $\arccos x = 2 \Rightarrow x = \cos 2$ ***[1 mark]*** $\Rightarrow x = -0.416$ ***[1 mark]***

10 a) $\text{cosec}\,\theta = \frac{5}{3} \Rightarrow \sin\theta = \frac{3}{5}$. Solving for θ gives $\theta = 0.64350...$,

$\theta = \pi - 0.64350... = 2.49809...$

So $\theta = 0.644, 2.50$ (both to 3 s.f.)

[1 mark for each correct answer].

Sketch the graph of y = sin x or use a CAST diagram to help you find the second solution.

b) (i) The identity $\text{cosec}^2\theta \equiv 1 + \cot^2\theta$ rearranges to give $\text{cosec}^2\theta - 1 \equiv \cot^2\theta$. Putting this into the equation:

$3\,\text{cosec}\,\theta = (\text{cosec}^2\theta - 1) - 17$

$18 + 3\,\text{cosec}\,\theta - \text{cosec}^2\theta = 0$ as required

[2 marks available — 1 mark for using correct identity, 1 mark for rearranging into required form]

(ii) To solve the equation in (i), use the substitution $x = \text{cosec}\,\theta$.

Then $18 + 3x - x^2 = 0$ ***[1 mark]*** $\Rightarrow x = 6$ and $x = -3$.

So $\text{cosec}\,\theta = 6$ and $\text{cosec}\,\theta = -3$ ***[1 mark]***.

$\text{cosec}\,\theta = \frac{1}{\sin\theta}$, so $\sin\theta = \frac{1}{6}$ and $\sin\theta = -\frac{1}{3}$ ***[1 mark]***.

$\sin\theta = \frac{1}{6} \Rightarrow \theta = \sin^{-1}\frac{1}{6} = 0.16744...$ or

$\theta = \pi - 0.16744... = 2.97414...$

$\sin\theta = -\frac{1}{3} \Rightarrow \theta = \sin^{-1}\left(-\frac{1}{3}\right) = -0.33983...$

but this is outside the required range.

So $\theta = 2\pi + (-0.33983...) = 5.94334...$ or

$\theta = \pi - (-0.33983...) = 3.48142...$

So $\theta = 0.167, 2.97$ ***[1 mark]*** and

$\theta = 3.48, 5.94$ ***[1 mark]*** (all to 3 s.f.).

You don't have to use x = cosec θ — it's just a little easier to factorise without all those pesky cosecs flying around.

11 Using the small angle approximations, $\sin\theta \approx \theta$, $\cos\theta \approx 1 - \frac{1}{2}\theta^2$ and $\tan\theta \approx \theta$. Substituting these values into the expression gives:

$4\sin\theta\tan\theta + 2\cos\theta \approx 4(\theta \times \theta) + 2(1 - \frac{1}{2}\theta^2)$

$= 4\theta^2 + 2 - \theta^2 = 2 + 3\theta^2$ ***[1 mark]***

12 $\tan 2\theta = \frac{1}{1 + \tan\theta}$

Using the double angle formula:

$\frac{2\tan\theta}{1 - \tan^2\theta} = \frac{1}{1 + \tan\theta}$ ***[1 mark]***

$2\tan\theta = \frac{(1 - \tan\theta)(1 + \tan\theta)}{1 + \tan\theta}$ ***[1 mark]***

$2\tan\theta = 1 - \tan\theta \Rightarrow \tan\theta = \frac{1}{3}$

So $\tan\theta = \frac{1}{3} = \frac{a}{2b} \Rightarrow b = \frac{3a}{2}$ ***[1 mark]***

Area $= a \times b = a \times \frac{3a}{2} = \frac{3a^2}{2}$ ***[1 mark]***

13 a) $\frac{1 + \cos x}{2} = \frac{1}{2}\left(1 + \cos 2\left(\frac{x}{2}\right)\right)$

$= \frac{1}{2}\left(1 + \left(2\cos^2\frac{x}{2} - 1\right)\right)$

$= \frac{1}{2}\left(2\cos^2\frac{x}{2}\right) = \cos^2\frac{x}{2}$

[2 marks available – 1 mark for using the correct identity, 1 mark for the correct rearrangement]

b) As $\cos^2\frac{x}{2} = 0.75$, $\frac{1 + \cos x}{2} = 0.75$.

So $1 + \cos x = 1.5$

$\cos x = 0.5$ ***[1 mark]*** $\Rightarrow x = \frac{\pi}{3}, \frac{5\pi}{3}$ ***[1 mark]***

You should know the solutions to cos x = 0.5 — it's one of the common angles.

14 a) The sound wave is a transformation of the curve $A = \sin t$ ***[1 mark]***

So compare $A = B\sin(kt)$ to $y = \sin x$:

$y = \sin x$ has a maximum at $y = 1$, and the sound wave has a maximum at $A = 6$, so the graph is stretched vertically by a factor of $6 \Rightarrow B = 6$ ***[1 mark]***

$y = \sin x = 0$ when $x = \pi, 2\pi, 3\pi$, etc.

$A = 0$ when $t = 0.004, 0.008, 0.012$, etc.

So if $A = 6\sin(kt)$,

$0.004k = \pi \Rightarrow k = \frac{\pi}{0.004} = 250\pi$ ***[1 mark]***

So the graph is squashed horizontally by a factor of 250π.

So, $A = 6\sin(250\pi t)$ as required.

b) Let $x = 250\pi t$, then:

$R\sin(x + \alpha) = 6\sin x + 2\sqrt{3}\cos x$

Expand LHS using the trigonometric addition formula:

$R\sin(x + \alpha) = R\sin x\cos\alpha + R\cos x\sin\alpha$

So $R\sin x\cos\alpha + R\cos x\sin\alpha = 6\sin x + 2\sqrt{3}\cos x$ ***[1 mark]***

Equating coefficients:

$R\cos\alpha = 6$, $R\sin\alpha = 2\sqrt{3}$ ***[1 mark]***

$\frac{R\sin\alpha}{R\cos\alpha} = \tan\alpha = \frac{2\sqrt{3}}{6} = \frac{\sqrt{3}}{3}$

$\Rightarrow \alpha = \tan^{-1}\left(\frac{\sqrt{3}}{3}\right) = \frac{\pi}{6}$ ***[1 mark]***

$(R\cos\alpha)^2 + (R\sin\alpha)^2 = 6^2 + (2\sqrt{3})^2 = R^2$

$\Rightarrow R = \sqrt{6^2 + (2\sqrt{3})^2} = \sqrt{48} = 4\sqrt{3}$ ***[1 mark]***

So the combined sound waves are modelled by

$A = 4\sqrt{3}\sin\left(x + \frac{\pi}{6}\right)$

15 $\sin 2\theta \equiv 2\sin\theta\cos\theta$, so $3\sin 2\theta\tan\theta \equiv 6\sin\theta\cos\theta\tan\theta$ ***[1 mark]***.

As $\tan\theta \equiv \frac{\sin\theta}{\cos\theta}$,

$6\sin\theta\cos\theta\tan\theta \equiv 6\sin\theta\cos\theta\frac{\sin\theta}{\cos\theta} \equiv 6\sin^2\theta$ ***[1 mark]***

so $3\sin 2\theta\tan\theta = 5 \Rightarrow 6\sin^2\theta = 5$ ***[1 mark]***

Then $\sin^2\theta = \frac{5}{6} \Rightarrow \sin\theta = \pm\sqrt{\frac{5}{6}} = \pm 0.9128...$ ***[1 mark]***

Solving this for θ gives $\theta = 1.15, 1.99, 4.29, 5.13$ ***[2 marks for all 4 correct answers, 1 mark for 2 correct answers]***

Don't forget the solutions for the negative square root as well — they're easy to miss. Drawing a sketch here is really useful — you can see that there are 4 solutions you need to find:

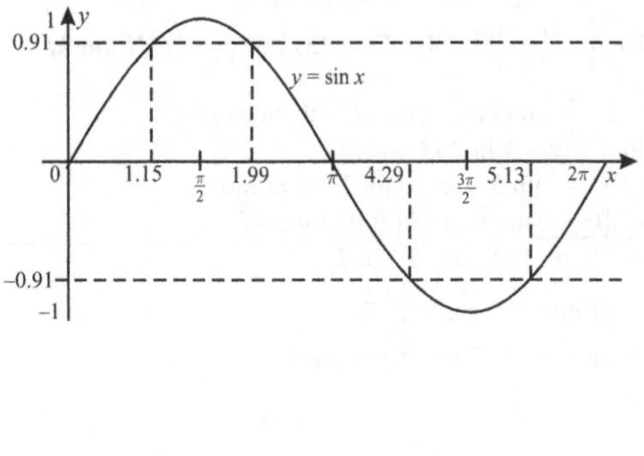

16 a) $\sqrt{2}\cos\theta - 3\sin\theta \equiv R\cos(\theta + \alpha)$. Using the cos addition rule, $R\cos(\theta + \alpha) \equiv R\cos\theta\cos\alpha - R\sin\theta\sin\alpha$,
so ① $R\cos\alpha = \sqrt{2}$ and ② $R\sin\alpha = 3$ ***[1 mark]***.
② ÷ ① gives $\tan a = \frac{3}{\sqrt{2}} \Rightarrow \alpha = 1.13$ (3 s.f.) ***[1 mark]***
①² + ②² gives:
$R^2\cos^2\alpha + R^2\sin^2\alpha = (\sqrt{2})^2 + 3^2 = 11 \Rightarrow R = \sqrt{11}$ ***[1 mark]***,
so $\sqrt{2}\cos\theta - 3\sin\theta = \sqrt{11}\cos(\theta + 1.13)$.

b) The equation you're trying to solve is $\sqrt{2}\cos\theta - 3\sin\theta = 3$ in the range $0 \le \theta \le 6$, so, from part a), $\sqrt{11}\cos(\theta + 1.13) = 3$.
So $\cos(\theta + 1.13) = \frac{3}{\sqrt{11}}$.
Solving this gives $\theta + 1.13 = 0.4405...$ ***[1 mark]***.
The range of solutions becomes $1.13 \le \theta + 1.13 \le 7.13$.
To find the other values of θ within the new range, $2\pi - 0.4405... = 5.842...$, $2\pi + 0.4405... = 6.723...$ ***[1 mark for both]***. Subtracting 1.13 gives $\theta = 4.712...$, $5.593...$ mins ***[1 mark for both]***. So the water reaches 3 feet to the right of the sprinkler at 4 minutes 43 seconds and at 5 minutes 36 seconds ***[1 mark for both]***.
You can sketch the graph to help you find all the values of θ.

c) Using part a), $d = (\sqrt{2}\cos\theta - 3\sin\theta)^4 = (\sqrt{11}\cos(\theta + 1.13))^4$
The maximum distances left and right occur at the minimum and maximum value of d (the minimum value corresponds to the maximum distance left). The maximum and minimum points of $\cos(\theta + 1.13)$ are ±1, so the maximum and minimum values of the function inside the brackets are $\pm\sqrt{11}$. This bracket is raised to the power 4, so the maximum distance right is: $(\pm\sqrt{11})^4 = 121$ feet ***[1 mark]***. Since $(\sqrt{11}\cos(\theta + 1.13))^4 \ge 0$, the maximum distance left is 0 feet ***[1 mark]***.
If you didn't realise that $(\sqrt{11}\cos(\theta + 1.13))^4$ is never negative, you'd have got the distance left wrong.

d) E.g. the sprinkler could be positioned against a wall, so it can never spray to the left ***[1 mark for a sensible comment]***.

17 $\text{cosec}\,2A \equiv \frac{1}{\sin 2A} \equiv \frac{1}{2\sin A\cos A}$

so $2\tan A\,\text{cosec}\,2A \equiv \frac{2\tan A}{2\sin A\cos A} \equiv \frac{2\frac{\sin A}{\cos A}}{2\sin A\cos A}$

$\equiv \frac{\sin A}{\sin A\cos^2 A} \equiv \frac{1}{\cos^2 A}$

$\equiv \sec^2 A \equiv 1 + \tan^2 A$

[3 marks available — 1 mark for using the double angle formula to expand sin 2A, 1 mark for rearranging and simplifying with the use of $\tan A \equiv \frac{\sin A}{\cos A}$, 1 mark for using $\sec^2 A \equiv 1 + \tan^2 A$ to get into the required form]

Pages 37-40: Exponentials and Logarithms

1 Rewrite all terms as powers of p and use the laws of logs to simplify:
$\log_p(p^4) + \log_p(p^{\frac{1}{2}}) - \log_p(p^{-\frac{1}{2}})$
$= 4\log_p p + \frac{1}{2}\log_p p - \left(-\frac{1}{2}\right)\log_p p$
$= 4 + \frac{1}{2} - \left(-\frac{1}{2}\right) = 4 + 1 = 5$ (as $\log_p p = 1$) ***[1 mark]***

2 $5^{(z^2-9)} = 2^{(z-3)}$, so taking logs of both sides gives:
$(z^2 - 9)\ln 5 = (z - 3)\ln 2$ ***[1 mark]***
$\Rightarrow (z + 3)(z - 3)\ln 5 - (z - 3)\ln 2 = 0$ ***[1 mark]***
$\Rightarrow (z - 3)[(z + 3)\ln 5 - \ln 2] = 0$ ***[1 mark]***
$\Rightarrow z - 3 = 0$ or $(z + 3)\ln 5 - \ln 2 = 0$
$\Rightarrow z = 3$ ***[1 mark]*** or $z = \frac{\ln 2}{\ln 5} - 3$
$\Rightarrow z = 3$ or $z = -2.57$ (3 s.f.) ***[1 mark]***

3 $3^{2x} = (3^x)^2$ (from the power laws), so let $y = 3^x$, then $y^2 = 3^{2x}$.
This gives a quadratic in y: $y^2 - 9y + 14 = 0$
$(y - 2)(y - 7) = 0$ ***[1 mark]***, so $y = 2$ or $y = 7$
$\Rightarrow 3^x = 2$ or $3^x = 7$ ***[1 mark for both]***
To solve these equations, take logs of both sides ***[1 mark]***.
$3^x = 2 \Rightarrow \log 3^x = \log 2 \Rightarrow x\log 3 = \log 2$
$\Rightarrow x = \frac{\log 2}{\log 3} = 0.631$ (3 s.f.) ***[1 mark]***
$3^x = 7 \Rightarrow \log 3^x = \log 7 \Rightarrow x\log 3 = \log 7$
$\Rightarrow x = \frac{\log 7}{\log 3} = 1.77$ (3 s.f.) ***[1 mark]***

4 a) $y = \ln(4x - 3)$, and $x = a$ when $y = 1$.
$1 = \ln(4a - 3) \Rightarrow e^1 = 4a - 3$ ***[1 mark]***
$\Rightarrow a = \frac{e^1 + 3}{4} = 1.43$ to 2 d.p. ***[1 mark]***

b) The curve can only exist when $4x - 3 > 0$ ***[1 mark]***
$\Rightarrow x > \frac{3}{4} \Rightarrow x > 0.75$, so $b = 0.75$ ***[1 mark]***.

5 a) A is the value of y when $x = 0$, so $A = 4$ ***[1 mark]***.
Now use this value to find b:
$\frac{4}{e} = 4e^{10b}$ ***[1 mark]*** $\Rightarrow 4e^{-1} = 4e^{10b}$
$\Rightarrow -1 = 10b \Rightarrow b = -0.1$ ***[1 mark]***

b) The gradient of $y = Ae^{bx}$ is bAe^{bx}. Here, $A = 4$ and $b = -0.1$, so the gradient is $-0.1 \times 4 \times e^{-0.1x} = -0.4e^{-0.1x}$
[1 mark for a correct gradient expression].
Set this equal to the value given and solve:
$-0.4e^{-0.1x} = -1$ ***[1 mark]*** $\Rightarrow e^{-0.1x} = 2.5$
$\Rightarrow -0.1x = \ln 2.5$ ***[1 mark]*** $\Rightarrow x = -10\ln 2.5$ ***[1 mark]***
When $x = -10\ln 2.5$, $y = 4e^{-0.1(-10\ln 2.5)} = 4e^{\ln 2.5} = 4 \times 2.5 = 10$
So the exact coordinates are $(-10\ln 2.5, 10)$ ***[1 mark]***.

6 $y = e^{ax} + b$
The sketch shows that when $x = 0$, $y = -6$, so:
$-6 = e^0 + b \Rightarrow -6 = 1 + b \Rightarrow b = -7$ ***[1 mark]***.
The sketch also shows that when $y = 0$, $x = \frac{1}{4}\ln 7$, so:
$0 = e^{(\frac{a}{4}\ln 7)} - 7$ ***[1 mark]*** $\Rightarrow e^{(\frac{a}{4}\ln 7)} = 7$
$\Rightarrow \frac{a}{4}\ln 7 = \ln 7 \Rightarrow \frac{a}{4} = 1 \Rightarrow a = 4$ ***[1 mark]***.
The asymptote occurs as $x \to -\infty$, so $e^{4x} \to 0$, and since $y = e^{4x} - 7$, $y \to -7$.
So the equation of the asymptote is $y = -7$ ***[1 mark]***.
You could also have solved this question by thinking about the series of transformations that would take you from the graph of $y = e^x$ to this one.

7 The value after the first year is $0.92 \times 8000 = £7360$ ***[1 mark]***.
You need to find n, the number of months after the first year when the value falls below £4000. So solve the equation:
$7360 \times e^{\frac{n}{12}\ln\left(1 - \frac{4}{100}\right)} = 4000$ ***[1 mark]*** $\Rightarrow e^{\frac{n}{12}\ln 0.96} = \frac{4000}{7360}$
$\Rightarrow \frac{n}{12}\ln 0.96 = \ln\left(\frac{4000}{7360}\right)$ ***[1 mark]***
$\Rightarrow n = 12\ln\frac{4000}{7360} \div \ln 0.96 = 179.246$ ***[1 mark]***
179 months after the first year the value is £4003.35 to the nearest penny (i.e. > 4000), so you need to round up to 180 months.
The total number of months is: 12 + 180 = 192 months ***[1 mark]***.
Don't forget to add the 12 at the end — that's the months from the first year (which had a different rate of depreciation).

8 a) You need to find t such that:
$2100 - 1500e^{-0.15t} > 5700e^{-0.15t}$ ***[1 mark]***
$2100 > 7200e^{-0.15t}$
$\frac{7}{24} > e^{-0.15t}$
$\ln\frac{7}{24} > -0.15t$ ***[1 mark]***
$\ln\frac{7}{24} \div -0.15 < t$
$t > 8.21429...$ ***[1 mark]***
So the population of Q first exceeds the population of P when $t > 8.21$ (3 s.f.), i.e. in the year 2018 ***[1 mark]***.
Don't forget to flip the inequality sign when you divide by −0.15.

b)

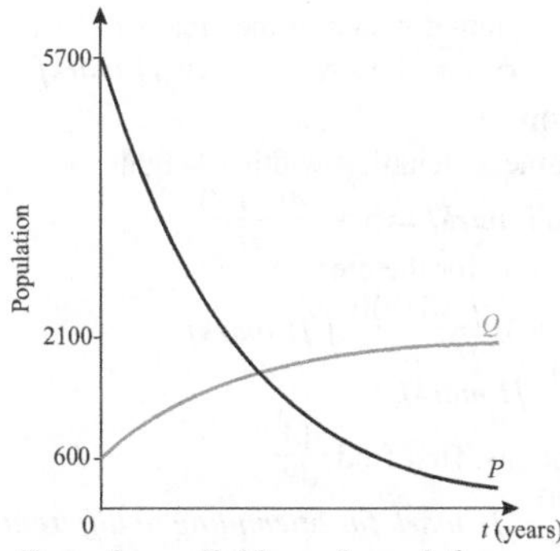

[2 marks available — 1 mark for correct shape of graph, 1 mark for (0, 5700) labelled]

c) Bird of prey — e.g. any one of:
- The model predicts the population of the birds of prey will increase, but will tend to a limit. This seems realistic, as the bird of prey will have to compete for the available sources of food as one source decreases.
- The population grows quite slowly (especially compared to the rate of decrease of the other species) — this seems more realistic than a rapid population growth.
- The rate of growth slows over time, which would be expected as food supplies dwindle.

[1 mark for a sensible comment about the birds of prey]

Endangered species — e.g. any one of:
- The model predicts the population will decrease, which seems realistic as the birds of prey will hunt them.
- The model predicts a very rapid decline at first, which does not seem realistic — you'd expect the rate of decrease to be slower at first.

[1 mark for a sensible comment about the endangered species]

d) You need to find t such that $5700e^{-0.15t} = 1000$ ***[1 mark]***

$\Rightarrow 1000 = \frac{5700}{e^{0.15t}} \Rightarrow e^{0.15t} = \frac{5700}{1000} = 5.7.$

$\Rightarrow 0.15t = \ln 5.7 \Rightarrow t = \frac{\ln 5.7}{0.15} = 11.6031...$ years ***[1 mark]***

So the population is predicted to drop below 1000 in the year 2021 ***[1 mark]***.

If you set up and solved an inequality that's fine — you'd still get the marks.

e) E.g. The function could be refined so that from 2021, the population is predicted to stop decreasing — it could either level out or start increasing ***[1 mark for a sensible comment]***.

9 a) $y = ab^t$, so take logs of both sides: $\log y = \log ab^t$

Then use the laws of logs: $\log y = \log a + \log b^t$ ***[1 mark]***

$\log y = \log a + t\log b$ ***[1 mark]***

$\log y = t\log b + \log a$, as required.

b) a is the average attendance in hundreds in the season where $t = 0$, i.e in the 2010/11 season ***[1 mark]***.

The attendance was around 50 supporters.

c) First find the values of a and b:

Comparing $\log y = t\log b + \log a$ to $y = mx + c$ gives $\log b = m$, the gradient of the graph, and $\log a = c$, the vertical-axis intercept of the graph.

Use points from the graph to calculate the gradient, m:

For example, using the points (2, 0.3) and (1, 0):

$$m = \frac{y_2 - y_1}{x_2 - x_1} = \frac{0.3 - 0}{2 - 1} = 0.3$$

So $\log b = 0.3 \Rightarrow b = 10^{0.3}$ ***[1 mark]***

Now estimate the vertical-axis intercept to find $\log_{10} a$:

$\log a = -0.3 \Rightarrow a = 10^{-0.3}$ ***[1 mark]***.

The equation is $y = 10^{-0.3} \times (10^{0.3})^t = 10^{0.3t - 0.3} = 10^{0.3(t-1)}$

y is the average attendance in hundreds, so the attendance exceeds 10 000 when $y > 100$, i.e. $10^{0.3(t-1)} > 100$ ***[1 mark]***

$0.3(t-1) > \log 100 \Rightarrow 0.3(t-1) > 2$

$\Rightarrow t > 7.666...$ years after the 2010/2011 season ***[1 mark]***.

This is during the 2017/2018 season ***[1 mark]***.

Don't worry if your values of a and b are slightly different — you should end up with the same answer though.

d) For the 2017/18 season, $t = 7$, which is beyond the values of t given on the graph ***[1 mark]***. This is extrapolation, so may not be reliable as the model might not hold beyond the value of $t = 5$ ***[1 mark]***.

Pages 41-44: Differentiation — 1

1 Using your calculator or an algebraic method:

At $x = 4$, $\frac{dy}{dx} = 39$ ***[1 mark]***

2 $\frac{dy}{dt} = 3t^2 - 14t + 8$ ***[1 mark]***

Solve when $\frac{dy}{dt} = 0$:

$3t^2 - 14t + 8 = 0 \Rightarrow (3t - 2)(t - 4) = 0$ ***[1 mark]***

$t = \frac{2}{3}$ s and $t = 4$ s ***[1 mark]***

3 a) The gradient of the normal at R is the same as the gradient of the line $4y + x = 24$. Rearrange this equation to find the gradient:

$4y + x = 24 \Rightarrow 4y = 24 - x \Rightarrow y = 6 - \frac{1}{4}x,$

so gradient of normal at R $= -\frac{1}{4}$

Gradient of curve at R $= -1 \div -\frac{1}{4} = 4$

Find an expression for the gradient of the curve by differentiating $y = kx^2 - 8x - 5$:

$\frac{dy}{dx} = 2kx - 8$

At R, gradient $= 2k(2) - 8 = 4k - 8$

Put this expression equal to the value of the gradient at R to find k:

$4k - 8 = 4 \Rightarrow 4k = 12 \Rightarrow k = 3$

[5 marks available — 1 mark for finding the gradient of the normal at R, 1 mark for finding the gradient of the curve at R, 1 mark for attempting to differentiate y, 1 mark for forming an equation for k, 1 mark for the correct value of k]

b) Gradient of tangent at R = gradient of curve = 4.

At R, $x = 2$, so $y = 3(2^2) - 8(2) - 5 = -9$ ***[1 mark]***

Use these values in $y - y_1 = m(x - x_1)$ to find the equation of the tangent:

$y + 9 = 4(x - 2) \Rightarrow y + 9 = 4x - 8 \Rightarrow y = 4x - 17$ ***[1 mark]***

Equate $y = 4x - 17$ and $y = 4x - \frac{1}{x^3} - 9$ to find S:

$4x - 17 = 4x - \frac{1}{x^3} - 9$ ***[1 mark]***

$-8 = -\frac{1}{x^3} \Rightarrow x = \frac{1}{2}$ and $y = 4(\frac{1}{2}) - 17 = -15$

So at S, $x = \frac{1}{2}$ ***[1 mark]*** and $y = -15$ ***[1 mark]***

4 $f'(x) = \lim_{h \to 0}\left(\frac{(8(x+h)^2 - 1) - (8x^2 - 1)}{h}\right)$ ***[1 mark]***

$= \lim_{h \to 0}\left(\frac{(8(x^2 + 2xh + h^2) - 1) - (8x^2 - 1)}{h}\right)$

$= \lim_{h \to 0}\left(\frac{8x^2 + 16xh + 8h^2 - 1 - 8x^2 + 1}{h}\right)$ ***[1 mark]***

$= \lim_{h \to 0}\left(\frac{16xh + 8h^2}{h}\right)$

$= \lim_{h \to 0}(16x + 8h)$ ***[1 mark]***

As $h \to 0$, $16x + 8h \to 16x$, so $f'(x) = 16x$

[1 mark for letting h → 0 and obtaining the correct limit]

5 a) Differentiate f(x) and set the derivative equal to zero:

$f'(x) = 8x^3 + 27$ ***[1 mark]***

$8x^3 + 27 = 0$ ***[1 mark]*** $\Rightarrow x^3 = -\frac{27}{8}$

$\Rightarrow x = \sqrt[3]{-\frac{27}{8}} = -\frac{3}{2} = -1.5$ ***[1 mark]***

When $x = -1.5$, $f(x) = 2(-1.5)^4 + 27(-1.5) = -30.375$ ***[1 mark]***

So the stationary point is at (−1.5, −30.375)

b) The function is increasing if the gradient is positive.

$f'(x) > 0$ if $8x^3 + 27 > 0 \Rightarrow x^3 > -\frac{27}{8} \Rightarrow x > \sqrt[3]{-\frac{27}{8}}$

$\Rightarrow x > -1.5$

The function is decreasing if the gradient is negative.

$f'(x) < 0$ if $8x^3 + 27 < 0 \Rightarrow x^3 < -\frac{27}{8} \Rightarrow x < \sqrt[3]{-\frac{27}{8}}$

$\Rightarrow x < -1.5$

[2 marks available — 1 mark for forming at least one correct inequality, 1 mark for both ranges of values correct]

c) You know from parts a) and b) that the function has a stationary point at (–1.5, –30.375) and that this is a minimum point because the function is decreasing to the left of this point and increasing to the right of it.
Find where the curve crosses the y-axis:
When $x = 0$, $f(x) = 0$, so the curve goes through the origin.
Find where the curve crosses the x-axis:
When $f(x) = 0$, $2x^4 + 27x = 0 \Rightarrow x(2x^3 + 27) = 0$
$\Rightarrow x = 0$ or $2x^3 + 27 = 0$
$\Rightarrow x^3 = -\frac{27}{2} \Rightarrow x = \sqrt[3]{-\frac{27}{2}} = -2.381$ (3 d.p.),
so the curve crosses the x-axis at $x = 0$ and $x = -2.381$.
Now use the information you've found to sketch the curve:

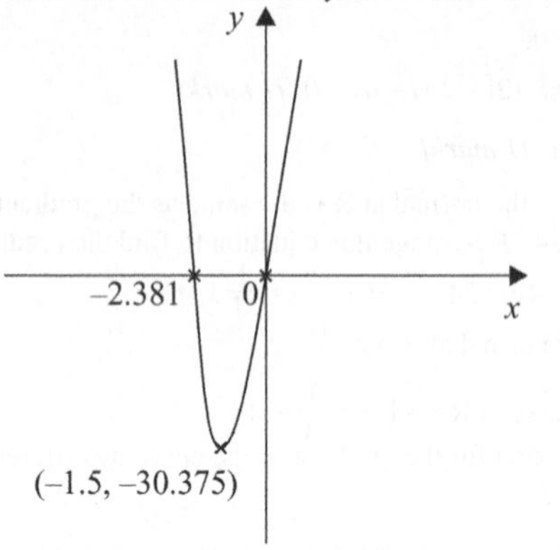

[3 marks available — 1 mark for a curve with the correct shape, 1 mark for the correct minimum point, 1 mark for the correct intercepts]

6 The graph is concave for $\frac{d^2y}{dx^2} < 0$.
$y = x^4 + 3x^3 - 6x^2 \Rightarrow \frac{dy}{dx} = 4x^3 + 9x^2 - 12x$ ***[1 mark]***
$\Rightarrow \frac{d^2y}{dx^2} = 12x^2 + 18x - 12$ ***[1 mark]***
$12x^2 + 18x - 12 < 0$ ***[1 mark]*** $\Rightarrow 2x^2 + 3x - 2 < 0$
$\Rightarrow (2x - 1)(x + 2) < 0$
$(2x - 1)(x + 2) < 0$ for $x < \frac{1}{2}$ and $x > -2$,
so the graph is concave for $-2 < x < \frac{1}{2}$ ***[1 mark]***.
To check your inequality think about the shape of the graph of $\frac{d^2y}{dx^2}$ – it's a positive quadratic, so is less than 0 between −2 and $\frac{1}{2}$.

7 a) At a point of inflection, $f''(x) = 0$, so find $f''(x)$.
$f(x) = 3x^3 + 9x^2 + 25x \Rightarrow f'(x) = 9x^2 + 18x + 25$ ***[1 mark]***
$\Rightarrow f''(x) = 18x + 18$ ***[1 mark]***
$f''(-1) = 18(-1) + 18 = 0$, so $f''(x) = 0$ at $x = -1$ ***[1 mark]***
To confirm that this is a point of inflection, you need to check what's happening either side of $x = -1$:
For $x < -1$, $f''(x) < 0$ and for $x > -1$, $f''(x) > 0$ ***[1 mark]***.
The curve changes from concave to convex, so $x = -1$ is a point of inflection ***[1 mark]***.

b) At a stationary point, $f'(x) = 0$.
$f'(x) = 9x^2 + 18x + 25$
$f'(-1) = 9(-1)^2 + 18(-1) + 25 = 16$. Since $16 \neq 0$, the point of inflection is not a stationary point. ***[2 marks available — 1 mark for finding f'(–1), 1 mark for a correct explanation of why this isn't a stationary point]***

c) $f(x)$ is an increasing function for all values of x if $f'(x) > 0$ for all x.
From a), $f'(x) = 9x^2 + 18x + 25$
Complete the square to show that $f'(x) > 0$:
$f'(x) = 9x^2 + 18x + 25$
$\Rightarrow f'(x) = 9(x^2 + 2x) + 25$
$\Rightarrow f'(x) = 9(x + 1)^2 - 9 + 25$
$\Rightarrow f'(x) = 9(x + 1)^2 + 16$ ***[1 mark]***
$(x + 1)^2 \geq 0$, so $f'(x)$ has a minimum value of 16
So $f'(x) > 0$ for all x, which means that $f(x)$ is an increasing function for all values of x ***[1 mark]***.

8 a) Surface area of the container = sum of the areas of all 5 faces $= x^2 + x^2 + xy + xy + xy = 2x^2 + 3xy$ ***[1 mark]***
40 litres = 40 000 cm^3
Volume of the container = length × width × height
$= x^2y = 40\,000$ cm^3 ***[1 mark]*** $\Rightarrow y = \frac{40\,000}{x^2}$
Put this into the formula for the area:
$A = 2x^2 + 3xy = 2x^2 + 3x\left(\frac{40\,000}{x^2}\right)$ ***[1 mark]***
$= 2x^2 + \frac{120\,000}{x}$ ***[1 mark]***

b) To find stationary points, first find $\frac{dA}{dx}$:
$\frac{dA}{dx} = 4x - \frac{120\,000}{x^2}$ ***[1 mark for attempting to differentiate, 1 mark for the correct function]***
Then find the value of x where $\frac{dA}{dx} = 0$:
$4x - \frac{120\,000}{x^2} = 0$ ***[1 mark]*** $\Rightarrow x^3 = 30\,000$
$\Rightarrow x = 31.07... = 31.1$ cm (3 s.f.) ***[1 mark]***
To check if it's a minimum, find $\frac{d^2A}{dx^2}$:
$\frac{d^2A}{dx^2} = 4 + \frac{240\,000}{x^3} = 12$ at $x = 31.07...$ ***[1 mark]***.
The second derivative is positive, so it's a minimum ***[1 mark]***

c) Put the value of x found in part b) into the formula for the area given in part a):
$A = 2(31.07...)^2 + \frac{120\,000}{31.07...}$ ***[1 mark]*** $= 5792.936...$
$= 5790$ cm^2 (3 s.f.) ***[1 mark]***

d) E.g. the model does not take into account the thickness of the steel, so the minimum area needed is likely to be slightly greater than this to create the required capacity
[1 mark for a sensible comment].

Pages 45-50: Differentiation — 2

1 a) $y = \frac{1}{\sqrt{2x - x^2}} = (2x - x^2)^{-\frac{1}{2}}$
Let $u = 2x - x^2$, so $y = u^{-\frac{1}{2}}$ ***[1 mark]***,
then $\frac{du}{dx} = 2 - 2x$ and $\frac{dy}{du} = -\frac{1}{2}u^{-\frac{3}{2}}$
Using the chain rule: $\frac{dy}{dx} = \frac{dy}{du} \times \frac{du}{dx} = -\frac{1}{2}u^{-\frac{3}{2}} \times (2 - 2x)$
$= -\frac{1}{2}(2x - x^2)^{-\frac{3}{2}} \times (2 - 2x)$ ***[1 mark]***
$= -\frac{2 - 2x}{2(\sqrt{2x - x^2})^3} = \frac{x - 1}{(\sqrt{2x - x^2})^3}$ ***[1 mark]***
So at (1, 1), $\frac{dy}{dx} = 0$ ***[1 mark]***.

b) $x = (4y + 10)^3$
Let $u = 4y + 10$, so $x = u^3$ ***[1 mark]***,
then $\frac{du}{dy} = 4$ and $\frac{dx}{du} = 3u^2$
Using the chain rule: $\frac{dx}{dy} = \frac{dx}{du} \times \frac{du}{dy} = 3u^2 \times 4$
$= 12(4y + 10)^2$ ***[1 mark]***
So $\frac{dy}{dx} = \frac{1}{\left(\frac{dx}{dy}\right)} = \frac{1}{12(4y + 10)^2}$ ***[1 mark]***
So at (8, –2), $\frac{dy}{dx} = \frac{1}{48}$ ***[1 mark]***
You could have found the answer by rearranging the equation to get y on its own and then differentiating normally.

2 a) Replace h with x in the height formula:
$x = \sqrt{\frac{2}{3}}a \Rightarrow a = \sqrt{\frac{3}{2}}x$ ***[1 mark]***
Now substitute $a = \sqrt{\frac{3}{2}}x$ into the expression for volume:
$V = \frac{\sqrt{2}}{12}\left(\sqrt{\frac{3}{2}}x\right)^3 = \frac{\sqrt{2}}{12} \times \frac{3\sqrt{3}}{2\sqrt{2}}x^3 = \frac{\sqrt{3}}{8}x^3$
[1 mark for substitution and correct simplification]

b) From the question, you know that the rate of change of volume with respect to time, $\frac{dV}{dt}$, is 240. And differentiating the expression for volume from part a) with respect to x gives

$\frac{dV}{dx} = \frac{3\sqrt{3}x^2}{8}$ ***[1 mark]***

Using the chain rule: $\frac{dx}{dt} = \frac{dx}{dV} \times \frac{dV}{dt}$ ***[1 mark]***

$= \frac{1}{\left(\frac{dV}{dx}\right)} \times \frac{dV}{dt} = \frac{8}{3\sqrt{3}x^2} \times 240 = \frac{640}{\sqrt{3}x^2}$ ***[1 mark]***

So when $x = 8$, $\frac{dx}{dt} = \frac{640}{64\sqrt{3}} = \frac{10}{\sqrt{3}} = \frac{10\sqrt{3}}{3}$ cm min^{-1}

[1 mark for substitution of x = 8, 1 mark for correct answer in surd form]

c) $\frac{dV}{dt} = \frac{dV}{dx} \times \frac{dx}{dt}$ ***[1 mark]***

$= \frac{3\sqrt{3}x^2}{8} \times \frac{32}{9\sqrt{3}} = \frac{4x^2}{3}$ ***[1 mark]***

So when $x = 12$, $\frac{dV}{dt} = \frac{4 \times 144}{3} = 192$ cm^3 min^{-1} ***[1 mark]***

3 a) $y = e^{2x} - 5e^x + 3x$, so using chain rule:

$\frac{dy}{dx} = 2e^{2x} - 5e^x + 3$

[1 mark for $2e^{2x}$, 1 mark for the other two terms correct]

b) Stationary points occur when $\frac{dy}{dx} = 0$, so:

$2e^{2x} - 5e^x + 3 = 0$ ***[1 mark]***.

This looks like a quadratic, so substitute $z = e^x$ and factorise:

$2z^2 - 5z + 3 = 0 \Rightarrow (2z - 3)(z - 1) = 0$ ***[1 mark]***

So the solutions are:

$2z - 3 = 0 \Rightarrow z = \frac{3}{2} \Rightarrow e^x = \frac{3}{2} \Rightarrow x = \ln\frac{3}{2}$ ***[1 mark]***, and

$z - 1 = 0 \Rightarrow z = 1 \Rightarrow e^x = 1 \Rightarrow x = \ln 1 = 0$ ***[1 mark]***.

c) To determine the nature of the stationary points, find $\frac{d^2y}{dx^2}$ at $x = 0$ and $x = \ln\frac{3}{2}$:

$\frac{d^2y}{dx^2} = 4e^{2x} - 5e^x$ ***[1 mark]***

When $x = 0$, $\frac{d^2y}{dx^2} = 4e^0 - 5e^0 = 4 - 5 = -1$,

so $\frac{d^2y}{dx^2} < 0$, which means the point is a maximum ***[1 mark]***.

When $x = \ln\frac{3}{2}$, $\frac{d^2y}{dx^2} = 4e^{2\ln\frac{3}{2}} - 5e^{\ln\frac{3}{2}} = 4\left(\frac{3}{2}\right)^2 - 5\left(\frac{3}{2}\right) = \frac{3}{2}$,

so $\frac{d^2y}{dx^2} > 0$, which means the point is a minimum ***[1 mark]***.

4 $f'(x) = \frac{2}{x} = 2x^{-1}$. $x > 0$, so $f'(x)$ is always positive — so $f(x)$ is increasing. $f''(x) = -2x^{-2}$, which is always negative. So $f(x)$ is concave ***[1 mark]***.

5 a) $y = \ln x\,(5x - 2)^3$, so use the product rule with $u = \ln x$ and $v = (5x - 2)^3$.

First use the chain rule to find $\frac{dv}{dx} = 15(5x - 2)^2$.

So $u = \ln x$, $\frac{du}{dx} = \frac{1}{x}$, $v = (5x - 2)^3$, $\frac{dv}{dx} = 15(5x - 2)^2$

Then $\frac{dy}{dx} = u\frac{dv}{dx} + v\frac{du}{dx} = \ln x \times 15(5x - 2)^2 + (5x - 2)^3 \times \frac{1}{x}$

$= 15\ln x\,(5x - 2)^2 + \frac{(5x - 2)^3}{x}$

$= (5x - 2)^2\left[15\ln x + \frac{(5x - 2)}{x}\right]$

$= (5x - 2)^2\left[15\ln x + 5 - \frac{2}{x}\right]$

So $a = 15$, $b = 5$ and $c = -2$.

[4 marks available — 1 mark each for finding expressions for du/dx and dv/dx, 1 mark for putting these expressions into the product rule, 1 mark for the answer in the correct form with correct a, b and c]

b) Evaluate $\frac{dy}{dx}$ when $x = 0.9$:

$\frac{dy}{dx} = (5 \times 0.9 - 2)^2\left[15\ln 0.9 + 5 - \frac{2}{0.9}\right]$

$= 7.483...$ ***[1 mark]***

Gradient of normal at point $= -1 \div \frac{dy}{dx}$

$= -1 \div 7.483...$

$= -0.1336...$

$= -0.134$ (3 s.f.) ***[1 mark]***

6 a) $y = 4x^2 \ln x$, so use the product rule to find $\frac{dy}{dx}$:

$u = 4x^2$ and $v = \ln x$, so $\frac{du}{dx} = 8x$ and $\frac{dv}{dx} = \frac{1}{x}$ ***[1 mark]***

So $\frac{dy}{dx} = \left(4x^2 \times \frac{1}{x}\right) + (\ln x \times 8x)$

$= 4x + 8x\ln x$ ***[1 mark]***

Now use the product rule with $u = 8x$ and $v = \ln x$ to find $\frac{d^2y}{dx^2}$:

$u = 8x$ and $v = \ln x$, so $\frac{du}{dx} = 8$ and $\frac{dv}{dx} = \frac{1}{x}$ ***[1 mark]***

So $\frac{d^2y}{dx^2} = 4 + \left(\left(8x \times \frac{1}{x}\right) + (\ln x \times 8)\right)$

$= 4 + 8 + 8\ln x$

$= 12 + 8\ln x$ ***[1 mark]***

You could have factorised $\frac{dy}{dx}$ to get $4x(1 + 2\ln x)$. This would make the following few steps a bit different, but the answer is the same.

b) The curve is concave for $\frac{d^2y}{dx^2} < 0$.

$12 + 8\ln x < 0$ ***[1 mark]*** $\Rightarrow \ln x < -1.5 \Rightarrow x < e^{-1.5}$

You know that $x > 0$, so the curve is concave for $0 < x < e^{-1.5}$ ***[1 mark]***.

The curve is convex for $\frac{d^2y}{dx^2} > 0$.

$12 + 8\ln x > 0$ ***[1 mark]*** $\Rightarrow \ln x > -1.5 \Rightarrow x > e^{-1.5}$, so the curve is convex for $x > e^{-1.5}$ ***[1 mark]***.

7 Use the chain rule to find $\frac{dy}{dx}$ for $y = \tan^2 x$.

Let $u = \tan x$ — then $y = u^2$.

$\frac{dy}{du} = 2u = 2\tan x$, and $\frac{du}{dx} = \sec^2 x$.

So $\frac{dy}{dx} = \frac{dy}{du} \times \frac{du}{dx} = 2\tan x \sec^2 x$ ***[1 mark]***

8 a) $y = \frac{4x - 1}{\tan x}$, so use the quotient rule:

$u = 4x - 1 \Rightarrow \frac{du}{dx} = 4$

$v = \tan x \Rightarrow \frac{dv}{dx} = \sec^2 x$

$\frac{dy}{dx} = \frac{v\frac{du}{dx} - u\frac{dv}{dx}}{v^2} = \frac{4\tan x - (4x - 1)\sec^2 x}{\tan^2 x}$

$= \frac{4}{\tan x} - \frac{(4x - 1)\sec^2 x}{\tan^2 x}$

Since $\frac{1}{\tan x} = \cot x$, $\sec^2 x = \frac{1}{\cos^2 x}$ and $\tan^2 x = \frac{\sin^2 x}{\cos^2 x}$:

$\frac{dy}{dx} = 4\cot x - \frac{(4x - 1)}{\cos^2 x\left(\frac{\sin^2 x}{\cos^2 x}\right)} = 4\cot x - \frac{(4x - 1)}{\sin^2 x}$

Since $\frac{1}{\sin^2 x} = \operatorname{cosec}^2 x$:

$\frac{dy}{dx} = 4\cot x - (4x - 1)\operatorname{cosec}^2 x$

[3 marks available — 1 mark for correct expressions for du/dx and dv/dx, 1 mark for correct use of the quotient rule, and 1 mark for reaching the correct expression for dy/dx]

Alternatively, you could have used the product rule with $y = (4x - 1)\cot x$.

b) Maximum point is when $\frac{dy}{dx} = 0$:
$4\cot x - (4x-1)\operatorname{cosec}^2 x = 0$ ***[1 mark]***
Dividing through by $\operatorname{cosec}^2 x$ gives
$\frac{4\cot x}{\operatorname{cosec}^2 x} - (4x-1) = 0$ ***[1 mark]***
$\frac{4\cot x}{\operatorname{cosec}^2 x} = \frac{4\cos x \sin^2 x}{\sin x} = 4\cos x \sin x$ ***[1 mark]***,
and using the double angle formula, $\sin 2x = 2\sin x\cos x$,
so $4\cos x\sin x = 2\sin 2x$.
So $2\sin 2x - 4x + 1 = 0$ ***[1 mark]***.
You're told that the point is a maximum, so you don't need to differentiate again to check.

9 $\frac{dx}{dt} = 2t$, $\frac{dy}{dt} = 3t^2 + 2$
So $\frac{dy}{dx} = \frac{dy}{dt} \div \frac{dx}{dt} = \frac{3t^2+2}{2t}$
Substitute $t = 1$ into this expression to find the gradient of the curve at $t = 1$:
$\frac{dy}{dx} = \frac{3(1)^2+2}{2(1)} = \frac{5}{2}$
Now find the coordinates of the point where $t = 1$:
$x = 1^2 + 1 = 2$ and $y = 1^3 + 2(1) = 3$
Now use the gradient at $t = 1$ and the point (2, 3) to find the equation of the tangent:
$y - 3 = \frac{5}{2}(x-2) \Rightarrow y - 3 = \frac{5}{2}x - 5 \Rightarrow y = \frac{5}{2}x - 2$
[5 marks available — 1 mark for a correct method to find dy/dx, 1 mark for a correct expression for dy/dx, 1 mark for substituting t = 1 to find the gradient, 1 mark for finding the coordinates when t = 1, 1 mark for the correct equation]

10 a) $\frac{dx}{d\theta} = \frac{\cos\theta}{2}$, $\frac{dy}{d\theta} = 2\sin 2\theta$
So $\frac{dy}{dx} = \frac{dy}{d\theta} \div \frac{dx}{d\theta}$
$= 2\sin 2\theta \div \frac{\cos\theta}{2} = \frac{4\sin 2\theta}{\cos\theta}$
[2 marks available — 1 mark for a correct method to find dy/dx, 1 mark for a correct expression for dy/dx]

b) When $\theta = \frac{\pi}{6}$, $\frac{dy}{dx} = \frac{4\sin\left(\frac{\pi}{3}\right)}{\cos\left(\frac{\pi}{6}\right)} = \frac{4\left(\frac{\sqrt{3}}{2}\right)}{\left(\frac{\sqrt{3}}{2}\right)} = 4$ ***[1 mark]***
$x = \frac{1}{2}\sin\frac{\pi}{6} - 3 = \frac{1}{2} \times \frac{1}{2} - 3 = \frac{1}{4} - 3 = -\frac{11}{4}$
$y = 5 - \cos\frac{\pi}{3} = 5 - \frac{1}{2} = \frac{9}{2}$
[1 mark for x and y values both correct]
So using $y - y_1 = m(x - x_1)$:
$y - \frac{9}{2} = 4\left(x + \frac{11}{4}\right) \Rightarrow 2y - 9 = 8x + 22$
So the equation in the correct form is $8x - 2y + 31 = 0$ ***[1 mark]***

c) Substitute $x = \frac{\sin\theta}{2} - 3$ and $y = 5 - \cos 2\theta$ into $y = -8x - 20$:
$5 - \cos 2\theta = -8\left(\frac{\sin\theta}{2} - 3\right) - 20$ ***[1 mark]***
$\Rightarrow 1 - \cos 2\theta + 4\sin\theta = 0$
Using the double angle identity, $\cos 2\theta \equiv 1 - 2\sin^2\theta$,
so $1 - (1 - 2\sin^2\theta) + 4\sin\theta = 0$ ***[1 mark]***
$\Rightarrow 1 - 1 + 2\sin^2\theta + 4\sin\theta = 0$
$\Rightarrow 2\sin^2\theta + 4\sin\theta = 0$
$\Rightarrow \sin^2\theta + 2\sin\theta = 0$ ***[1 mark]***
$\Rightarrow \sin\theta(\sin\theta + 2) = 0$
This gives $\sin\theta = 0$ or $\sin\theta = -2$ ***[1 mark]***.
Since $\sin\theta$ must be between –1 and 1, $\sin\theta = -2$ is not valid.
So substitute $\sin\theta = 0$ into the expression for x:
$x = \frac{\sin\theta}{2} - 3 \Rightarrow x = 0 - 3 = -3$ ***[1 mark]***
Substitute $x = -3$ into $y = -8x - 20$
to get $y = -8(-3) - 20 = 4$ ***[1 mark]***
So P is the point (–3, 4).

d) Rewrite the equation for y using the identity $\cos 2\theta \equiv 1 - 2\sin^2\theta$:
$y = 5 - \cos 2\theta = 5 - (1 - 2\sin^2\theta) = 4 + 2\sin^2\theta$ ***[1 mark]***
Now rearrange the equation for x to make $\sin\theta$ the subject:
$x = \frac{\sin\theta}{2} - 3 \Rightarrow 2x + 6 = \sin\theta$ ***[1 mark]***
Substitute this into the equation for y:
$y = 4 + 2\sin^2\theta = 4 + 2(2x+6)^2$
$\Rightarrow y = 4 + 2(4x^2 + 24x + 36)$
$\Rightarrow y = 8x^2 + 48x + 76$ ***[1 mark]***

11 $y = \cos^{-1} x \Rightarrow \cos y = x$ ***[1 mark]***
Differentiate with respect to x:
$-\sin y \times \frac{dy}{dx} = 1 \Rightarrow \frac{dy}{dx} = -\frac{1}{\sin y}$ ***[1 mark]***
Using the identity $\cos^2 y + \sin^2 y = 1$,
$\sin^2 y = 1 - \cos^2 y \Rightarrow \sin y = \sqrt{1 - \cos^2 y}$
So $\frac{dy}{dx} = -\frac{1}{\sqrt{1-\cos^2 y}}$ ***[1 mark]***
As $\cos y = x$, this expression becomes $\frac{dy}{dx} = -\frac{1}{\sqrt{1-x^2}}$ ***[1 mark]***
You could have differentiated x with respect to y then used $\frac{dy}{dx} = \frac{1}{\left(\frac{dx}{dy}\right)}$ *instead of using implicit differentiation here.*

12 a) Use implicit differentiation to find $\frac{dy}{dx}$:
$\frac{d}{dx}x^3 + \frac{d}{dx}x^2y = \frac{d}{dx}y^2 - \frac{d}{dx}1$
$3x^2 + \frac{d}{dx}x^2y = \frac{d}{dx}y^2 - 0$
$3x^2 + \frac{d}{dx}x^2y = \frac{d}{dy}y^2\frac{dy}{dx}$
$3x^2 + \frac{d}{dx}x^2y = 2y\frac{dy}{dx}$
$3x^2 + x^2\frac{d}{dx}y + y\frac{d}{dx}x^2 = 2y\frac{dy}{dx}$
$3x^2 + x^2\frac{dy}{dx} + 2xy = 2y\frac{dy}{dx}$
Rearrange to make $\frac{dy}{dx}$ the subject:
$(2y - x^2)\frac{dy}{dx} = 3x^2 + 2xy$
$\frac{dy}{dx} = \frac{3x^2 + 2xy}{2y - x^2}$
[4 marks available — 1 mark for the correct differentiation of x^3 and –1, 1 mark for the correct differentiation of y^2, 1 mark for the correct differentiation of x^2y and 1 mark for rearranging to find the correct answer]

b) Substitute $x = 1$ into the original equation:
$x = 1 \Rightarrow (1)^3 + (1)^2y = y^2 - 1$ ***[1 mark]***
$\Rightarrow y^2 - y - 2 = 0$
$\Rightarrow (y-2)(y+1) = 0$
$\Rightarrow y = 2$ or $y = -1$
$a > b$, so $a = 2$, $b = -1$ ***[1 mark]***

c) At Q (1, –1),
$\frac{dy}{dx} = \frac{3(1)^2 + 2(1)(-1)}{2(-1) - (1)^2} = \frac{3-2}{-2-1} = -\frac{1}{3}$ ***[1 mark]***
So the gradient of the normal at Q is $-1 \div -\frac{1}{3} = 3$ ***[1 mark]***
$y - y_1 = m(x - x_1)$
$\Rightarrow y + 1 = 3(x-1)$
$\Rightarrow y = 3x - 4$ ***[1 mark]***

13 a) Use implicit differentiation to find an expression for $\frac{dy}{dx}$:
$\frac{d}{dx}(y^2 - 6xy + 9y + 2x) = \frac{d}{dx}(7 - 9x^2)$
$\Rightarrow 2y\frac{dy}{dx} - \frac{d}{dx}6xy + 9\frac{dy}{dx} + 2 = -18x$ ***[1 mark]***
$\Rightarrow 2y\frac{dy}{dx} - 6x\frac{dy}{dx} - 6y + 9\frac{dy}{dx} + 2 = -18x$ ***[1 mark]***
$\Rightarrow \frac{dy}{dx}(2y - 6x + 9) = 6y - 18x - 2$
$\Rightarrow \frac{dy}{dx} = \frac{6y - 18x - 2}{2y - 6x + 9}$ ***[1 mark]***

b) A vertical tangent occurs when $\frac{dy}{dx}$ is undefined, i.e. when the denominator = 0.

So $2y - 6x + 9 = 0 \Rightarrow y = 3x - \frac{9}{2}$ ***[1 mark]***

Substitute this into the original equation, and solve for x:

$\left(3x - \frac{9}{2}\right)^2 - 6x\left(3x - \frac{9}{2}\right) + 9\left(3x - \frac{9}{2}\right) + 2x = 7 - 9x^2$ ***[1 mark]***

$\Rightarrow 9x^2 - 27x + \frac{81}{4} - 18x^2 + 27x + 27x - \frac{81}{2} + 2x = 7 - 9x^2$

$\Rightarrow 29x = \frac{109}{4}$

$\Rightarrow x = \frac{109}{116}$ ***[1 mark]***

So the equation of the vertical tangent to the curve is $x = \frac{109}{116}$.

Remember — a tangent just touches the curve at a point, and that's still true for vertical tangents. The tangent here touches the curve at the point $\left(\frac{109}{116}, -\frac{195}{116}\right)$.

14 Use implicit differentiation to find $\frac{dy}{dx}$:

$\frac{d}{dx}(\sin \pi x) - \frac{d}{dx}\left(\cos \frac{\pi y}{2}\right) = \frac{d}{dx}(0.5)$

$\pi \cos \pi x - \frac{d}{dx}\left(\cos \frac{\pi y}{2}\right) = 0$ ***[1 mark]***

$\pi \cos \pi x - \frac{d}{dy}\left(\cos \frac{\pi y}{2}\right)\frac{dy}{dx} = 0$

$\pi \cos \pi x + \left(\frac{\pi}{2}\sin \frac{\pi y}{2}\right)\frac{dy}{dx} = 0$ ***[1 mark]***

Rearrange to make $\frac{dy}{dx}$ the subject:

$\frac{dy}{dx} = -\frac{\pi \cos \pi x}{\frac{\pi}{2}\sin \frac{\pi y}{2}} = -\frac{2\cos \pi x}{\sin \frac{\pi y}{2}}$ ***[1 mark]***

The stationary point is where the gradient is zero.

$\frac{dy}{dx} = 0 \Rightarrow -\frac{2\cos \pi x}{\sin \frac{\pi y}{2}} = 0 \Rightarrow \cos \pi x = 0$ ***[1 mark]***

$\Rightarrow x = \frac{1}{2}$ or $x = \frac{3}{2}$ in the range $0 \le x \le 2$ ***[1 mark]***

Put these values in the equation of the curve:

$x = \frac{3}{2} \Rightarrow \sin \frac{3\pi}{2} - \cos \frac{\pi y}{2} = 0.5$

$\Rightarrow -1 - \cos \frac{\pi y}{2} = 0.5$

$\Rightarrow \cos \frac{\pi y}{2} = -1.5$

So y has no solutions when $x = \frac{3}{2}$ ***[1 mark]***

$x = \frac{1}{2} \Rightarrow \sin \frac{\pi}{2} - \cos \frac{\pi y}{2} = 0.5$

$\Rightarrow 1 - \cos \frac{\pi y}{2} = 0.5$

$\Rightarrow \cos \frac{\pi y}{2} = 0.5$

$\Rightarrow \frac{\pi y}{2} = \frac{\pi}{3}$

$\Rightarrow y = \frac{2}{3}$ in the range $0 \le y \le 2$ ***[1 mark]***

So the stationary point of the graph of $\sin \pi x - \cos \frac{\pi y}{2} = 0.5$ for the given ranges of x and y is at $\left(\frac{1}{2}, \frac{2}{3}\right)$.

Pages 51-54: Integration — 1

1 $\int \left(2\sqrt{x} + \frac{1}{x^3}\right)dx = \int (2x^{\frac{1}{2}} + x^{-3})\,dx = \frac{4}{3}x^{\frac{3}{2}} - \frac{1}{2}x^{-2} + C$

$= \frac{4}{3}\sqrt{x^3} - \frac{1}{2x^2} + C$ ***[1 mark]***

2 $\int y^2\,dx = \int \left(\frac{x^2+3}{\sqrt[3]{x}}\right)^2 dx = \int (x^{\frac{5}{3}} + 3x^{-\frac{1}{3}})^2\,dx$

$= \int (x^{\frac{10}{3}} + 6x^{\frac{4}{3}} + 9x^{-\frac{2}{3}})\,dx = \frac{x^{\frac{13}{3}}}{\left(\frac{13}{3}\right)} + \frac{6x^{\frac{7}{3}}}{\left(\frac{7}{3}\right)} + \frac{9x^{\frac{1}{3}}}{\left(\frac{1}{3}\right)} + C$

$= \frac{3}{13}x^{\frac{13}{3}} + \frac{18}{7}x^{\frac{7}{3}} + 27x^{\frac{1}{3}} + C$

[4 marks available — 1 mark for expanding and writing all terms as powers of x, 1 mark for increasing the power of one term by 1, 1 mark for two correct simplified terms, 1 mark for the third correct integrated term and adding C]

3 To find f(x), integrate f'(x):

$f(x) = \int \left(2x + 5\sqrt{x} + \frac{6}{x^2}\right)dx = \int (2x + 5x^{\frac{1}{2}} + 6x^{-2})\,dx$

$= \frac{2x^2}{2} + 5\left(\frac{x^{\frac{3}{2}}}{\left(\frac{3}{2}\right)}\right) + \left(\frac{6x^{-1}}{-1}\right) + C$

$f(x) = x^2 + \frac{10\sqrt{x^3}}{3} - \frac{6}{x} + C$

You've been given a point on the curve so calculate the value of C:
If $y = 7$ when $x = 3$, then

$3^2 + \frac{10\sqrt{3^3}}{3} - \frac{6}{3} + C = 7$

$9 + 10\sqrt{3} - 2 + C = 7$

$7 + 10\sqrt{3} + C = 7 \Rightarrow C = -10\sqrt{3}$

$f(x) = x^2 + \frac{10\sqrt{x^3}}{3} - \frac{6}{x} - 10\sqrt{3}$

[6 marks available — 1 mark for writing all terms as powers of x, 1 mark for increasing the power of one term by 1, 1 mark for two correct simplified terms, 1 mark for the third correct integrated term and adding C, 1 mark for substituting in the coordinates of the point, 1 mark for the correct answer]

4 To find the area of region A, you need to integrate the function between $x = 2$ and $x = 4$:

Area $= \int_2^4 \frac{2}{\sqrt{x^3}}\,dx = \int_2^4 2x^{-\frac{3}{2}}\,dx = [-2(2x^{-\frac{1}{2}})]_2^4 = \left[\frac{-4}{x^{\frac{1}{2}}}\right]_2^4 = \left[\frac{-4}{\sqrt{x}}\right]_2^4$

$= \left(\frac{-4}{\sqrt{4}}\right) - \left(\frac{-4}{\sqrt{2}}\right) = \frac{-4}{2} + \frac{4}{\sqrt{2}} = -2 + \frac{4\sqrt{2}}{2}$

$= 2\sqrt{2} - 2$ as required

[5 marks available — 1 mark for writing down the correct integral to find, 1 mark for integrating correctly, 1 mark for correct handling of the limits, 1 mark for rationalising the denominator, 1 mark for rearranging to give the answer in the correct form]

5 $\int_p^{4p} \left(\frac{1}{\sqrt{x}} - 4x^3\right)dx = \int_p^{4p} (x^{-\frac{1}{2}} - 4x^3)\,dx = \left[\frac{x^{\frac{1}{2}}}{\left(\frac{1}{2}\right)} - \frac{4x^4}{4}\right]_p^{4p}$

$= [2x^{\frac{1}{2}} - x^4]_p^{4p} = [2\sqrt{x} - x^4]_p^{4p}$

$= (2\sqrt{4p} - (4p)^4) - (2\sqrt{p} - p^4)$

$= (4\sqrt{p} - 256p^4) - (2\sqrt{p} - p^4)$

$= 2\sqrt{p} - 255p^4$

[4 marks available — 1 mark for increasing the power of one term by 1, 1 mark for the correct integrated terms, 1 mark for correct handling of the limits, 1 mark for simplifying to get the final answer]

6 To find the shaded area, you need to integrate the function between −1 and 0.5 and add it to the integral of the function between 0.5 and 2 (making this value positive first).

$\int_{-1}^{0.5} (2x^3 - 3x^2 - 11x + 6)\,dx = \left[\frac{2x^4}{4} - \frac{3x^3}{3} - \frac{11x^2}{2} + 6x\right]_{-1}^{0.5}$

$= \left[\frac{x^4}{2} - x^3 - \frac{11}{2}x^2 + 6x\right]_{-1}^{0.5}$

$= \left(\frac{(0.5)^4}{2} - (0.5)^3 - \frac{11}{2}(0.5)^2 + 6(0.5)\right)$

$- \left(\frac{(-1)^4}{2} - (-1)^3 - \frac{11}{2}(-1)^2 + 6(-1)\right)$

$= 1.53125 - (-10) = 11.53125$

So the area between −1 and 0.5 is 11.53125.

$\int_{0.5}^{2} (2x^3 - 3x^2 - 11x + 6)\,dx = \left[\frac{x^4}{2} - x^3 - \frac{11}{2}x^2 + 6x\right]_{0.5}^{2}$

$= \left(\frac{(2)^4}{2} - (2)^3 - \frac{11}{2}(2)^2 + 6(2)\right) - 1.53125$

$= -10 - 1.53125 = -11.53125$

So the area between 0.5 and 2 is 11.53125.

So area = 11.53125 + 11.53125 = 23.0625

[6 marks available — 1 mark for considering the area above and below the x-axes separately, 1 mark for increasing the power of one term by 1, 1 mark for the correct integral, 1 mark for finding the area between −1 and 0.5, 1 mark for finding the area between 0.5 and 2, 1 mark for adding the areas to get the correct answer]

If you'd just integrated between −1 and 2, you'd have ended up with an answer of 0, as the areas cancel each other out.

7 Evaluate the integral, treating k as a constant:

$$\int_{\sqrt{2}}^{2}(8x^3 - 2kx)\,dx = \left[\frac{8x^4}{4} - \frac{2kx^2}{2}\right]_{\sqrt{2}}^{2} = [2x^4 - kx^2]_{\sqrt{2}}^{2}$$
$$= (2(2)^4 - k(2)^2) - (2(\sqrt{2})^4 - k(\sqrt{2})^2)$$
$$= (32 - 4k) - (8 - 2k) = 24 - 2k$$

You know that the value of this integral is $2k^2$, so set this expression equal to $2k^2$ and solve to find k:

$24 - 2k = 2k^2$

$0 = 2k^2 + 2k - 24 \Rightarrow k^2 + k - 12 = 0 \Rightarrow (k + 4)(k - 3) = 0$

So $k = -4$ or $k = 3$

[5 marks available — 1 mark for increasing the power of one term by 1, 1 mark for the correct integrated terms, 1 mark for substituting in the limits, 1 mark for setting this expression equal to $2k^2$, 1 mark for solving the quadratic to find both values of k]

8 Integrate the curve $y = \dfrac{2}{3(\sqrt[3]{5x-2})}$ with respect to x between 2 and 5.8 to find the shaded region:

$$\int_2^{5.8}\frac{2}{3(\sqrt[3]{5x-2})}\,dx = \int_2^{5.8}\frac{2}{3}(5x-2)^{-\frac{1}{3}}\,dx \text{ [1 mark]}$$
$$= \left[\frac{1}{5}\cdot\frac{2}{3}\cdot\frac{3}{2}(5x-2)^{\frac{2}{3}}\right]_2^{5.8} \text{ [1 mark]}$$
$$= \left[\frac{1}{5}(\sqrt[3]{5x-2})^2\right]_2^{5.8}$$
$$= \frac{1}{5}(\sqrt[3]{27})^2 - \frac{1}{5}(\sqrt[3]{8})^2 \text{ [1 mark]}$$
$$= \frac{3^2}{5} - \frac{2^2}{5} = \frac{5}{5} = 1 \text{ [1 mark]}$$

9 a) A and B are the points where the two lines intersect, so

$\frac{8}{x^2} = 9 - x^2$ ***[1 mark]*** $\Rightarrow 8 = 9x^2 - x^4$

$\Rightarrow x^4 - 9x^2 + 8 = 0$

$\Rightarrow (x^2 - 8)(x^2 - 1) = 0$ ***[1 mark]***

$x^2 = 8 \Rightarrow x = \pm\sqrt{8} = \pm 2\sqrt{2} = 2\sqrt{2}$ as $x \geq 0$

$x^2 = 1 \Rightarrow x = \pm 1 = 1$ as $x \geq 0$ ***[1 mark for both values of x]***

So $x = 1$ at A and $x = 2\sqrt{2}$ at B.

Then the shaded region is the area under $y = 9 - x^2$ minus the area under $y = \frac{8}{x^2}$ from $x = 1$ to $x = 2\sqrt{2}$, so the area is:

$\int_1^{2\sqrt{2}}\left(9 - x^2 - \frac{8}{x^2}\right)dx$ ***[1 mark]***

b) Using the result from part a):

$$\int_1^{2\sqrt{2}}\left(9 - x^2 - \frac{8}{x^2}\right)dx = \left[9x - \frac{x^3}{3} + \frac{8}{x}\right]_1^{2\sqrt{2}}$$
$$= \left(18\sqrt{2} - \frac{(2\sqrt{2})^3}{3} + \frac{8}{2\sqrt{2}}\right) - \left(9 - \frac{1}{3} + 8\right)$$
$$= 18\sqrt{2} - \frac{16\sqrt{2}}{3} + 2\sqrt{2} - 9 + \frac{1}{3} - 8$$
$$= -\frac{50}{3} + \frac{44}{3}\sqrt{2}$$

[4 marks available — 1 mark for increasing the power of one term by 1, 1 mark for the correct integral, 1 mark for correct handling of the limits, 1 mark for simplifying to get the final answer]

10 $\int_0^2(2x + x^2 - x^3)\,dx$ ***[1 mark]***

You might find it useful to quickly sketch the curves here — you can see that $y = x^2 + 2$ is above $y = x^3 - 2x + 2$ between the two given points, so you then find the area by integrating $(x^2 + 2) - (x^3 - 2x + 2) = 2x + x^2 - x^3$.

11 Line N is a normal to the curve C, so differentiate:

$\frac{dy}{dx} = \frac{1}{2}x^{-\frac{1}{2}} - x$ ***[1 mark]***

When $x = 1$, $\frac{dy}{dx} = \frac{1}{2} - 1 = -\frac{1}{2}$, so the gradient of the normal to the curve at this point is $-1 \div -\frac{1}{2} = 2$ ***[1 mark]***.

So the equation of the normal is:

$y - \frac{3}{2} = 2(x - 1) \Rightarrow y = 2x - \frac{1}{2}$ ***[1 mark]***.

So the area of A is $\int_0^1\left[\left(\sqrt{x} - \frac{1}{2}x^2 + 1\right) - \left(2x - \frac{1}{2}\right)\right]dx$ ***[1 mark]***.

Using the result from part a):

$$\int_0^1\left[\left(\sqrt{x} - \frac{1}{2}x^2 + 1\right) - \left(2x - \frac{1}{2}\right)\right]dx$$
$$= \int_0^1\left(x^{\frac{1}{2}} - \frac{1}{2}x^2 - 2x + \frac{3}{2}\right)dx$$
$$= \left[\frac{2}{3}x^{\frac{3}{2}} - \frac{1}{6}x^3 - x^2 + \frac{3}{2}x\right]_0^1 \text{ [1 mark]}$$
$$= \left(\frac{2}{3} - \frac{1}{6} - 1 + \frac{3}{2}\right) - 0 = 1$$

[1 mark for substituting in the limits correctly, 1 mark for the correct answer]

You could have done this one by working out each bit separately.

12 Find the value of the integral in terms of p:

$$\int_{2p}^{6p}\frac{x^3 + 4x^2}{x^3}\,dx = \int_{2p}^{6p}\left(1 + \frac{4}{x}\right)dx = [x + 4\ln x]_{2p}^{6p}$$
$$= (6p + 4\ln 6p) - (2p + 4\ln 2p)$$
$$= 4p + 4\ln\frac{6p}{2p} = 4p + 4\ln 3$$

You know the value of the integral, so set these expressions equal to each other and solve for p:

$4p + 4\ln 3 = 4\ln 12$

$p = \ln 12 - \ln 3 = \ln\frac{12}{3} = \ln 4$

[4 marks available — 1 mark for simplifying the fraction and integrating, 1 mark for the correct integral, 1 mark for substituting in the limits correctly and simplifying, 1 mark for setting the expressions equal to each other and solving to find p]

13 a) $4x^2 + 4x - 3 = (2x + 3)(2x - 1)$, so $g(x) = \dfrac{4x - 10}{(2x+3)(2x-1)}$

Rewrite this as partial fractions:

$\frac{4x - 10}{(2x+3)(2x-1)} \equiv \frac{A}{2x+3} + \frac{B}{2x-1}$

$\Rightarrow 4x - 10 \equiv A(2x - 1) + B(2x + 3)$

Substituting $x = \frac{1}{2}$ gives $B = -2$

Substituting $x = -\frac{3}{2}$ gives $A = 4$

$\Rightarrow g(x) = \frac{4}{(2x+3)} - \frac{2}{(2x-1)}$

[4 marks available — 1 mark for factorising the denominator, 1 mark for writing as partial fractions with the correct denominators, 1 mark for finding A or B, 1 mark for the correct partial fractions]

b)
$$\int_{-1}^{0}\frac{4x-10}{4x^2+4x-3}\,dx = \int_{-1}^{0}\left(\frac{4}{(2x+3)} - \frac{2}{(2x-1)}\right)dx$$
$$= [2\ln|2x+3| - \ln|2x-1|]_{-1}^{0}$$
$$= (2\ln 3 - \ln|-1|) - (2\ln 1 - \ln|-3|)$$
$$= 2\ln 3 + \ln 3 = 3\ln 3 = \ln 3^3 = \ln 27$$

[3 marks available — 1 mark for the correct integral, 1 mark for substituting in the limits, 1 mark for simplifying to give the answer in the correct form]

Pages 55-59: Integration — 2

1
$$\int_{\frac{\pi}{12}}^{\frac{\pi}{8}}\sin 2x\,dx = \left[-\frac{1}{2}\cos 2x\right]_{\frac{\pi}{12}}^{\frac{\pi}{8}}$$
$$= \left(-\frac{1}{2}\cos\left(\frac{\pi}{4}\right)\right) - \left(-\frac{1}{2}\cos\left(\frac{\pi}{6}\right)\right)$$
$$= -\frac{1}{2\sqrt{2}} + \frac{\sqrt{3}}{4} = \frac{\sqrt{3} - \sqrt{2}}{4}$$

[3 marks available — 1 mark for integrating correctly, 1 mark for substituting in the limits, 1 mark for the correct answer in surd form]

2 a) $\frac{d}{dx}(e^{\tan x}) = \sec^2 x\, e^{\tan x}$, so the integral is of the form $\int\frac{du}{dx}g'(u)\,dx = g(u) + C$.

So $\int f(x)\,dx = \int\sec^2 x\, e^{\tan x}\,dx = e^{\tan x} + C$

[2 marks available — 1 mark for attempting to use the formula, 1 mark for the correct answer including + C]

b) $\int_0^{\frac{\pi}{3}}\left(f(x)+3\tan^2\left(\frac{x}{2}\right)+3\right)dx$

$= \int_0^{\frac{\pi}{3}} f(x)\,dx + 3\int_0^{\frac{\pi}{3}}\left(\tan^2\left(\frac{x}{2}\right)+1\right)dx$

Use the identity $\sec^2 x \equiv 1+\tan^2 x$ to write $\tan^2\frac{x}{2}+1$ as $\sec^2\frac{x}{2}$.
Using the result from part a) as well:

$\int_0^{\frac{\pi}{3}} f(x)\,dx + 3\int_0^{\frac{\pi}{3}}\left(\tan^2\left(\frac{x}{2}\right)+1\right)dx = [e^{\tan x}]_0^{\frac{\pi}{3}} + 3\int_0^{\frac{\pi}{3}}\sec^2\left(\frac{x}{2}\right)dx$

$= e^{\tan\frac{\pi}{3}} - e^{\tan 0} + 3\left[2\tan\left(\frac{x}{2}\right)\right]_0^{\frac{\pi}{3}} = e^{\sqrt{3}} - e^0 + 3\left[2\tan\left(\frac{\pi}{6}\right) - 2\tan 0\right]$

$= e^{\sqrt{3}} - 1 + 6\frac{\sqrt{3}}{3} - 0 = e^{\sqrt{3}} + 2\sqrt{3} - 1$

[5 marks available — 1 mark for substituting in the result from part a), 1 mark for rewriting the integral in terms of sec² $\frac{x}{2}$, 1 mark for integrating correctly, 1 mark for substituting the limits correctly, 1 mark for the correct answer]

3 As $u = \ln x$, $\frac{du}{dx} = \frac{1}{x}$, so $x\,du = dx$ ***[1 mark]***. The limits $x = 1$ and $x = 2$ become $u = \ln 1 = 0$ and $u = \ln 2$ ***[1 mark]***.

$\left(\frac{\ln x}{\sqrt{x}}\right)^2 = \frac{(\ln x)^2}{x}$. So the integral is:

$\int_0^{\ln 2}\frac{u^2}{x}x\,du = \int_0^{\ln 2} u^2\,du$ ***[1 mark]***

$= \left[\frac{u^3}{3}\right]_0^{\ln 2}$ ***[1 mark]***

$= \frac{(\ln 2)^3}{3} - \frac{0^3}{3} = 0.111$ (3 s.f.) ***[1 mark]***

4 $u = x^2 - 2$
When $x = 2$, $u = 2^2 - 2 = 2$. When $x = \sqrt{2}$, $u = 2 - 2 = 0$.
So the limits are 0 and 2 ***[1 mark]***.

5 a) If $x = \sin\theta$, then $\frac{dx}{d\theta} = \cos\theta$, so $dx = d\theta\cos\theta$ ***[1 mark]***.
Putting all this into the integral gives:

$\int\frac{x}{1-x^2}dx = \int\frac{\sin\theta}{1-\sin^2\theta}\cos\theta\,d\theta$ ***[1 mark]***

Using the identity $\sin^2\theta + \cos^2\theta \equiv 1$, replace $1 - \sin^2\theta$:

$\int\frac{\sin\theta\cos\theta}{\cos^2\theta}d\theta = \int\frac{\sin\theta}{\cos\theta}d\theta = \int\tan\theta\,d\theta$ ***[1 mark]***

$= -\ln|\cos\theta| + C$ ***[1 mark]***

$= -\ln\sqrt{\cos^2\theta} + C$ ***[1 mark]***

$= -\ln\sqrt{1-\sin^2\theta} + C$

$= -\ln\sqrt{1-x^2} + C$ ***[1 mark]***

b) The area bounded by the graphs is the area under $y = -x^2 + 2$ minus the area under $y = \frac{x}{1-x^2}$ from $x = 0$ to $x = \frac{1}{2}$.

So the area is $\int_0^{\frac{1}{2}}\left(-x^2+2-\frac{x}{1-x^2}\right)dx$

$= \int_0^{\frac{1}{2}}(-x^2+2)\,dx - \int_0^{\frac{1}{2}}\left(\frac{x}{1-x^2}\right)dx$ ***[1 mark]***

$= \left[-\frac{1}{3}x^3+2x\right]_0^{\frac{1}{2}} - \left[-\ln\sqrt{1-x^2}\right]_0^{\frac{1}{2}}$ ***[1 mark]***

$= \left[-\frac{1}{3}\left(\frac{1}{2}\right)^3+2\left(\frac{1}{2}\right)\right] - \left[-\frac{1}{3}(0)^3+2(0)\right]$

$-\left[-\ln\sqrt{1-\left(\frac{1}{2}\right)^2} + \ln\sqrt{1-0^2}\right]$ ***[1 mark]***

$= -\frac{1}{24} + 1 + \ln\frac{\sqrt{3}}{2} - \ln 1$

$= \ln\frac{\sqrt{3}}{2} + \frac{23}{24}$, as required. ***[1 mark]***

It might be easier to picture what's going on if you add the second curve and the line to the sketch given in the question.

6 From the chain rule, $\int y\,dx = \int y\frac{dx}{dt}\,dt$.

Find $\frac{dx}{dt}$: $x = -2\cos t$, so $\frac{dx}{dt} = 2\sin t$ ***[1 mark]***

At $x = -2$: $-2 = -2\cos t \Rightarrow 1 = \cos t \Rightarrow t = 0$

At $x = 0$: $0 = -2\cos t \Rightarrow 0 = \cos t \Rightarrow t = \frac{\pi}{2}$

[1 mark for both correct]

So the area of A is: $\int_0^{\frac{\pi}{2}}(3\cos t\sin t)(2\sin t)\,dt = \int_0^{\frac{\pi}{2}} 6\cos t\sin^2 t\,dt$

Let $u = \sin t$, so $\frac{du}{dt} = \cos t$ ***[1 mark]***. So $dt = \frac{du}{\cos t}$.

The limits $t = 0$ and $t = \frac{\pi}{2}$ become $u = \sin 0 = 0$ and $u = \sin\frac{\pi}{2} = 1$.

Putting this all into the integral gives:

$\int_0^{\frac{\pi}{2}} 6\cos t\sin^2 t\,dt = \int_0^1 6u^2\cos t\frac{du}{\cos t} = \int_0^1 6u^2\,du$ ***[1 mark]***

$= [2u^3]_0^1$ ***[1 mark]*** $= 2(1)^3 - 2(0)^3 = 2$ ***[1 mark]***

You might have been tempted to convert the parametric equations into a Cartesian equation to integrate — this method is usually much harder. You may have spotted that $6\cos t\sin^2 t = \frac{d}{dt}(2\sin^3 t)$ and integrated using the fundamental theorem of calculus.

7 a) Integrating the rate at which water is flowing gives the total amount of water that has flowed.
So the amount of water that has flowed into the container after x seconds (i.e. from 0 to x seconds) is given by $\int_0^x 4te^{-2t}\,dt$.

Let $u = 4t$, so $\frac{du}{dt} = 4$. Let $\frac{dv}{dt} = e^{-2t}$, so $v = -\frac{1}{2}e^{-2t}$.

Using integration by parts:

$\int u\frac{dv}{dt}dt = uv - \int v\frac{du}{dt}dt$

$\int_0^x 4te^{-2t}\,dt = \left[4t\left(-\frac{1}{2}e^{-2t}\right)\right]_0^x - \int_0^x 4\left(-\frac{1}{2}e^{-2t}\right)dt$

$= [-2te^{-2t}]_0^x + \int_0^x 2e^{-2t}\,dt = -2xe^{-2x} + 0 + [-e^{-2t}]_0^x$

$= -2xe^{-2x} - e^{-2x} + e^0 = -2xe^{-2x} - e^{-2x} + 1$

$= -e^{-2x}(2x+1) + 1$

[5 marks available — 1 mark for correct choice of u and dv/dt, 1 mark for correct differentiation and integration to obtain du/dt and v, 1 mark for correct integration by parts method, 1 mark for substituting in the limits, 1 mark for the correct answer]

b) Let $f(x) = -e^{-2x}(2x+1) + 1$. Then the amount of water that flowed into the container during the first second is $f(1)$ and the amount that flowed in after that is $f(6) - f(1)$. So the difference is:

$f(1) - (f(6) - f(1)) = 2f(1) - f(6)$

$= 2(-e^{-2\times 1}(2\times 1+1)+1) + e^{-2\times 6}(2\times 6+1) + 1$

$= -6e^{-2} + 2 + 13e^{-12} + 1 = (13e^{-12} - 6e^{-2} + 3)$ ml

[2 marks available — 1 mark for substituting x = 1 and x = 6 correctly, 1 mark for the correct answer]

8 Let $u = \ln x$, so $\frac{du}{dx} = \frac{1}{x}$.

Let $\frac{dv}{dx} = \frac{1}{2x^2} = \frac{1}{2}x^{-2}$, so $v = -\frac{1}{2}x^{-1}$

Using integration by parts,

$\int_1^4\frac{\ln x}{2x^2}dx = \left[-\frac{\ln x}{2x}\right]_1^4 - \int_1^4 -\frac{1}{2x^2}dx = \left[-\frac{\ln x}{2x}\right]_1^4 - \left[\frac{1}{2x}\right]_1^4$

$= \left[-\frac{\ln 4}{8} - -\frac{\ln 1}{2}\right] - \left[\frac{1}{8} - \frac{1}{2}\right] = \frac{3}{8} - \frac{\ln 4}{8}\ \left(= \frac{3-\ln 4}{8}\right)$

[6 marks available — 1 mark for correct choice of u and dv/dx, 1 mark for correct differentiation and integration to obtain du/dx and v, 1 mark for correct integration by parts method, 1 mark for correct integral, 1 mark for substituting in the limits, 1 mark for answer]

9 a) $\frac{dN}{dt} = k\sqrt{N}, k > 0$ ***[1 mark for LHS, 1 mark for RHS]***
When $N = 36$, $\frac{dN}{dt} = 0.36$. Putting these values into the equation gives $0.36 = k\sqrt{36}$ ***[1 mark]*** $= 6k \Rightarrow k = 0.06$ (the population is increasing so ignore the negative square root).
So the differential equation is $\frac{dN}{dt} = 0.06\sqrt{N}$ ***[1 mark]***.

b) (i) $\frac{dN}{dt} = \frac{kN}{\sqrt{t}} \Rightarrow \int \frac{1}{N}\, dN = \int \frac{k}{\sqrt{t}}\, dt$
$\ln|N| = 2k\sqrt{t} + C$ ***[1 mark]***
$\Rightarrow N = e^{2k\sqrt{t}+C} = Ae^{2k\sqrt{t}}$, where $A = e^C$ ***[1 mark]***
For the initial population, $t = 0$, so $N = 25$ when $t = 0$.
Putting these values into the equation: $25 = Ae^0 \Rightarrow 25 = A$, so the equation for N is: $N = 25e^{2k\sqrt{t}}$ ***[1 mark]***.

(ii) When initial population has doubled, $N = 50$ ***[1 mark]***.
Put this value and the value for k into the equation and solve for t:
$50 = 25e^{2(0.05)\sqrt{t}} \Rightarrow 2 = e^{0.1\sqrt{t}} \Rightarrow \ln 2 = 0.1\sqrt{t}$ ***[1 mark]***
$10\ln 2 = \sqrt{t} \Rightarrow (10\ln 2)^2 = t \Rightarrow t = 48.045$
So it will take 48 weeks ***[1 mark]*** (to the nearest week) for the population to double.

10 a) First solve the differential equation to find S:
$\frac{dS}{dt} = k\sqrt{S} \Rightarrow \frac{1}{\sqrt{S}}\, dS = k\, dt$
$\Rightarrow \int S^{-\frac{1}{2}}\, dS = \int k\, dt$
$\Rightarrow 2S^{\frac{1}{2}} = kt + C$ ***[1 mark]***
$\Rightarrow S = \left(\frac{1}{2}(kt + C)\right)^2 = \frac{1}{4}(kt + C)^2$ ***[1 mark]***
At the start of the campaign, $t = 0$.
Putting $t = 0$ and $S = 81$ into the equation gives:
$81 = \frac{1}{4}(0 + C)^2 \Rightarrow 324 = C^2 \Rightarrow C = 18$ (C must be positive, otherwise the sales would be decreasing).
This gives the equation $S = \frac{1}{4}(kt + 18)^2$ ***[1 mark]***.

b) When $t = 0$, $S = 81$ and $\frac{dS}{dt} = 18$.
Substituting this into $\frac{dS}{dt} = k\sqrt{S}$ gives $k = 2$.
Using $S = \frac{1}{4}(kt + 18)^2$ with $t = 5$ and $k = 2$ gives $\frac{1}{4}((5 \times 2) + 18)^2 = 196$ kg sold.
[3 marks available — 1 mark for finding the value of k, 1 mark for substituting correct values of t and k, 1 mark for answer]

c) To find the value of t when $S = 225$, solve the equation $225 = \frac{1}{4}(2t + 18)^2$ ***[1 mark]***:
$225 = \frac{1}{4}(2t + 18)^2 \Rightarrow 900 = (2t + 18)^2$
$\Rightarrow 30 = 2t + 18 \Rightarrow 12 = 2t \Rightarrow 6 = t$
So it will be 6 days ***[1 mark]*** before 225 kg of cheese is sold.

11 a) (i) $\frac{dr}{dt} = -krt, k > 0$ ***[1 mark for RHS, 1 mark for LHS]***

(ii) S = area of curved surface + area of circular surface
$= \frac{1}{2}(4\pi r^2) + \pi r^2 = 3\pi r^2$ ***[1 mark]***
So $\frac{dS}{dr} = 6\pi r$ ***[1 mark]***
$\frac{dS}{dt} = \frac{dS}{dr} \times \frac{dr}{dt}$ ***[1 mark]***
$= 6\pi r \times -krt = -6\pi kr^2 t = -2kt(3\pi r^2) = -2ktS$
[1 mark for correct substitution and simplification to required answer]

b) (i) $\frac{dS}{dt} = -2ktS \Rightarrow \frac{dS}{S} = -2kt\, dt$
$\Rightarrow \int \frac{1}{S}\, dS = \int -2kt\, dt$
$\Rightarrow \ln S = -kt^2 + \ln A$
[1 mark for correct integration of both sides, plus a constant term]
$\Rightarrow S = e^{-kt^2 + \ln A} = Ae^{-kt^2}$ ***[1 mark]***
$S = 200$ at $t = 10 \Rightarrow 200 = Ae^{-100k}$
$S = 50$ at $t = 30 \Rightarrow 50 = Ae^{-900k}$
$\Rightarrow Ae^{-100k} = 4Ae^{-900k}$ ***[1 mark]***
$\Rightarrow e^{-100k} = 4e^{-900k}$
$\Rightarrow -100k = \ln 4 - 900k$
$\Rightarrow 800k = \ln 4$
$\Rightarrow k = 0.00173$ (3 s.f.) ***[1 mark]***
So $200 = Ae^{-100k} = Ae^{-0.173} = 0.841A$
$\Rightarrow A = 238$ (3 s.f.) ***[1 mark]***
So $S = 238e^{-0.00173t^2}$

(ii) The initial surface area is given when $t = 0$
$\Rightarrow S = 238e^0 = 238$ cm^2 (3 s.f.) ***[1 mark]***

c) E.g. The differential equation for the hemisphere was calculated using an expression for its surface area.
The expression for the surface area of a full sphere will be different to the expression for a hemisphere of the same radius, so this differential equation will not be appropriate ***[1 mark for a sensible comment]***.

Pages 60-64: Numerical Methods

1 When $x = -0.5$, $y = 4.51...$
When $x = 0$, $y = 3$
When $x = 0.5$, $y = 1.51...$
When $x = 1.0$, $y = -5$
There is a change of sign between $x = 0.5$ and $x = 1.0$, so there is a root in the interval $0.5 < x < 1.0$ ***[1 mark]***

2 a) To find the inverse, let $y = f(x)$, so $y = 4(x^2 - 1)$.
Now make x the subject:
$y = 4(x^2 - 1) \Rightarrow \frac{y}{4} = x^2 - 1 \Rightarrow \frac{y}{4} + 1 = x^2$
So $x = \sqrt{\frac{y}{4} + 1}$ ***[1 mark]*** (you can ignore the negative square root, as the domain of f(x) is $x \geq 0$).
Finally, replace y with x and x with $f^{-1}(x)$:
$f^{-1}(x) = \sqrt{\frac{x}{4} + 1}$ ***[1 mark for correct inverse]***.
$y = f^{-1}(x)$ is a reflection of $y = f(x)$ in the line $y = x$ ***[1 mark]***, so the point at which the lines $y = f(x)$ and $y = f^{-1}(x)$ meet is also the point where $y = f^{-1}(x)$ meets the line $y = x$.
At this point, $x = \sqrt{\frac{x}{4} + 1}$, so $\sqrt{\frac{x}{4} + 1} - x = 0$
[1 mark for setting $f^{-1}(x)$ equal to x and rearranging].

b) Let $g(x) = \sqrt{\frac{x}{4} + 1} - x$
If there is a root in the interval $1 < x < 2$ then there will be a change of sign for $g(x)$ between 1 and 2:
$g(1) = \sqrt{\frac{1}{4} + 1} - 1 = 0.1180...$
$g(2) = \sqrt{\frac{2}{4} + 1} - 2 = -0.7752...$ ***[1 mark for both]***
There is a change of sign and the function is continuous over this interval, so there is a root in the interval $1 < x < 2$ ***[1 mark]***.

c) $x_{n+1} = \sqrt{\frac{x_n}{4} + 1}$, and $x_0 = 1$, so:
$x_1 = \sqrt{\frac{1}{4} + 1} = 1.1180...$ ***[1 mark]***
$x_2 = \sqrt{\frac{1.1180...}{4} + 1} = 1.1311...$
$x_3 = \sqrt{\frac{1.1311...}{4} + 1} = 1.1326...$
$x_4 = \sqrt{\frac{1.1326...}{4} + 1} = 1.1327...$ ***[1 mark]***
So $x \approx 1.13$ to 3 s.f. ***[1 mark]***.

d) No. If you sketch the line $y = x$ on the graph, you can see that it does not cross the curve $y = f^{-1}(x)$ more than once, so there is only one root of the equation $\sqrt{\frac{x}{4}+1} - x = 0$.
[1 mark for 'No' with suitable explanation]

3 a) When the curve and line intersect, $6^x = x + 2 \Rightarrow 6^x - x - 2 = 0$. Let $f(x) = 6^x - x - 2$. If there is a root in the interval [0.5, 1] then there will be a change of sign for f(x) between 0.5 and 1:
$f(0.5) = 6^{0.5} - 0.5 - 2 = -0.0505...$
$f(1) = 6^1 - 1 - 2 = 3$ ***[1 mark for both]***
There is a change of sign and the function is continuous over this interval, so there is a root in the interval [0.5, 1] ***[1 mark]***.

b) Substitute $f(x) = 6^x - x - 2$ into the Newton-Raphson formula:

$$x_{n+1} = x_n - \frac{f(x_n)}{f'(x_n)} = x_n - \frac{6^{x_n} - x_n - 2}{6^{x_n}\ln 6 - 1}$$
$$= \frac{x_n(6^{x_n}\ln 6 - 1)}{6^{x_n}\ln 6 - 1} - \frac{6^{x_n} - x_n - 2}{6^{x_n}\ln 6 - 1}$$
$$= \frac{x_n 6^{x_n}\ln 6 - x_n - 6^{x_n} + x_n + 2}{6^{x_n}\ln 6 - 1}$$
$$= \frac{6^{x_n}(x_n \ln 6 - 1) + 2}{6^{x_n}\ln 6 - 1} \text{ as required}$$

[4 marks available — 1 mark for differentiating f(x) correctly, 1 mark for substituting everything into the Newton-Raphson formula, 1 mark for putting x_n and $f(x_n)$ over a common denominator, 1 mark for factorising the numerator]

c) $x_0 = 0.5$

$$x_1 = \frac{6^{(0.5)}((0.5)\ln 6 - 1) + 2}{6^{(0.5)}\ln 6 - 1} = 0.514904...$$ ***[1 mark]***

$x_2 = 0.514653...$
$x_3 = 0.514653...$
So the x-coordinate of P is approximately 0.5147 (4 s.f.). ***[1 mark]***
If you put 0.5 into your calculator and press =, then input (6^{ANS} × (ANS × ln 6 − 1) + 2) ÷ (6^{ANS} × ln 6 − 1) and keep pressing =, you'll get the iterative sequence without having to type it in each time.

d) From part c), $x \approx 0.5147$ to 4 s.f.
If this is accurate, then $x = 0.5147$ to 4 s.f., so the upper and lower bounds are 0.51475 and 0.51465 ***[1 mark]***
— any value in this range would be rounded to 0.5147.
$f(x) = 6^x - x - 2$, and at point P, $f(x) = 0$.
$f(0.51475) = 0.000338...$ and $f(0.51465) = -0.0000116...$
[1 mark for both f(0.51475) positive and f(0.51465) negative].
There is a change of sign, and since f(x) is continuous there must be a root in this interval ***[1 mark]***.

e) E.g. If the tangent has a gradient of 0, the denominator of the fraction in the iteration formula will be 0 so the Newton-Raphson method will fail for this starting value as no value of x_1 can be found. ***[1 mark for any suitable explanation]***

4 a) Substitute the values you're given for x_0, $f(x_0)$ and $f'(x_0)$ into the Newton-Raphson formula:

$$x_1 = x_0 - \frac{f(x_0)}{f'(x_0)} = -1.5 - \frac{-1.625}{9.75}$$
$$= -1.33333... = -1.333 \text{ (4 s.f.)}$$

[2 marks available — 1 mark for substituting the values into the Newton-Raphson formula correctly, 1 mark for the correct answer]

b) If $x = -1.315$ to 4 s.f., the upper and lower bounds are −1.3145 and −1.3155 ***[1 mark]*** — any value in this range would be rounded to −1.315. $f(x) = x^3 - x^2 + 4$.
$f(-1.3145) = 0.00075...$ and $f(-1.3155) = -0.00706...$
[1 mark for both f(−1.3145) positive and f(−1.3155) negative].
There is a change of sign, and since f(x) is continuous there must be a root in this interval, so the value of b must be correct to 4 s.f. ***[1 mark]***.

c) The denominator of the fraction in the Newton-Raphson formula is $f'(x) = 3x^2 - 2x$ ***[1 mark]***.
When $x = \frac{2}{3}$, $3x^2 - 2x = 3(\frac{2}{3})^2 - 2(\frac{2}{3}) = 0$
— so the denominator is 0, which means the Newton-Raphson method fails as no value of x_1 can be found ***[1 mark]***.

5 a) The trapezium rule is given by:

$$\int_a^b y\,dx \approx \frac{h}{2}[y_0 + 2(y_1 + y_2 + ...y_{n-1}) + y_n]$$

where n is the number of intervals (in this case 4), and h is the width of each strip:

$$h = \frac{b-a}{n} = \frac{2-0}{4} = 0.5$$ ***[1 mark]***

Work out each y value:
$x_0 = 0$ $\quad y_0 = 2^{0^2} = 2^0 = 1$
$x_1 = 0.5$ $\quad y_1 = 2^{0.5^2} = 2^{0.25} = 1.189$ (3 d.p.)
$x_2 = 1$ $\quad y_2 = 2^{1^2} = 2^1 = 2$
$x_3 = 1.5$ $\quad y_3 = 2^{1.5^2} = 2^{2.25} = 4.757$ (3 d.p.)
$x_4 = 2$ $\quad y_4 = 2^{2^2} = 2^4 = 16$ ***[1 mark for all values correct]***
Now put all these values into the formula:

$$\int_0^2 2^{x^2} dx \approx \frac{0.5}{2}[1 + 2(1.189 + 2 + 4.757) + 16]$$ ***[1 mark]***
$$= \frac{1}{4}(17 + 15.892) = 8.22 \text{ (3 s.f.)}$$ ***[1 mark]***

b) E.g. The curve is convex, so a trapezium on each strip has a greater area than that under the curve. So the trapezium rule gives an overestimate for the area.
[1 mark for a correct answer with an explanation relating to the shape of the graph].

c) To improve the accuracy of the estimate, increase the number of intervals used in the trapezium rule ***[1 mark]***.

6 a) When $x = \frac{\pi}{2}$, $y = \frac{\pi}{2}\sin\frac{\pi}{2} = \frac{\pi}{2} = 1.5708$ (5 s.f.),
and when $x = \frac{3\pi}{4}$, $y = \frac{3\pi}{4}\sin\frac{3\pi}{4} = 1.6661$ (5 s.f.)
[1 mark for both]

b) The width of each strip (h) is $\frac{\pi}{4}$, so the trapezium rule gives:

$$\text{Area of } R \approx \frac{1}{2} \times \frac{\pi}{4}[0 + 2(0.55536 + 1.5708 + 1.6661) + 0]$$
$$= \frac{\pi}{8}[2(3.79226)] = 2.97843... = 2.978 \text{ (4 s.f.)}$$

[3 marks available — 1 mark for correct value of h, 1 mark for using the formula correctly, 1 mark for correct answer]

c) Let $u = x$, so $\frac{du}{dx} = 1$. Let $\frac{dv}{dx} = \sin x$, so $v = -\cos x$
[1 mark for correct choice of u and dv/dx, 1 mark for correct du/dx and v]
Using integration by parts,

$$\int_0^\pi x\sin x\,dx = [-x\cos x]_0^\pi - \int_0^\pi -\cos x\,dx$$ ***[1 mark]***
$$= [-x\cos x]_0^\pi + [\sin x]_0^\pi$$ ***[1 mark]***
$$= (-\pi\cos\pi + 0\cos 0) + (\sin\pi - \sin 0)$$ ***[1 mark]***
$$= (\pi - 0) + (0) = \pi$$ ***[1 mark]***

If you'd tried to use u = sin x, you'd have ended up with a more complicated function to integrate ($x^2\cos x$).

d) To find the percentage error, divide the difference between the approximate answer and the exact answer by the exact answer and multiply by 100:

$$\left|\frac{\pi - 2.97843...}{\pi}\right| \times 100 = 5.2\% \text{ (2 s.f.)}$$

[2 marks available — 1 mark for appropriate method, 1 mark for correct answer]

7 $n = 5,\ h = \frac{4 - 1.5}{5} = 0.5$

Work out the x- and y-values (y-values given to 5 s.f. where appropriate):

$x_0 = 1.5 \quad y_0 = 2.8182$
$x_1 = 2.0 \quad y_1 = 4$
$x_2 = 2.5 \quad y_2 = 5.1216$
$x_3 = 3.0 \quad y_3 = 6.1716$
$x_4 = 3.5 \quad y_4 = 7.1364$
$x_5 = 4.0 \quad y_5 = 8$

$$\int_{1.5}^{4} y\,dx \approx \frac{0.5}{2}[2.8182 + 2(4 + 5.1216 + 6.1716 + 7.1364) + 8]$$

$= 13.91935 = 13.92$ to 4 s.f.

[4 marks available — 1 mark for the correct value of h, 1 mark for correct x- and y-values, 1 mark for using the formula correctly, 1 mark for the correct answer]

8 a) $n = 5,\ h = \frac{3 - 2.5}{5} = 0.1$

Work out the x- and y-values (y-values given to 6 s.f.):

$x_0 = 2.5 \quad y_0 = 0.439820$
$x_1 = 2.6 \quad y_1 = 0.424044$
$x_2 = 2.7 \quad y_2 = 0.408746$
$x_3 = 2.8 \quad y_3 = 0.393987$
$x_4 = 2.9 \quad y_4 = 0.379802$
$x_5 = 3.0 \quad y_5 = 0.366204$

$$\int_{2.5}^{3} y\,dx \approx \frac{0.1}{2}[0.439820 + 2(0.424044 + 0.408746 + 0.393987 + 0.379802) + 0.366204]$$

$= 0.2009591... = 0.2010$ (4 s.f.)

[4 marks available — 1 mark for the correct value of h, 1 mark for correct x- and y-values, 1 mark for using the formula correctly, 1 mark for the correct answer]

b) The area of a rectangle with base 0.5 and height f(2.5) will be an overestimate of area R as the top of the rectangle will be above the top of the curve.
This rectangle has area $0.5 \times 0.439820 = 0.21991$ ***[1 mark]***.
The area of a rectangle with base 0.5 and height f(3) will be an underestimate as the top of the rectangle will be below the top of the curve.
This rectangle has area $0.5 \times 0.366204 = 0.183102$ ***[1 mark]***.
So the actual area of R lies between these two values, i.e. $0.183102 < R < 0.21991$. Both the upper and lower limits round to 0.2, so $R = 0.2$ correct to 1 d.p. ***[1 mark]***

Pages 65-67: Vectors

1

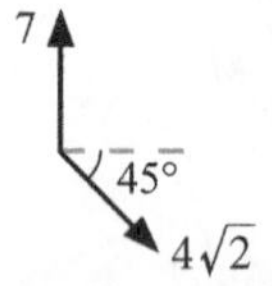

Use trigonometry to find the horizontal and vertical components of the magnitude $4\sqrt{2}$ vector:
Horizontal component: $4\sqrt{2}\cos 315° = 4\mathbf{i}$
Vertical component: $4\sqrt{2}\sin 315° = -4\mathbf{j}$
So the resultant velocity is $7\mathbf{j} + (4\mathbf{i} - 4\mathbf{j}) = (4\mathbf{i} + 3\mathbf{j})$ ms^{-1} ***[1 mark]***.

Remember — angles are normally measured anticlockwise from the positive x-axis, so here, 360° – 45° = 315°

2 $\overrightarrow{XY} = \overrightarrow{OY} - \overrightarrow{OX} = (2\mathbf{i} - \mathbf{j} + 3\mathbf{k}) - (5\mathbf{i} - 2\mathbf{j} - 6\mathbf{k}) = -3\mathbf{i} + \mathbf{j} + 9\mathbf{k}$

$|\overrightarrow{XY}| = \sqrt{(-3)^2 + 1^2 + 9^2} = \sqrt{91}$ ***[1 mark]***

3 $\overrightarrow{AB} = \overrightarrow{OB} - \overrightarrow{OA} = (5\mathbf{i} - 3\mathbf{j} + 6\mathbf{k}) - (-\mathbf{i} + 7\mathbf{j} - 2\mathbf{k})$
$= 6\mathbf{i} - 10\mathbf{j} + 8\mathbf{k}$ ***[1 mark]***

$\overrightarrow{AM} = \frac{1}{2}\overrightarrow{AB} = 3\mathbf{i} - 5\mathbf{j} + 4\mathbf{k}$

Use this to find $\overrightarrow{CM}$:

$\overrightarrow{CM} = -\overrightarrow{OC} + \overrightarrow{OA} + \overrightarrow{AM}$
$= -(5\mathbf{i} + 4\mathbf{j} + 3\mathbf{k}) + (-\mathbf{i} + 7\mathbf{j} - 2\mathbf{k}) + (3\mathbf{i} - 5\mathbf{j} + 4\mathbf{k})$
$= -3\mathbf{i} - 2\mathbf{j} - \mathbf{k}$

[1 mark for a correct method, 1 mark for the correct vector]

$|\overrightarrow{CM}| = \sqrt{(-3)^2 + (-2)^2 + (-1)^2} = \sqrt{14}$

$|\overrightarrow{AB}| = \sqrt{6^2 + (-10)^2 + 8^2} = \sqrt{200}$

$k = \frac{|\overrightarrow{CM}|}{|\overrightarrow{AB}|} = \frac{\sqrt{14}}{\sqrt{200}}$ ***[1 mark]***

$= \sqrt{\frac{7}{100}} = \frac{1}{10}\sqrt{7}$ ***[1 mark]***

4 $\overrightarrow{AB} = \overrightarrow{OB} - \overrightarrow{OA}$
$= (14\mathbf{i} + 12\mathbf{j} - 9\mathbf{k}) - (-2\mathbf{i} + 4\mathbf{j} - 5\mathbf{k}) = (16\mathbf{i} + 8\mathbf{j} - 4\mathbf{k})$ ***[1 mark]***

$\overrightarrow{AC} = \overrightarrow{OC} - \overrightarrow{OA}$
$= (2\mathbf{i} + \mu\mathbf{j} + \lambda\mathbf{k}) - (-2\mathbf{i} + 4\mathbf{j} - 5\mathbf{k}) = 4\mathbf{i} + (\mu - 4)\mathbf{j} + (\lambda + 5)\mathbf{k}$ ***[1 mark]***

$\overrightarrow{AB}$ and $\overrightarrow{AC}$ both share the point A, so to show they're collinear you need to show that the vectors are parallel i.e. $\overrightarrow{AB} = k\overrightarrow{AC}$ for some constant k. So $(16\mathbf{i} + 8\mathbf{j} - 4\mathbf{k}) = k(4\mathbf{i} + (\mu - 4)\mathbf{j} + (\lambda + 5)\mathbf{k})$ ***[1 mark]***

Equate coefficients of **i**, **j**, **k** separately:

$16 = 4k \Rightarrow k = 4$ ***[1 mark]***
$8 = k(\mu - 4) \Rightarrow \mu = 6$
$-4 = k(\lambda + 5) \Rightarrow \lambda = -6$ ***[1 mark for both μ and λ correct]***

5 $\overrightarrow{AB} = \overrightarrow{OB} - \overrightarrow{OA} = \begin{pmatrix}4\\-12\\8\end{pmatrix} - \begin{pmatrix}1\\-3\\2\end{pmatrix} = \begin{pmatrix}3\\-9\\6\end{pmatrix}$ ***[1 mark]***

D is $\frac{2}{3}$ of the way along $\overrightarrow{AB}$, so $\overrightarrow{AD} = \frac{2}{3}\overrightarrow{AB}$

$= \frac{2}{3}\begin{pmatrix}3\\-9\\6\end{pmatrix} = \begin{pmatrix}2\\-6\\4\end{pmatrix}$ ***[1 mark]***

$\overrightarrow{OD} = \overrightarrow{OA} + \overrightarrow{AD} = \begin{pmatrix}1\\-3\\2\end{pmatrix} + \begin{pmatrix}2\\-6\\4\end{pmatrix} = \begin{pmatrix}3\\-9\\6\end{pmatrix}$ ***[1 mark]***

Now, $\overrightarrow{OD} = -\frac{1}{2}\overrightarrow{CE}$

$\Rightarrow \overrightarrow{CE} = -2\overrightarrow{OD} = -2\begin{pmatrix}3\\-9\\6\end{pmatrix} = \begin{pmatrix}-6\\18\\-12\end{pmatrix}$ ***[1 mark]***

So $\overrightarrow{OE} = \overrightarrow{OC} + \overrightarrow{CE} = \begin{pmatrix}-3\\9\\-6\end{pmatrix} + \begin{pmatrix}-6\\18\\-12\end{pmatrix} = \begin{pmatrix}-9\\27\\-18\end{pmatrix}$ ***[1 mark]***

6 $\overrightarrow{PS} = \overrightarrow{QR}$ as $PQRS$ is a parallelogram, so

$\overrightarrow{PS} = \overrightarrow{PR} - \overrightarrow{PQ} = \begin{pmatrix}2\\-9\\3\end{pmatrix} - \begin{pmatrix}-14\\-6\\-7\end{pmatrix} = \begin{pmatrix}16\\-3\\10\end{pmatrix}$ ***[1 mark]***

$|\overrightarrow{PS}| = \sqrt{16^2 + (-3)^2 + 10^2} = \sqrt{365}$

$|\overrightarrow{PR}| = \sqrt{2^2 + (-9)^2 + 3^2} = \sqrt{94}$

$|\overrightarrow{RS}| = |\overrightarrow{PQ}| = \sqrt{(-14)^2 + (-6)^2 + (-7)^2} = \sqrt{281}$

[1 mark for attempting to find magnitudes using Pythagoras, 1 mark for all 3 magnitudes correct]

Find $\angle RPS$ using the cosine rule:

$\cos\angle RPS = \frac{94 + 365 - 281}{2 \times \sqrt{94} \times \sqrt{365}} = 0.48048...$ ***[1 mark]***

$\angle RPS = \cos^{-1} 0.48048...$
$= 61.282...° = 61.3°$ (1 d.p.) ***[1 mark]***

7 a) Position vector of drone A:
$\mathbf{a}+\mathbf{b}+\mathbf{c} = (4\mathbf{i}+6\mathbf{j}+5\mathbf{k}) + (-\mathbf{i}-2\mathbf{j}-2\mathbf{k}) + (-3\mathbf{j}+\mathbf{k})$
$= (3\mathbf{i}+\mathbf{j}+4\mathbf{k})$ ***[1 mark]***
Position vector of drone B:
$2\mathbf{a}+\mathbf{b}-3\mathbf{c} = 2(4\mathbf{i}+6\mathbf{j}+5\mathbf{k}) + (-\mathbf{i}-2\mathbf{j}-2\mathbf{k}) - 3(-3\mathbf{j}+\mathbf{k})$
$= (7\mathbf{i}+19\mathbf{j}+5\mathbf{k})$ ***[1 mark]***
So the distance between drones A and B is:
$\sqrt{(7-3)^2+(19-1)^2+(5-4)^2}$ ***[1 mark]***
$= \sqrt{341} = 18.466... = 18.5$ m (3 s.f.) ***[1 mark]***

b) Vector from drone A to drone B is:
$(7\mathbf{i}+19\mathbf{j}+5\mathbf{k}) - (3\mathbf{i}+\mathbf{j}+4\mathbf{k}) = 4\mathbf{i}+18\mathbf{j}+\mathbf{k}$
So the vector to take drone A to 2 m below drone B is:
$(4\mathbf{i}+18\mathbf{j}+\mathbf{k}) - 2\mathbf{k} = (4\mathbf{i}+18\mathbf{j}-\mathbf{k})$ m
[2 marks available — 1 mark for a correct method, 1 mark for the correct answer]

c) The position vector of drone B as it moves in the positive $\mathbf{j}$ direction can be described by:
$(7\mathbf{i}+(19+\lambda)\mathbf{j}+5\mathbf{k})$ m for $\lambda \geq 0$ ***[1 mark]***
So at the limit of the drone's range:
$|7\mathbf{i}+(19+\lambda)\mathbf{j}+5\mathbf{k}| = 50$ m
$\Rightarrow \sqrt{7^2+(19+\lambda)^2+5^2} = 50$ ***[1 mark]***
$\Rightarrow (19+\lambda)^2 = 2500-49-25 = 2426$
$\Rightarrow \lambda^2+38\lambda+361 = 2426$
$\Rightarrow \lambda^2+38\lambda-2065 = 0$ ***[1 mark]***
Solve for λ using the quadratic formula:
$\lambda = \dfrac{-38 \pm \sqrt{38^2-4(1)(-2065)}}{2(1)}$ ***[1 mark]***
$\Rightarrow \lambda = \dfrac{-38 \pm \sqrt{9704}}{2}$
$\Rightarrow \lambda = 30.25444...$ (ignore the $-$ ve solution as $\lambda \geq 0$)
$\Rightarrow \lambda = 30.3$ m (3 s.f) ***[1 mark]***
OK I won't lie, that last part was pretty nasty. But actually... once you've got the initial equation written down, it's just standard algebra that you've been doing since GCSE.

Section Two — Statistics

Pages 68-73: Data Presentation and Interpretation

1 $1085 \div 135.625 = 8$ ***[1 mark]***

2 a) mean $= \dfrac{\sum x}{n} = \dfrac{500}{10} = 50$ ***[1 mark]***
variance $= \dfrac{\sum x^2}{10} - 50^2 = \dfrac{25\,622}{10} - 2500$ ***[1 mark]*** $= 62.2$
So standard deviation $= \sqrt{62.2} = 7.89$ ***[1 mark]***

b) (i) The mean will be unchanged ***[1 mark]***, because the new value is equal to the original mean ***[1 mark]***.
(ii) The standard deviation will decrease ***[1 mark]***. This is because the standard deviation measures the deviation of values from the mean. So by adding a new value that's equal to the mean, you're not adding to the total deviation from the mean, but as you have an extra reading, you now have to divide by 11 (not 10) when you work out the variance ***[1 mark]***.
Understanding what the standard deviation actually is can help you get your head round questions like this.

3 The area of the $1300 \leq m < 1350$ bar is $1.25 \times 8 = 10$ cm^2 and the frequency (i.e. number of groups) is 4. So each group is represented by an area of $10 \div 4 = 2.5$ cm^2. The $1500 \leq m < 1700$ bar has frequency 3, so its area is 2.5 cm$^2 \times 3 = 7.5$ cm^2 ***[1 mark]***.
The $1500 \leq m < 1700$ class is four times the width of the $1300 \leq m < 1350$ class so: width $= 4 \times 1.25 = 5$ cm ***[1 mark]***, height $= 7.5 \div 5 = 1.5$ cm ***[1 mark]***.

4 a) The ordered list of the 12 data points is:
3.8, 4.1, 4.2, 4.6, 4.9, 5.5, 5.8, 5.9, 6.0, 6.2, 6.4, 9.1.
n is even and $\frac{n}{2} = 6$, so take the average of the 6th and 7th values. So the median (Q_2) is:
$\frac{1}{2}(5.5+5.8) = 5.65$, which represents £5650 ***[1 mark]***.
Since $12 \div 4 = 3$, the lower quartile is the average of the 3rd and 4th values. So the lower quartile (Q_1) is:
$\frac{1}{2}(4.2+4.6) = 4.4$, which represents £4400 ***[1 mark]***.
Since $12 \div 4 \times 3 = 9$, the upper quartile is the average of the 9th and 10th values. So the upper quartile (Q_3) is:
$\frac{1}{2}(6.0+6.2) = 6.1$, which represents £6100 ***[1 mark]***.

b) The lower fence is given by:
$Q_1 - 1.5 \times (Q_3 - Q_1) = 4.4 - 1.5 \times (6.1 - 4.4) = 1.85$.
So there are no outliers below the lower fence.
The upper fence is given by:
$Q_3 + 1.5 \times (Q_3 - Q_1) = 6.1 + 1.5 \times (6.1 - 4.4) = 8.65$.
So there is one outlier — the value of 9.1.
[2 marks available — 1 mark for calculating fences, 1 mark for finding the correct outlier]

c) E.g. the manager should not include this outlier in his analysis as it might be caused by an outside factor, e.g. Christmas, so including it would not accurately reflect normal sales. /
The manager should include this outlier in his analysis as it accurately reflects actual sales for this period, even if one week was unusually high. ***[1 mark for a sensible comment]***

d) E.g. the mean and standard deviation are affected by outliers, whereas the median and IQR are not. So as this set of data includes an outlier, the median and IQR are more useful. /
The mean and standard deviation take into account all data values, so are more useful as they reflect the actual data.
[2 marks available — 2 marks for stating which values are more useful with a sensible explanation, otherwise 1 mark for a sensible comment]

e) Weeks 5-6 ***[1 mark]***
E.g. The jewellery sales for weeks 5-6 make up a higher proportion of the total sales for each week than in other weeks
[1 mark for a sensible comment].

5 a) Use the frequency density axis and the formula frequency = frequency density × class width to work out the missing values in the table:

Monthly phone bill, £b	Frequency
$0 \le b < 10$	12
$10 \le b < 15$	23
$15 \le b < 18$	$5 \times 3 = 15$
$18 \le b < 20$	$5 \times 2 = 10$
$20 \le b < 25$	18
$25 \le b < 35$	6

[2 marks available — 1 mark for using frequency = frequency density × class width, 1 mark for both entries in table correct]

b) £12.50 is halfway through the $10 \le b < 15$ class, so there are approximately $23 \div 2 = 11.5$ students that pay between £12.50 and £15. £17.50 is $\frac{5}{6}$ of the way through the $15 \le b < 18$ class, so there are $\frac{5}{6} \times 15 = 12.5$ students that pay between £15 and £17.50. So an estimate for the number of students that have a monthly phone bill of between £12.50 and £17.50 is $11.5 + 12.5 = 24$.

[2 marks available — 1 mark for a correct method, 1 mark for the correct answer]

c) Add columns to the table showing the class midpoint and the midpoint × frequency:

Monthly phone bill, £b	Frequency, f	Class midpoint, x	$f \times x$
$0 \le b < 10$	12	5	60
$10 \le b < 15$	23	12.5	287.5
$15 \le b < 18$	15	16.5	247.5
$18 \le b < 20$	10	19	190
$20 \le b < 25$	18	22.5	405
$25 \le b < 35$	6	30	180

There are $12 + 23 + 15 + 10 + 18 + 6 = 84$ students in total, and $\sum fx = 60 + 287.5 + 247.5 + 190 + 405 + 180 = 1370$.

So mean $= \frac{\sum fx}{\sum f} = \frac{1370}{84} = 16.309... = £16.31$ to 2 d.p.

[3 marks available — 1 mark for use of class midpoints, 1 mark for $\sum fx$, 1 mark for the correct answer]

d) Add columns for x^2 and fx^2:

Monthly phone bill, £b	Frequency, f	x^2	$f \times x^2$
$0 \le b < 10$	12	25	300
$10 \le b < 15$	23	156.25	3593.75
$15 \le b < 18$	15	272.25	4083.75
$18 \le b < 20$	10	361	3610
$20 \le b < 25$	18	506.25	9112.5
$25 \le b < 35$	6	900	5400

$\sum fx^2 = 26\,100$

Standard deviation $= \sqrt{\frac{\sum fx^2}{\sum f} - \bar{x}^2} = \sqrt{\frac{26\,100}{84} - 16.309...^2}$

$= 6.68683... = £6.69$ (2 d.p.)

[3 marks available — 1 mark for calculating $\sum fx^2$, 1 mark for substituting into the formula for standard deviation, 1 mark for the correct answer]

e) E.g. The monthly phone bills for the Year 12 students are generally higher, as they have a higher mean ***[1 mark]***.
E.g. The monthly phone bills for the Year 7 students are less varied, because their standard deviation is smaller ***[1 mark]***.

6 a) Isaac: Outliers are below 5850 – (2 × 7360) = –8870 miles (impossible) or above 5850 + (2 × 7360) = 20 570 miles. The value 29 000 miles (in 2001) is above 20 570 miles, so it is an outlier and should be circled ***[1 mark]***.
Niamh: Outliers are below 7480 – (2 × 8380) = –9280 miles (impossible) or above 7480 + (2 × 8380) = 24 240 miles. The value 27 000 miles (in 2001) is above 24 240 miles so it is an outlier and should be circled ***[1 mark]***.

b) E.g. The outliers for both Isaac and Niamh occurred in the same year so their company may have been pushing for more door-to-door satellite television sales that year. / 2001 may have been a good year for satellite television sales generally ***[1 mark for a sensible comment]***.
Although outliers can be down to recording errors, in this case it wouldn't appear to be an error as the data for both Isaac and Niamh follows a similar pattern.

c) E.g. Khalid's claim is not correct. The data only describes how far they travelled for their work, not how successful they were in making sales ***[1 mark for a sensible comment]***.

7 a) Median position is $30 \div 2 = 15$
Q_1 position is $30 \div 4 = 7.5$
Q_3 position is $(3 \times 30) \div 4 = 22.5$
So, using the graph, median ≈ 3.8 m ***[1 mark]***,
$Q_1 \approx 3.25$ m ***[1 mark]*** and $Q_3 \approx 4.45$ m ***[1 mark]***
The interquartile range is 4.45 – 3.25 = 1.2 m ***[1 mark]***

b) Outliers would be below 3.25 – 1.5 × 1.2 = 1.45 m or above 4.45 + 1.5 × 1.2 = 6.25 m ***[1 mark for both]***.
From the graph you can see that the minimum and maximum possible values are 2 m and 6 m, so this data set contains no outliers ***[1 mark]***.

c) Subtract the cumulative frequency at the upper class boundary from the cumulative frequency at the lower class boundary:

Height, h (metres)	$0 < h \le 2$	$2 < h \le 3$	$3 < h \le 4$	$4 < h \le 5$	$5 < h \le 6$
Frequency	0	5	17 – 5 = 12	27 – 17 = 10	30 – 27 = 3

[2 marks available — 1 mark for any two answers correct, 2 mark for all answers correct]

d) The giraffes in the zoo are generally taller, as they have a higher median ***[1 mark]***.
Two giraffes in the nature reserve have extreme heights that are outliers, but there are no outliers in the zoo ***[1 mark]***.
The two populations seem similarly varied, since they have similar ranges (the range for the zoo is 2.86 m and, ignoring the outliers, the range for the nature reserve is 2.8 m), although the IQR for the giraffes in the zoo is slightly greater than for the giraffes in the nature reserve ***[1 mark]***.

8 a) 280 minutes ***[1 mark]***

b) If the runners were in the 21-25 age group in 2000, then they would be in the 31-35 age group in 2010. The graph shows that the 31-35 age group's mean time to finish the race was higher in 2010 than the 21-25 age group's times in 2000, which would mean the runners were slower, so the graph does not suggest these runners' times improved.
[2 marks available — 1 mark for sensible explanation and 1 mark for the correct conclusion]

c) E.g. That the same runners participated in the 2010 marathon and the 2000 marathon ***[1 mark for a sensible comment]***.

d) E.g. If there were different numbers of runners in each age category, the value calculated by Serj would not take this into account ***[1 mark for a sensible explanation]***. To calculate a more accurate value, he should multiply the mean for each age category by the number of runners in that category, add these values up then divide by the total number of runners ***[1 mark for a suitable method]***.

Pages 74-77: Probability

1 a) A and B are mutually exclusive, so $P(A \cap B) = 0$.
This means the circles don't intersect.
B and C are independent, so
$P(B \cap C) = P(B) \times P(C) = 0.4 \times 0.3 = 0.12$
$P(A \cap C) = 0.06$
Use this to fill in the Venn diagram:

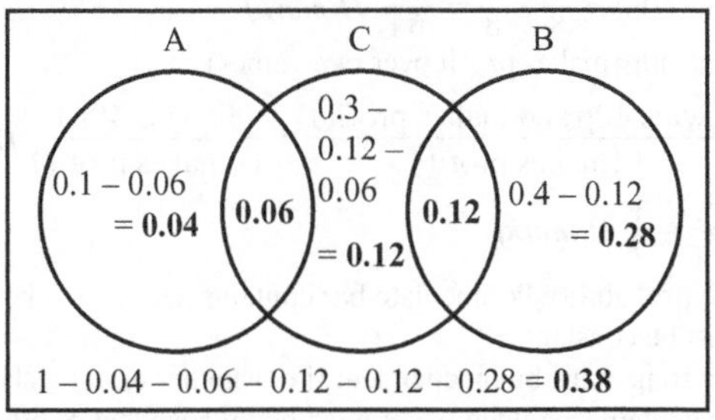

[5 marks available — 1 mark for circles overlapping correctly, 1 mark for calculating P(B ∩ C), 1 mark for calculating the remaining probabilities in both circles A and B, 1 mark for calculating the remaining probability in circle C, 1 mark for the correct probability outside the circles]

b) $P(A) \times P(C) = 0.1 \times 0.3 = 0.03$
$P(A \cap C) = 0.06 \neq P(A) \times P(C)$,
so events A and C are not independent.
[2 marks available — 1 mark for finding P(A) × P(C) and stating P(A ∩ C), 1 mark for the correct conclusion]

c) $P(B \cup C) = 0.06 + 0.12 + 0.12 + 0.28 = 0.58$ ***[1 mark]***

d) $P(A' \cap B') = 0.12 + 0.38 = 0.5$ ***[1 mark]***

e) $P(B'|A') = \frac{P(B' \cap A')}{P(A')} = \frac{0.5}{0.9} = \frac{5}{9} = 0.56$ (2 d.p.)
[2 marks available — 1 mark for using the conditional probability formula, 1 mark for the correct answer]
Use the numbers in the Venn diagram to answer parts c)-e).

2 As L and M are independent, $P(L \cap M) = P(L) \times P(M)$ ***[1 mark]***
$P(L) = 0.1 + 0.4 = 0.5$ and $P(M) = 2x + 0.4$ ***[1 mark]***
$P(L \cap M) = 0.4 = 0.5 \times (2x + 0.4) = x + 0.2 \Rightarrow x = 0.2$ ***[1 mark]***
So this means $P(L \cup M) = 0.1 + 0.4 + 0.4 = 0.9$
$\Rightarrow P(L' \cap M') = 1 - 0.9 = 0.1$ ***[1 mark]***

3 Draw a tree diagram:

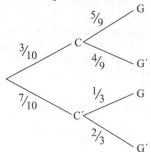

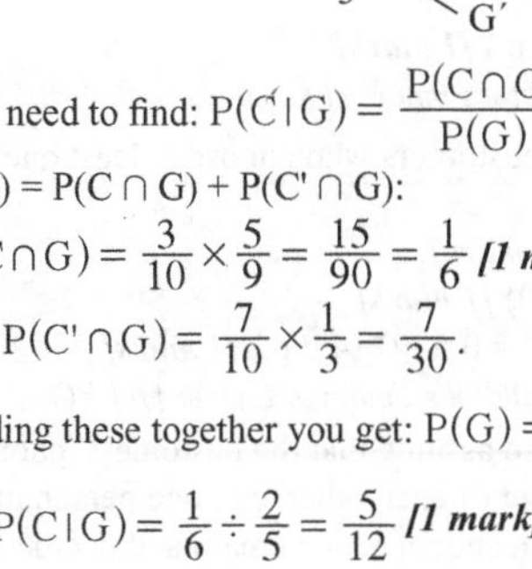

You need to find: $P(C|G) = \frac{P(C \cap G)}{P(G)}$ ***[1 mark]***.
$P(G) = P(C \cap G) + P(C' \cap G)$:
$P(C \cap G) = \frac{3}{10} \times \frac{5}{9} = \frac{15}{90} = \frac{1}{6}$ ***[1 mark]***,
and $P(C' \cap G) = \frac{7}{10} \times \frac{1}{3} = \frac{7}{30}$.
Adding these together you get: $P(G) = \frac{1}{6} + \frac{7}{30} = \frac{2}{5}$ ***[1 mark]***.
So $P(C|G) = \frac{1}{6} \div \frac{2}{5} = \frac{5}{12}$ ***[1 mark]***.

4 a) Let U be the event 'selected fan is under 18'.
There are 1945 males, of which 305 are under 18,
so $P(U \mid M) = \frac{305}{1945} = \frac{61}{389}$.
[2 marks available — 1 mark for a correct method, 1 mark for the correct answer]
You could have found this using the formula for conditional probability.

b) E.g. Alan has assumed that the fans at the next match will have the same mix of ages and genders, but many factors affect the attendance at a game, and different opponents may have a different age or gender balance in their fans.
[2 marks available — 1 mark for an assumption, 1 mark for a sensible reason why this may not be valid]

5 a) Draw a tree diagram. Let C = 'pick a heart from the complete pack':

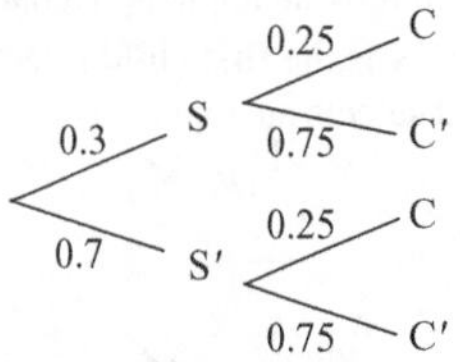

The probability of at least one event happening is the same as 1 minus the probability of neither event happening:
$P(S \cup C) = 1 - P(S' \cap C')$
$= 1 - (0.7 \times 0.75) = 1 - 0.525 = 0.475$
[2 marks available — 1 mark for a correct method, 1 mark for the correct answer]
You could also get the answer by doing $P(S \cap C) + P(S \cap C') + P(S' \cap C)$.

b) Let P(H) be the probability of drawing at least two hearts, and let C_1, C_2 and C_3 be the event of selecting a heart with the first, second and third card respectively.
Draw a tree diagram to calculate the probability of $P(H \cap C_1)$:

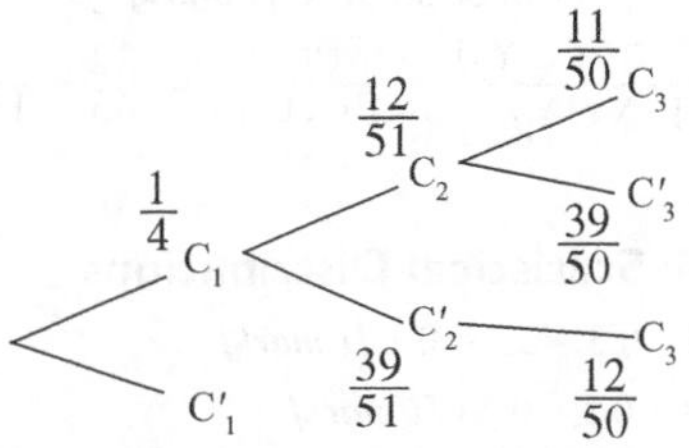

The branches of this tree diagram that are labelled with probabilities are the only ones where both a heart is selected first and at least two hearts are selected, so:

$$P(H \cap C_1) = \left(\frac{1}{4} \times \frac{12}{51} \times \frac{11}{50}\right) + \left(\frac{1}{4} \times \frac{12}{51} \times \frac{39}{50}\right) + \left(\frac{1}{4} \times \frac{39}{51} \times \frac{12}{50}\right) = \frac{89}{850}$$

So, $P(H \mid C_1) = \frac{P(H \cap C_1)}{P(C_1)} = \frac{89}{850} \div \frac{1}{4} = \frac{356}{850}$
$= 0.419$ (3 s.f.)
[3 marks available — 1 mark for a correct method to find P(H ∩ C₁), 1 mark for P(H ∩ C₁) correct and 1 mark for the correct answer]
You could also get this answer without using the formula, by just considering the tree diagram from the point after C_1 has happened.

c) E.g. I have assumed that Jessica is equally likely to select any of the cards in the complete pack of cards.
[1 mark for any sensible comment]

6 a) $P(B|A) \neq P(B)$, so A and B are not independent ***[1 mark]***

b) $P(A) = \frac{P(A \cap B)}{P(B|A)} = \frac{P(A|B)P(B)}{P(B|A)}$
$= \frac{0.31 \times 0.4}{0.25} = 0.496$ ***[1 mark]***

7 a) Draw a Venn diagram using the information you know:

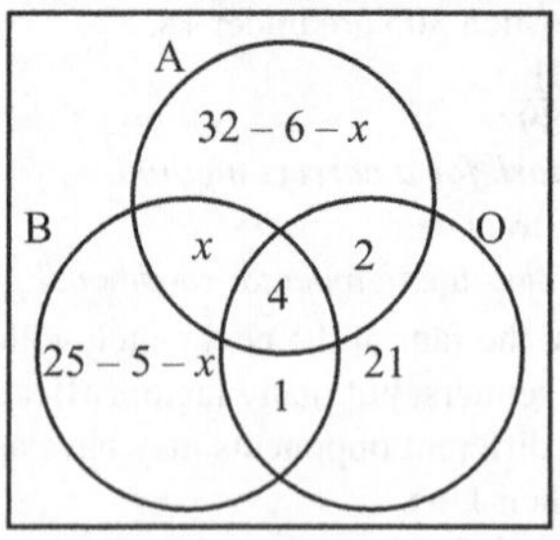

[1 mark]

Everything inside the circles should add up to 65:
$(32 - 6 - x) + x + 4 + 2 + (25 - 5 - x) + 1 + 21 = 65$ ***[1 mark]***
$74 - x = 65 \Rightarrow x = 9$ ***[1 mark]***
So $x + 4 = 13$ children took an apple and a banana ***[1 mark]***

b) Draw a tree diagram (X is the first child selects an apple, Y is the second child selects an apple):

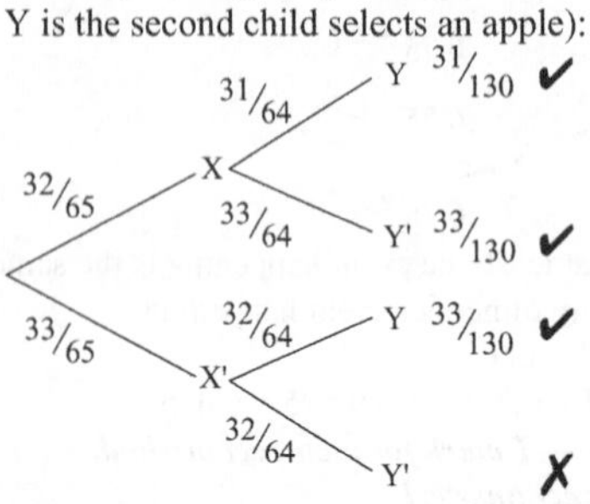

The ticked outcomes are those where at least one person takes an apple. So $P(X \cup Y) = \frac{31}{130} + \frac{33}{130} + \frac{33}{130} = \frac{97}{130}$ ***[1 mark]***

$P(X | X \cup Y) = \frac{P(X \cap (X \cup Y))}{P(X \cup Y)}$ ***[1 mark]***

As all of X is contained within X ∪ Y,
X ∩ (X ∪ Y) will be all of X. ***[1 mark]***

So $\frac{P(X \cap (X \cup Y))}{P(X \cup Y)} = \frac{P(X)}{P(X \cup Y)} = \frac{32}{65} \div \frac{97}{130} = \frac{64}{97}$ ***[1 mark]***

Pages 78-84: Statistical Distributions

1 a) $1 - 0.4 - 0.3 - 0.2 = 0.1$ ***[1 mark]***

b) $2 \times 0.4 \times 0.3 = 0.24$ ***[1 mark]***
To score a total of 1, one contestant must score 0 and the other scores 1. There are 2 possible ways that this can happen.

2 a) x can only take the values 1 to 6, so $P(X = 10) = 0$ ***[1 mark]***.

b) The total probability must be 1, so go through all the possible values of x and add the probabilities:
$$\frac{k}{6} + \frac{2k}{6} + \frac{3k}{6} + \frac{3k}{6} + \frac{2k}{6} + \frac{k}{6} = \frac{12k}{6} = 2k$$ ***[1 mark]***.
This must equal 1, so k must be $\frac{1}{2}$ ***[1 mark]***.

c) $P(1 < X \leq 4) = P(X = 2) + P(X = 3) + P(X = 4)$ ***[1 mark]***
$= \frac{1}{6} + \frac{1}{4} + \frac{1}{4} = \frac{2}{3}$ ***[1 mark]***

3 a) The probability of getting 3 heads is: $\frac{1}{2} \times \frac{1}{2} \times \frac{1}{2} = \frac{1}{8}$

The probability of getting 2 heads is: $3 \times \frac{1}{2} \times \frac{1}{2} \times \frac{1}{2} = \frac{3}{8}$
(multiply by 3 because any of the three coins could be the tail — the order of the heads and the tail isn't important).
The probability of getting 1 or 0 heads
$= 1 - P(\text{2 heads}) - P(\text{3 heads}) = 1 - \frac{3}{8} - \frac{1}{8} = \frac{1}{2}$
Hence the probability distribution of X is:

x	20p	10p	nothing
$P(X = x)$	$\frac{1}{8}$	$\frac{3}{8}$	$\frac{1}{2}$

[3 marks for a completely correct table, otherwise 1 mark for drawing a table with the correct values of x and 1 mark for any one correct probability]

b) There are three ways to make a profit over two games: win 20p and 10p, win 10p and 20p, or win 20p and 20p.
So P(makes profit over 2 games)
$= \left(\frac{1}{8} \times \frac{3}{8}\right) + \left(\frac{3}{8} \times \frac{1}{8}\right) + \left(\frac{1}{8} \times \frac{1}{8}\right)$
$= \frac{3}{64} + \frac{3}{64} + \frac{1}{64} = \frac{7}{64}$ ***[1 mark]***
$P(\text{wins 40p}) = \frac{1}{8} \times \frac{1}{8} = \frac{1}{64}$ ***[1 mark]***
P(wins 40p | makes profit over two games)
$= \frac{P(\text{wins 40p and makes profit})}{P(\text{makes profit})} = \frac{P(\text{wins 40p})}{P(\text{makes profit})}$ ***[1 mark]***
$= \frac{1/64}{7/64} = \frac{1}{7}$ ***[1 mark]***

4 a) - The probability P(chocolate bar contains a golden ticket) must be constant.
- The trials must be independent (i.e. whether or not a chocolate bar contains a golden ticket must be independent of other chocolate bars). ***[1 mark for each correct condition]***

b) $P(X > 1) = 1 - P(X \leq 1)$ ***[1 mark]***
$= 1 - 0.3990... = 0.6009$ (4 d.p.) ***[1 mark]***.

c) If more than 35 bars do not contain a golden ticket, then the student finds 4 or fewer golden tickets.
So find $P(X \leq 4)$ ***[1 mark]*** $= 0.9520$ (4 d.p.) ***[1 mark]***

5 a) Let the random variable X represent the number of cars in the sample of 20 that develop the rattle.
Then $X \sim B(20, 0.65)$ ***[1 mark]***,
and you need to find $P(12 \leq X < 15)$.
$P(12 \leq X < 15) = P(X \leq 14) - P(X \leq 11)$
$= 0.7546... - 0.2376...$ ***[1 mark for either]***
$= 0.5170$ (4 d.p.) ***[1 mark]***

b) $P(X > 10) = 1 - P(X \leq 10)$ ***[1 mark]***
$= 1 - 0.1217...$
$= 0.8782... = 0.8782$ (4 d.p.) ***[1 mark]***.

c) The probability of more than half of a sample of 20 cars having the rattle is 0.8782... (from part b).
Let Q be the number of samples containing more than 10 rattling cars. Then $Q \sim B(5, 0.8782...)$ ***[1 mark]***.
$$P(Q = 3) = \binom{5}{3} \times 0.8782...^3 \times (1 - 0.8782...)^2$$ ***[1 mark]***
$= 0.1005$ (to 4 d.p.) ***[1 mark]***
You could use your calculator's binomial p.d.f. to find P(Q = 3).

6 a) Let X be the number of customers in the sample of 20 who chose a sugar cone. Then $X \sim B(n, p)$ where $n = 20$, but you need to find p (the probability of choosing a sugar cone).
p is equal to the proportion of customers on the 1st July who chose a sugar cone, so:
$p = \frac{880}{1100} = 0.8$ ***[1 mark]***, so $X \sim B(20, 0.8)$ ***[1 mark]***
$P(X = 12) = \binom{20}{12} \times 0.8^{12} \times 0.2^{8}$ ***[1 mark]***
$= 0.0222$ (4 d.p.) ***[1 mark]***
You could use your calculator's binomial functions to find P(X = 12).

b) Let Y be the number of customers who choose at least one scoop of chocolate ice cream.
Then $Y \sim B(75, 0.42)$ ***[1 mark]***.
$P(Y > 30) = 1 - P(Y \leq 30)$ ***[1 mark]***
$= 1 - 0.4099... = 0.5901$ (4 d.p.) ***[1 mark]***
You need to use your calculator's binomial c.d.f. to find P(Y ≤ 30).

c) E.g. it is not reasonable to assume that the customers' choices of ice cream are independent of each other, e.g. one person might see another person with a chocolate ice cream and decide to get one too, so the 75 trials are not independent. / The probability of choosing chocolate ice cream may not be constant, e.g. it might run out. Therefore the model may not be valid.
[1 mark for a sensible comment]

7 a) E.g. The model is appropriate because (any two of):
- The histogram is roughly the shape of a normal distribution (i.e. bell-shaped).
- The histogram is roughly symmetrical about the mean.
- All the data lies between 2.0 kg and 5.0 kg (and 3 standard deviations from the mean is the range 2.05-5.05 kg).

[2 marks for stating the model is appropriate and giving two sensible reasons, otherwise 1 mark for a sensible comment]

b) Let M represent the masses of the newborn babies.
$M \sim N(3.55, 0.5^2)$
$P(M < 2.5) = 0.0179$ (4 d.p.)
[2 marks available — 1 mark for setting up the calculation correctly, 1 mark for the correct answer]

8 a) The mean lies halfway between the points of inflection,
so $\mu = \frac{5940 + 6030}{2} = 5985$ ml ***[1 mark]***
The points of inflection occur at $\mu \pm \sigma$,
so $6030 = 5985 + \sigma \Rightarrow \sigma = 45$ ml ***[1 mark]***
You could have found μ and σ by setting up and solving two simultaneous equations ($\mu + \sigma = 6030$ and $\mu - \sigma = 5940$), or by finding σ first.

b) $v \sim N(5985, 45^2)$
$P(5900 \leq v \leq 6100) = 0.9652$ (4 d.p.)
[2 marks available — 1 mark for setting up the calculation correctly, 1 mark for the correct answer]

9 a) Let X represent the exam marks. Then $X \sim N(50, 15^2)$.
$P(X < 30) = 0.0912$ (4 d.p.)
[2 marks available — 1 mark for setting up the calculation correctly, 1 mark for the correct answer]

b) $P(X \geq 41) = 0.7257...$ (4 d.p.) ***[1 mark]***
$0.7257... \times 1000 = 725.7... \approx 726$ candidates passed the exam ***[1 mark]***

c) You need to find x such that $P(X \geq x) = 0.1$
Using the inverse normal function, $x = 69$ marks (to the nearest whole number).
[2 marks available — 1 mark for a correct calculation, 1 mark for the correct answer]

10 a) Let X represent the base diameters. Then $X \sim N(12, \sigma^2)$.
$P(X > 13) = 0.05 \Rightarrow P(X \leq 13) = 0.95$ ***[1 mark]***
So $P\left(Z \leq \frac{13 - 12}{\sigma}\right) = P\left(Z \leq \frac{1}{\sigma}\right) = 0.95$
Using the inverse normal function,
$\Rightarrow \frac{1}{\sigma} = 1.6448...$ ***[1 mark]***
$\Rightarrow \sigma = 1 \div 1.6448... = 0.6079... = 0.608$ inches (to 3 s.f.) ***[1 mark]***

b) $X \sim N(12, 0.6079...^2)$ ***[1 mark]***
$P(X < 10.8) = 0.0242...$ ***[1 mark]***
So you'd expect $0.0242... \times 100 \approx 2$ pizza bases to be discarded ***[1 mark]***.

c) P(at least 1 base too small) = 1 – P(no bases too small)
P(base not too small) = 1 – 0.0242... = 0.9757...
P(no bases too small) = $0.9757...^3 = 0.9291...$ ***[1 mark]***
P(at least 1 base too small) = 1 – 0.9291... ***[1 mark]***
= 0.0709 (4 d.p.) ***[1 mark]***

11 a) $X \sim N(4, 1.1^2)$
$P(X < 3.5) = 0.3247$ (4 d.p.)
[2 marks available — 1 mark for setting up the calculation correctly, 1 mark for the correct answer]

b) 'Deviates from the mean by more than 1 minute' means the window cleaner takes less than 4 – 1 = 3 minutes or more than 4 + 1 = 5 minutes, so you need to find:
$P(X < 3) + P(X > 5) = 0.1816... + 0.1816... = 0.3633$ (4 d.p.)
[3 marks available — 1 mark for finding the values either side of the mean, 1 mark for setting up the calculation correctly, 1 mark for the correct answer]
Here, you could have worked out $1 - P(3 < X < 5)$ instead.

c) You need to find t such that $P(X > t) = 0.01$
Using the inverse normal function, $t = 6.6$ mins (1 d.p.) (in minutes and seconds, this is 6 min and 36 seconds).
[2 marks available — 1 mark for a correct calculation, 1 mark for the correct answer]

12 a) $M \sim N(93, \sigma^2)$ and $P(M \geq 95) = 0.2$ ***[1 mark]***.
So $P(M < 95) = 0.8$.
Transform this to a statement about the standard normal variable Z by subtracting the mean and dividing by the standard deviation:
$P\left(Z < \frac{95 - 93}{\sigma}\right) = 0.8 \Rightarrow P\left(Z < \frac{2}{\sigma}\right) = 0.8$
Using the inverse normal function: $\frac{2}{\sigma} = 0.8416...$ ***[1 mark]***.
So $\sigma = \frac{2}{0.8416...} = 2.3763...$ ***[1 mark]***.
So $M \sim N(93, 2.3763...^2)$, and you need to find $P(M < 88)$.
So the probability that a packet cannot be sold is
$P(M < 88)$ ***[1 mark]*** = 0.0176... = 0.0177 (4 d.p.) ***[1 mark]***.

b) First, you need to set up a binomial distribution for P, the number of packets that cannot be sold.
So $P \sim B(20, 0.0176...)$ ***[1 mark]***. You need to find
$P(P = 1) = \binom{20}{1} \times 0.0176...^1 \times (1 - 0.0176...)^{19}$ ***[1 mark]***
= 0.2520 (4 d.p.) ***[1 mark]***
Here, you had to spot that you needed to set up a binomial distribution — otherwise you'd have been a bit stuck.

13 a) S represents the number of sampled customers at Soutergate Cinema who went to see the superhero film,
so $S \sim B(200, 0.48)$ ***[1 mark]***.

b) A normal approximation is appropriate here because n is large (here, it's 200) ***[1 mark]*** and p is close to 0.5 (it's 0.48) ***[1 mark]***.

c) mean $\approx 200 \times 0.48 = 96$ ***[1 mark]***
(standard deviation)$^2 \approx 200 \times 0.48 \times (1 - 0.48) = 49.92$,
so standard deviation $\approx \sqrt{49.92} = 7.07$ (3 s.f.) ***[1 mark]***
$S \sim B(200, 0.48)$ can be approximated by $C \sim N(96, 49.92)$.

d) A normal approximation would not be appropriate in this situation ***[1 mark]***, as p is not close to 0.5 (it's 0.03) ***[1 mark]***.
You could also say that $np = 90 \times 0.03 = 2.7 < 5$.

e) Let V represent the number of sampled customers at Vulcan Cinema who went to see the horror film. Then $V \sim B(90, 0.03)$.
$P(V > 4) = 1 - P(V \leq 4) = 1 - 0.86588... = 0.1341$ (4 d.p.)
[3 marks available — 1 mark for setting up the correct binomial distribution, 1 mark for a correct calculation, 1 mark for the correct answer]

Pages 85-88: Statistical Hypothesis Testing

1 Quota sampling ***[1 mark]***

2 a) All the pupils in her school ***[1 mark]***.

b) Opportunity (or convenience) sampling ***[1 mark]***
It is unlikely to be representative because, e.g: the members of the sample are all in the same age group, so won't represent the whole school / older pupils are likely to have different views on politics to younger pupils / A-level politics students might be biased towards certain views / all the pupils who aren't in Josie's A-level politics class are excluded from the sample.
[1 mark for a sensible explanation]

3 a) E.g. people in different age groups may be likely to receive higher or lower pay rises, so it is important that the proportion in each age group in the sample is representative of the proportion in the population.
[1 mark for a sensible explanation]

b) Total population of working adults
= 1200 + 2100 + 3500 + 3200 + 1500 = 11 500
18-27 years: $\frac{1200}{11\,500} \times 50 = 5.217... \approx 5$
28-37 years: $\frac{2100}{11\,500} \times 50 = 9.130... \approx 9$
38-47 years: $\frac{3500}{11\,500} \times 50 = 15.217... \approx 15$
48-57 years: $\frac{3200}{11\,500} \times 50 = 13.913... \approx 14$
Over 57 years: $\frac{1500}{11\,500} \times 50 = 6.521... \approx 7$
[3 marks available — 1 mark for using the correct total in the calculations, 1 mark for at least 2 correct values, 1 mark for all 5 correct values]

c) Jamila can't use her data to draw conclusions about the whole population because, e.g: she only has data for one small town in one location / the types of employment in her town might not be representative of the whole of the UK / the age distribution of the working adults in Jamila's town might not be representative of the whole of the UK.
[1 mark for a sensible explanation]

4 a) If p = proportion of days on which it usually rains, then H_0: $p = 0.5$ and H_1: $p \neq 0.5$ ***[1 mark]***.
Let X = number of sampled days on which it rained.
Under H_0, $X \sim B(20, 0.5)$. ***[1 mark]***
Under H_0, you'd expect there to be $20 \times 0.5 = 10$ days on which it rained. The observed value of 4 is less than this, so you're interested in the lower tail.
Find the p-value of obtaining 4 or less:
$P(X \leq 4) = 0.0059$ (4 d.p.) ***[1 mark]***
It's a 2-tail test, so the probability in each tail is 0.005.
$0.0059 > 0.005$ ***[1 mark]***, so the result is not significant ***[1 mark]***.
There is insufficient evidence at the 1% level to suggest that the proportion of days on which it rained in the year Adil is investigating has changed ***[1 mark]***.
0.0059 is only just bigger than 0.005 — at the 5% level of significance there is sufficient evidence to reject H_0.
If you prefer, you can carry out the test in part a) by finding the critical region. You get a critical region of $X \leq 3$ or $X \geq 17$.

b) The probability of incorrectly rejecting the null hypothesis equals the actual significance level of the test. The critical region for this test is in two parts.
The first part is $X \leq 5$, since $P(X \leq 5) = 0.02069...$
(and $P(X \leq 6) = 0.0576... > 0.025$) ***[1 mark]***.
The second part is $X \geq 15$, since $P(X \geq 15) = 0.02069...$
(and $P(X \geq 14) = 0.0576... > 0.025$) ***[1 mark]***.
So the actual significance level and the probability of incorrectly rejecting the null hypothesis is
$0.02069... + 0.02069... = 0.04138... = 0.0414$ (3 s.f.) ***[1 mark]***.

5 a) If p = proportion of students who have done judo for at least two years, then H_0: $p = 0.2$ and H_1: $p \neq 0.2$. ***[1 mark for both]***.
Let X = number of students in the sample of 20 who have done judo for at least two years. Under H_0, $X \sim B(20, 0.2)$ ***[1 mark]***, and you'd expect there to be $20 \times 0.2 = 4$ students in the sample who have done judo for at least two years. The observed value of 7 is more than this, so you're interested in the upper tail, i.e. when $X \geq 7$ ***[1 mark]***.
Find the probability of a value of 7 or more:
$P(X \geq 7) = 1 - P(X \leq 6)$
$= 1 - 0.9133... = 0.0867$ (4 d.p.) ***[1 mark]***
It's a 2-tail test, so there's a probability of 0.025 in each tail.
$0.0867 > 0.025$, so the result is not significant ***[1 mark]***.
There is insufficient evidence at the 5% level to suggest that the percentage who have done judo for at least two years is different ***[1 mark]***.
You might have chosen to find the critical region instead of the p-value. Here's the working you'd need — you can either generate these values one by one or you might be able to use your calculator to generate a table of values for the distribution.
It's a 2-tail test, so the critical region is split into two, with a probability of ≤ 0.025 in each tail.
For the lower tail:
$P(X \leq 0) = 0.0115$ and $P(X \leq 1) = 0.0692$
For the upper tail:
$P(X \geq 9) = 1 - 0.9900 = 0.0100$ and
$P(X \geq 8) = 1 - 0.9679 = 0.0321$
So the critical region is $X = 0$ or $X \geq 9$.
7 does not lie in the critical region, so do not reject H_0.

b) E.g. One assumption is that the sample members are independent of each other, so that one member having done judo for at least two years doesn't affect whether another member has. This is likely to be true for Nate's test as he has chosen sample members randomly from all his students.
A second assumption is that there is a constant probability of students having done judo for at least two years. This is likely to be true for Nate's test as by randomly selecting the sample from the whole population, he will avoid selecting only 'basic' or 'advanced' students.
[4 marks available — 1 mark each for two suitable assumptions, 1 mark each for two sensible comments that show that the assumptions are likely to be correct]

6 If p = proportion of gym members who use the pool, then H_0: $p = 0.45$ and H_1: $p < 0.45$ ***[1 mark]***.
Let X be the number of people in a sample of 50 who use the pool. Then under H_0, $X \sim B(50, 0.45)$ and the result of the test is that the manager rejects H_0, so you're looking for the biggest possible value x such that $P(X \leq x) \leq 0.05$ ***[1 mark]***.
$P(X \leq 16) = 0.0427$ and $P(X \leq 17) = 0.0765$
[1 mark for both probabilities].
So the maximum possible number in the sample who use the pool is 16 ***[1 mark]***.
You might be able to use your calculator to generate a table of values for the distribution, rather than working them out one at a time.

7 Let X represent the mass (in g) of a chocolate muffin and let μ = mean mass (in g) of the chocolate muffins.
Then H_0: $\mu = 110$ and H_1: $\mu < 110$ ***[1 mark]***.
Under H_0, $X \sim N(110, 3^2)$, so $\overline{X} \sim N(110, 0.6)$
(since $\frac{\sigma^2}{n} = \frac{3^2}{15} = 0.6$). Find the probability of a value of $\overline{X}$ at least as extreme as the observed value:
$$P(\overline{X} < 108.5) = P\left(Z < \frac{108.5 - 110}{\sqrt{0.6}}\right)$$
$$= P(Z < -1.9364...) = 0.0264 \text{ (4 d.p.)}$$
[1 mark for both $\overline{X} \sim N(110, 0.6)$ and $\overline{X} < 108.5$, 1 mark for the correct probability]
$0.0264 < 0.1$, so the result is significant ***[1 mark]***.
There is sufficient evidence at the 10% level to suggest that the mean mass of the chocolate muffins is less than 110 g ***[1 mark]***.
If you chose to find the critical region for this test, you should have found a CR of $\overline{X} < 109.2$ g.

8 Let X represent the height (in cm) of a sunflower in the second field and let μ = mean height (in cm) of the sunflowers in the second field.
Then H_0: $\mu = 150$ and H_1: $\mu \neq 150$ ***[1 mark]***.
Under H_0, $X \sim N(150, 20)$, so $\overline{X} \sim N\left(150, \frac{20}{6}\right)$ ***[1 mark]***.
$$\overline{x} = 140, \text{ so } z = \frac{140 - 150}{\sqrt{20}/\sqrt{6}} = -5.4772... \text{ [1 mark]}$$
It's a 2-tail test at the 1% level, so the critical region is given by $P(Z > z) = 0.005$ or $P(Z < -z) = 0.005$.
Using your calculator, $P(Z > 2.5758) = 0.005$, so the critical region is $Z < -2.5758$ or $Z > 2.5758$.
$-5.4772... < -2.5758$, so it lies in the critical region and the result is significant ***[1 mark]***. There is sufficient evidence at the 1% level to suggest that the mean height of the sunflowers in the second field is different from the first field ***[1 mark]***.
If you chose to find the p-value instead of the critical region, you should have calculated $P(\overline{X} \leq 140)$ or $P(Z \leq -5.4772...) = 2.16023 \times 10^{-8}$, which is less than 0.005, so the result is significant.

9 a) Let μ = mean car wash duration (in minutes).
Then H_0: $\mu = 8$ and H_1: $\mu < 8$ ***[1 mark]***.
Under H_0, $X \sim N(8, 1.2)$, so $\overline{X} \sim N(8, 0.06)$.
Find the probability of a value of $\overline{X}$ at least as extreme as the observed value:

$$P(\overline{X} \leq 7.8) = P\left(Z \leq \frac{7.8 - 8}{\sqrt{0.06}}\right)$$
$$= P(Z \leq -0.8164...) = 0.2071 \text{ (4 d.p.)}$$

[1 mark for both $\overline{X} \sim N(8, 0.06)$ and $\overline{X} \leq 7.8$, 1 mark for the correct probability]

0.2071 > 0.05, so the result is not significant ***[1 mark]***.
There is insufficient evidence at the 5% level to suggest that the mean car wash duration has fallen ***[1 mark]***.

b) To fail to reject the null hypothesis requires z such that $P(Z < z) = 0.05$. $P(Z < -1.6449) = 0.05$, so $z = -1.6449$.

$$z = \frac{\overline{x} - 8}{\sqrt{0.06}} = -1.6449 \text{ [1 mark]} \Rightarrow \overline{x} = 7.597...$$

So the least value is 7.60 minutes (3 s.f.) ***[1 mark]***.

10 a) Let X represent the journey time (in minutes).
Assuming $X \sim N(27, 6.1^2)$, then $\overline{X} \sim N\left(27, \frac{6.1^2}{45}\right)$ ***[1 mark]***.

$$P(\overline{X} \leq 24.8) = P\left(Z \leq \frac{24.8 - 27}{6.1/\sqrt{45}}\right) \text{ [1 mark]}$$
$$= P(Z \leq -2.419...) = 0.00777 \text{ (3 s.f.) [1 mark]}$$

b) E.g. The probability must be compared to a given significance level to draw a valid conclusion to the hypothesis test. ***[1 mark]***

c) E.g. The data was collected on a single day, so it may not be a representative sample (e.g. if the traffic was particularly good or bad on this day). ***[1 mark]***

Pages 89-91: Correlation and Regression

1 0.799 ***[1 mark]***
A correlation coefficient is always between –1 and 1, and 1 corresponds to a strong positive correlation.

2 a)

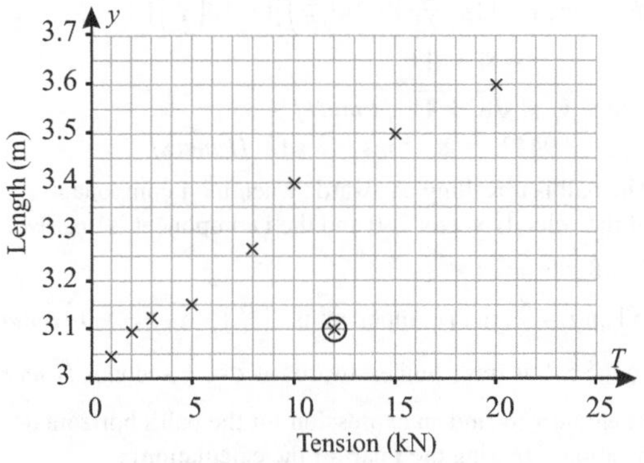

[1 mark for correctly circled point]

b) Strong positive correlation — as the tension (T) increases, the length of the cable (y) also increases ***[1 mark]***.

c) a represents the length of the cable when it is not under tension, so when $T = 0$, the cable is 3 m long ***[1 mark]***.
b represents the extension of the cable, so for every 1 kN increase in tension, the length of the cable increases by 0.03 m ***[1 mark]***.

d) The estimate for 50 kilonewtons may be unreliable as it involves extrapolating beyond the range of the experimental data ***[1 mark]***.

3 a) E.g. The diagram does show negative correlation overall, so Jiao's claim seems reasonable ***[1 mark]***. However, the data is clearly grouped into two clusters (possibly one for rural locations and one for urban locations), with little correlation within each cluster ***[1 mark]***.

b) E.g. Although correlation doesn't necessarily mean causation, in this case it seems reasonable that Killian is correct, as a habitat where reindeer thrive (e.g. a woodland) will not be densely populated — if it were, it would no longer be woodland so the deer population would decrease. / No, Killian is not likely to be correct — there could be a third factor affecting both populations (e.g. climate — reindeer prefer a colder climate, whereas population density for people is higher in more temperate regions.) ***[1 mark for a suitable statement, 1 mark for a sensible explanation]***

4 Call the PMCC for the whole population ρ.
Then H_0: $\rho = 0$, H_1: $\rho > 0$ ***[1 mark for both]*** (so this is a 1-tail test).
The test statistic is $r = 0.634$.
The significance level is $\alpha = 0.05$.
The critical value for a sample size of 10 is 0.5494.
Since 0.634 > 0.5494, the result is significant and there is evidence at the 5% level of significance to reject H_0 and to support the alternative hypothesis. There is evidence that the PMCC between floor area and advertised price of houses on the website is positive ***[1 mark]***.

5 a) (Moderate) positive correlation — the greater the engine size, the greater the amount of carbon dioxide emissions produced ***[1 mark]***.

b) E.g. Sammi's claim is not supported because the correlation shown in the graph is just for Volkswagen vehicles.
It doesn't say anything about cars of other makes.
[2 marks available — 1 mark for identifying that the claim is not supported, 1 mark for a suitable explanation]

c) Call the PMCC for the whole population ρ. Then H_0: $\rho = 0$, H_1: $\rho \neq 0$ ***[1 mark for both]*** (so this is a 2-tail test).
The test statistic is $r = 0.3371$.
The significance level is $\alpha = 0.01$.
The critical value for a sample size of 17 is 0.6055.
Since 0.3371 < 0.6055, the result is not significant and there is insufficient evidence at the 1% level of significance to reject H_0 and to support the alternative hypothesis that the engine sizes of the Volkswagen vehicles and the hydrocarbon emissions produced by them are correlated ***[1 mark]***.

Section Three — Mechanics

Pages 92-96: Kinematics — 1

1 Displacement (S) is given by the area under the graph.
The area under the line is the area of a trapezium:
area under the line = $\frac{U+V}{2} \times T$
So $S = \frac{1}{2}(U + V)T$, as required.
[3 marks available — 1 mark for stating that displacement is the area under the graph, 1 mark for a using a suitable method to find the area under the line, 1 mark for the correct conclusion]

2 a) $u = 5, v = 0, a = -9.8, t = ?$
Using $v = u + at$: $0 = 5 - 9.8t \Rightarrow t = 5 \div 9.8 = 0.5102...$
$t = 0.51$ s (2 s.f.)
[3 marks available — 1 mark for using appropriate equation, 1 mark for correct workings, 1 mark for correct value of t]

b) $s = -2, u = 5, v = ?, a = -9.8$
Using $v^2 = u^2 + 2as$:
$v^2 = 5^2 + 2(-9.8 \times -2) = 64.2 \Rightarrow v = -8.0124...$
$= -8.0$ ms^{-1} (2 s.f.)
The velocity is negative when it reaches B as the ball is travelling in the negative direction (you can also see this from the graph).
[3 marks available — 1 mark for using appropriate equation, 1 mark for correct workings, 1 mark for correct value of v]

c) E.g. The graph shows the ball instantaneously changing velocity from point B to point C, which is unrealistic.
[1 mark for any sensible comment]

3 From passing the sign to entering the tunnel:
$s = ut + \frac{1}{2}at^2 \Rightarrow 110 = 8u + \frac{1}{2}(a \times 8^2)$ ***[1 mark]***
$\Rightarrow 110 = 8u + 32a$ ① ***[1 mark]***
From passing the sign to leaving the tunnel:
$s = ut + \frac{1}{2}at^2 \Rightarrow 870 = 32u + \frac{1}{2}(a \times 32^2)$ ***[1 mark]***
$\Rightarrow 870 = 32u + 512a$ ② ***[1 mark]***
② – 4 × ① gives:
$430 = 384a \Rightarrow a = 1.119... = 1.12$ ms^{-2} (3 s.f.) ***[1 mark]***
Substitute back into ① to find u:
$110 = 8u + 32a$
$u = \frac{110 - 32(1.119...)}{8} = 9.270... = 9.27$ ms^{-1} (3 s.f.) ***[1 mark]***

4 Using $\mathbf{v} = \mathbf{u} + \mathbf{a}t$:
$\mathbf{v} = (7\mathbf{i} - 3\mathbf{j}) + 2(\mathbf{i} + 4\mathbf{j}) = (9\mathbf{i} + 5\mathbf{j})$ ms^{-1} ***[1 mark]***

5 $s = \int v \, dt = \frac{11}{2}t^2 - \frac{2}{3}t^3 + c$ for $0 \le t \le 5$.
When $t = 0, s = 0 \Rightarrow c = 0$, so $s = \frac{11}{2}t^2 - \frac{2}{3}t^3$
So when $t = 5$:
$s = \frac{11}{2}(25) - \frac{2}{3}(125) = 54.16... = 54.2$ m (3 s.f.)
[4 marks available — 1 mark for integrating with respect to time, 1 mark for obtaining an expression for s, 1 mark for finding c, 1 mark for correct final answer]

6 a) $a = \frac{dv}{dt}$ ***[1 mark]***
$a = 2 - 3(-2)e^{-2t} = (2 + 6e^{-2t})$ ms^{-2} ***[1 mark]***

b) t must be greater than or equal to 0.
When $t = 0$, $a = 2 + 6e^{-2\times 0} = 8$ ms^{-2} ***[1 mark]***
As $t \to \infty, 6e^{-2t} \to 0$, so $a \to 2$ ms^{-2} ***[1 mark]***
So, $2 < a \le 8$ ***[1 mark]***

c) $s = \int v \, dt$ ***[1 mark]***
$s = t^2 + \frac{3}{2}e^{-2t} + 4t + c$ ***[1 mark]***
When $t = 0$, the particle is at the origin (i.e. $s = 0$):
$0 = 0 + \frac{3}{2} + c \Rightarrow c = -\frac{3}{2}$
So, $s = \left(t^2 + \frac{3}{2}e^{-2t} + 4t - \frac{3}{2}\right)$ m ***[1 mark]***

7 a) Find the acceleration using the displacement at $t = 3$:
$\mathbf{u} = 0\mathbf{i} + 0\mathbf{j}, \mathbf{a} = \mathbf{a}, \mathbf{s} = (9\mathbf{i} - 18\mathbf{j}), t = 3$
$\mathbf{s} = \mathbf{u}t + \frac{1}{2}\mathbf{a}t^2$
$(9\mathbf{i} - 18\mathbf{j}) = \frac{1}{2} \times \mathbf{a} \times 3^2$ ***[1 mark]***
$(9\mathbf{i} - 18\mathbf{j}) = 4.5\mathbf{a} \Rightarrow \mathbf{a} = (2\mathbf{i} - 4\mathbf{j})$ ms^{-2} ***[1 mark]***
The particle starts at O, so its position vector at time t is equal to its displacement:
So $\mathbf{p} = \mathbf{s} = \frac{1}{2}(2\mathbf{i} - 4\mathbf{j})t^2$ ***[1 mark]***
$\mathbf{p} = (\mathbf{i} - 2\mathbf{j})t^2$ m ***[1 mark]***

b) Find an expression for the second particle's displacement after t seconds:
$\mathbf{s} = \mathbf{v}t$
$\mathbf{s} = (3\mathbf{i} - 5\mathbf{j})t$ ***[1 mark]***
So the second particle's position vector at time t is:
$\mathbf{q} = (a\mathbf{i} + b\mathbf{j}) + (3\mathbf{i} - 5\mathbf{j})t$
When they collide, their position vectors are equal:
$(\mathbf{i} - 2\mathbf{j})t^2 = (a\mathbf{i} + b\mathbf{j}) + (3\mathbf{i} - 5\mathbf{j})t$
$t = 8$, so:
$64(\mathbf{i} - 2\mathbf{j}) = (a\mathbf{i} + b\mathbf{j}) + 8(3\mathbf{i} - 5\mathbf{j})$ ***[1 mark]***
$64\mathbf{i} - 128\mathbf{j} - 24\mathbf{i} + 40\mathbf{j} = a\mathbf{i} + b\mathbf{j}$
$40\mathbf{i} - 88\mathbf{j} = a\mathbf{i} + b\mathbf{j}$
So $a = 40$ and $b = -88$ ***[1 mark for both]***

8 Integrate the acceleration to find an expression for the velocity.
a is a constant, so $v = \int a \, dt = at + c$ ***[1 mark]***.
When $t = 0$, $v = u$, so $u = c$ and this gives $v = at + u$ ***[1 mark]***.
Integrate again to find an expression for the object's displacement:
$s = \int v \, dt = \int at + u \, dt = \frac{1}{2}at^2 + ut + k$ ***[1 mark]***.
The object sets off from the origin, so setting $t = 0, s = 0 \Rightarrow k = 0$ which gives $s = ut + \frac{1}{2}at^2$ as required ***[1 mark]***.

9 $\mathbf{v} = \frac{d\mathbf{s}}{dt} = (15t^2 + 14t)\mathbf{i} + 10t\mathbf{j}$ ***[1 mark]***
If $\tan\theta = \frac{1}{2}$, then the **i**-component is double the **j**-component:
$15t^2 + 14t = 2 \times 10t \Rightarrow 15t^2 - 6t = 0$ ***[1 mark]***
$\Rightarrow 3t(5t - 2) = 0 \Rightarrow t = 0$ (reject) or $t = \frac{2}{5}$ ***[1 mark]***
When $t = \frac{2}{5}$, $\mathbf{v} = \left(15\left(\frac{4}{25}\right) + 14\left(\frac{2}{5}\right)\right)\mathbf{i} + 10\left(\frac{2}{5}\right)\mathbf{j}$
$= 8\mathbf{i} + 4\mathbf{j}$
so speed $= |\mathbf{v}| = \sqrt{8^2 + 4^2}$ ***[1 mark]***
$= 8.9442... = 8.94$ ms^{-1} (3 s.f.) ***[1 mark]***

10 a) The ball is travelling eastwards when the **j** component of the velocity vector is 0 and the **i** component is positive.
$3t - 8 = 0 \Rightarrow t = \frac{8}{3}$.
When $t = \frac{8}{3}$, the **i** component is $2\left(\frac{8}{3}\right) - 5 = \frac{1}{3} > 0$ ***[1 mark]***,
so the ball is travelling eastwards at $t = \frac{8}{3}$ seconds ***[1 mark]***.

b) Integrate **v** to find an expression for the ball's horizontal position (ignoring the **j** part of the calculation) :
$\int \mathbf{v}_i \, dt = \mathbf{s}_i = \int (2t - 5)\mathbf{i} \, dt$ ***[1 mark]***
$= (t^2 - 5t)\mathbf{i} + \mathbf{c}$ ***[1 mark]***
When $t = 2$, $\mathbf{s} = -2\mathbf{i} + 10\mathbf{j}$. Use this to find **c**:
$(4 - 10)\mathbf{i} + \mathbf{c} = -2\mathbf{i} \Rightarrow \mathbf{c} = 4\mathbf{i}$ ***[1 mark]***
So, $\mathbf{s}_i = (t^2 - 5t + 4)\mathbf{i}$.
The ball is west of the origin whenever
$t^2 - 5t + 4 < 0 \Rightarrow (t - 1)(t - 4) < 0 \Rightarrow 1 < t < 4$. ***[1 mark]***

11 a) Robot 2: $\mathbf{u} = 0\mathbf{i} + 0\mathbf{j}, \mathbf{v} = \mathbf{v}, \mathbf{a} = (0.4\mathbf{i} + 0.2\mathbf{j}), t = 6$
Using $\mathbf{v} = \mathbf{u} + \mathbf{a}t$:
$\mathbf{v} = 0\mathbf{i} + 0\mathbf{j} + (0.4\mathbf{i} + 0.2\mathbf{j}) \times 6 = (2.4\mathbf{i} + 1.2\mathbf{j})$ ms^{-1}
So speed $= \sqrt{2.4^2 + 1.2^2} = 2.68$ ms^{-1} (3 s.f.)
[3 marks available — 1 mark for a correct method, 1 mark for the correct velocity, 1 mark for the correct answer]

b) Robot 1: $\mathbf{s} = \overrightarrow{AC}$, $\mathbf{u} = (\mathbf{i} + 3\mathbf{j})$, $\mathbf{a} = 0\mathbf{i} + 0\mathbf{j}$, $t = 6$

Using $\mathbf{s} = \mathbf{u}t + \frac{1}{2}\mathbf{a}t^2$:

$\overrightarrow{AC} = ((\mathbf{i} + 3\mathbf{j}) \times 6) + 0 = (6\mathbf{i} + 18\mathbf{j})$ m

Robot 2: $\mathbf{s} = \overrightarrow{BC}$, $\mathbf{u} = 0\mathbf{i} + 0\mathbf{j}$, $\mathbf{a} = (0.4\mathbf{i} + 0.2\mathbf{j})$, $t = 6$

Using $\mathbf{s} = \mathbf{u}t + \frac{1}{2}\mathbf{a}t^2$:

$\overrightarrow{BC} = 0\mathbf{i} + 0\mathbf{j} + \left(\frac{1}{2}(0.4\mathbf{i} + 0.2\mathbf{j}) \times 6^2\right) = (7.2\mathbf{i} + 3.6\mathbf{j})$ m

Then $\overrightarrow{AB} = \overrightarrow{AC} + \overrightarrow{CB} = \overrightarrow{AC} - \overrightarrow{BC}$

$= (6\mathbf{i} + 18\mathbf{j}) - (7.2\mathbf{i} + 3.6\mathbf{j}) = (-1.2\mathbf{i} + 14.4\mathbf{j})$ m

[4 marks available — 1 mark for using suitable suvat equations, 1 mark for finding $\overrightarrow{AC}$, 1 mark for finding $\overrightarrow{BC}$, 1 mark for the correct answer]

c) E.g. That the robots act as particles, that no other external forces act on the robots.

[2 marks in total — 1 mark for each valid answer]

12 $\mathbf{a} = \dot{\mathbf{v}} = [(-6\sin 3t + 5)\mathbf{i} + 2\mathbf{j}]$ ms^{-2}

[1 mark for attempting to differentiate the velocity vector, 1 mark for correctly differentiating both components]

The **j**-component of the acceleration is constant, so the **i**-component is the only one which can be maximised.
To do this, set $\sin 3t = -1$.

sin 3t only takes values between –1 and 1. Choose the value which will give the greatest i-component — you're multiplying it by a negative number, so you want to use –1.

$\mathbf{a} = ((-6 \times -1) + 5)\mathbf{i} + 2\mathbf{j} = 11\mathbf{i} + 2\mathbf{j}$ ***[1 mark]***

Magnitude $= |\mathbf{a}| = \sqrt{11^2 + 2^2}$ ***[1 mark]*** $= \sqrt{121 + 4}$

$= \sqrt{125} = 5\sqrt{5}$ ms^{-2} ***[1 mark]***

Pages 97-98: Kinematics — 2

1 a) Need to find the times when the stone is 22 m above the ground (i.e. when it is at the level of projection), so consider vertical motion, taking up as positive: ***[1 mark]***

$s = 0$, $u = 14\sin 46°$, $a = -9.81$, $t = ?$

Acceleration is constant, so use a constant acceleration formula, e.g. $s = ut + \frac{1}{2}at^2$

$0 = 14\sin 46t° - 4.905t^2$ ***[1 mark]***

$0 = (14\sin 46° - 4.905t)t$

So, $t = 0$ (i.e. when the stone is thrown) or

$14\sin 46° - 4.905t = 0 \Rightarrow t = 2.0531...$ s ***[1 mark]***

So the stone is at least 22 m above the ground for:

$2.0531... - 0 = 2.05$ s (3 s.f.) ***[1 mark]***

b) No acceleration horizontally, so the horizontal component of velocity remains constant at $14\cos 46°$ ms^{-1}. ***[1 mark]***

Consider vertical motion once more, taking up as positive to find the vertical component of the stone's final velocity:

$s = -22$, $u = 14\sin 46°$, $a = -9.81$, $v = ?$

$v^2 = u^2 + 2as = (14\sin 46°)^2 + (2 \times -9.81 \times -22)$ ***[1 mark]***

$= 533.06...$ ***[1 mark]***

Don't bother finding the square root, as you'd only have to square it again in the next bit of the answer.

Speed $= \sqrt{(14\cos 46)^2 + 533.06...}$ ***[1 mark]***

$= 25.052... = 25.1$ ms^{-1} (3 s.f.) ***[1 mark]***

2 a) Let the horizontal displacement when the golf ball hits the ground be X m and the vertical displacement be Y m (up is positive). Then using trigonometry:

$\tan 10° = \frac{Y}{X} \Rightarrow Y = X\tan 10°$ ***[1 mark]***

So the position vector of the golf ball when it hits the ground is:

$(X\mathbf{i} + X\tan 10°\mathbf{j})$ ***[1 mark]***

Now, use **suva**t:

$\mathbf{s} = (X\mathbf{i} + X\tan 10°\mathbf{j})$, $\mathbf{u} = (29\mathbf{i} + 24\mathbf{j})$, $\mathbf{a} = (-9.8\mathbf{j})$, $t = t$

Using $\mathbf{s} = \mathbf{u}t + \frac{1}{2}\mathbf{a}t^2$:

$(X\mathbf{i} + X\tan 10°\mathbf{j}) = (29\mathbf{i} + 24\mathbf{j})t + \frac{1}{2}(-9.8\mathbf{j})t^2$

$\Rightarrow X\mathbf{i} + X\tan 10°\mathbf{j} = 29t\mathbf{i} + (24t - 4.9t^2)\mathbf{j}$ ***[1 mark]***

b) $X\mathbf{i} + X\tan 10°\mathbf{j} = 29t\mathbf{i} + (24t - 4.9t^2)\mathbf{j}$

$\Rightarrow X = 29t \Rightarrow t = \frac{X}{29}$ and $X\tan 10° = 24t - 4.9t^2$ ***[1 mark]***

So $X\tan 10° = 24\left(\frac{X}{29}\right) - 4.9\left(\frac{X}{29}\right)^2$

$\Rightarrow X\tan 10° = \left(\frac{24}{29}\right)X - \left(\frac{4.9}{841}\right)X^2$

$\Rightarrow \left(\frac{4.9}{841}\right)X^2 - \left(\frac{24}{29}\right)X + X\tan 10° = 0$ ***[1 mark]***

$\Rightarrow X\left(\left(\frac{4.9}{841}\right)X - \left(\frac{24}{29}\right) + \tan 10°\right) = 0$

$\Rightarrow X = 0$ (reject)

or $\left(\frac{4.9}{841}\right)X - \left(\frac{24}{29}\right) + \tan 10° = 0 \Rightarrow X = 111.777...$ ***[1 mark]***

So the position vector of the golf ball when it hits the ground is $(X\mathbf{i} + X\tan 10°\mathbf{j}) = (110\mathbf{i} + 20\mathbf{j})$ m (2 s.f.)

[1 mark for each correct component]

3 a) Consider motion vertically, taking up as positive:

$s = ?$, $u = 10\sin 20°$, $v = 0$, $a = -9.8$. ***[1 mark]***

Use $v^2 = u^2 + 2as$:

$0 = (10\sin 20°)^2 - 19.6s$ ***[1 mark]***

$\Rightarrow s = (10\sin 20°)^2 \div 19.6 = 0.59682...$ m ***[1 mark]***

The stone is thrown from 1 m above the ground, so the maximum height reached is $1 + 0.59682... = 1.6$ m (2 s.f.) ***[1 mark]***

b) Again consider vertical motion:

$s = -1$, $u = 10\sin 20°$, $a = -9.8$, $t = ?$.

Use $s = ut + \frac{1}{2}at^2$

$-1 = (10\sin 20°)t - 4.9t^2$ ***[1 mark]***

$\Rightarrow 4.9t^2 - (10\sin 20°)t - 1 = 0$.

Use the quadratic formula to find t:

$t = \dfrac{10\sin 20° + \sqrt{(-10\sin 20°)^2 + (4 \times 4.9 \times 1)}}{9.8}$ ***[1 mark]***

$= 0.91986... = 0.92$ s (2 s.f.) ***[1 mark]***

You don't need to worry about the other value of t that the formula gives you as it will be negative, and the equation isn't valid for t < 0.

c) E.g. Air resistance acting on the stone (affecting acceleration) has not been included in the model, so it may be inaccurate.

[1 mark for any suitable modelling assumption that may affect the accuracy of the model]

Pages 99-104: Forces and Newton's Laws

1 Resolving horizontally:

$P\sin 40° = 20\cos(105° - 90°) \Rightarrow P = 30.1$ N (3 s.f.) ***[1 mark]***

2 Resolving vertically:

$T_1\sin 47° + T_2\sin 32° = 5.2$ ① ***[1 mark]***

Resolving horizontally:

$T_1\cos 47° = T_2\cos 32° \Rightarrow T_2 = \dfrac{T_1\cos 47°}{\cos 32°}$ ② ***[1 mark]***

Substituting ② into ①,

$T_1\sin 47° + T_1\tan 32°\cos 47° = 5.2$ ***[1 mark]***

$T_1 = \dfrac{5.2}{\sin 47° + \tan 32°\cos 47°} = 4.492... = 4.49$ N (3 s.f.) ***[1 mark]***

$T_2 = \dfrac{(4.492...)\cos 47°}{\cos 32°} = 3.612... = 3.61$ N (3 s.f.) ***[1 mark]***

3 If the resultant force is **R** then

$\mathbf{R} = \mathbf{A} + \mathbf{B} = (2\mathbf{i} - 11\mathbf{j}) + (7\mathbf{i} + 5\mathbf{j}) = (9\mathbf{i} - 6\mathbf{j})$ N ***[1 mark]***

Using $\mathbf{F} = m\mathbf{a}$:

$(9\mathbf{i} - 6\mathbf{j}) = 0.5\mathbf{a} \Rightarrow \mathbf{a} = (18\mathbf{i} - 12\mathbf{j})$ ms^{-2} ***[1 mark]***

$\mathbf{v} = \mathbf{u} + \mathbf{a}t = 0 + \mathbf{a} \times 4 = (72\mathbf{i} - 48\mathbf{j})$ ms^{-1} ***[1 mark]***

4 Resolving horizontally: $S\cos 40° = F$ ***[1 mark]***

Resolving vertically: $R = 2g + S\sin 40°$ ***[1 mark]***

The ring is stationary, so $F \leq \mu R$ ***[1 mark]***.

So, $S\cos 40° \leq 0.3(2g + S\sin 40°)$ ***[1 mark]***

$S\cos 40° \leq 0.6g + 0.3S\sin 40°$

$S\cos 40° - 0.3S\sin 40° \leq 0.6g$

$S(\cos 40° - 0.3\sin 40°) \leq 0.6g$

$S \leq 10.3$ N (3 s.f.) ***[1 mark]***

5 a)

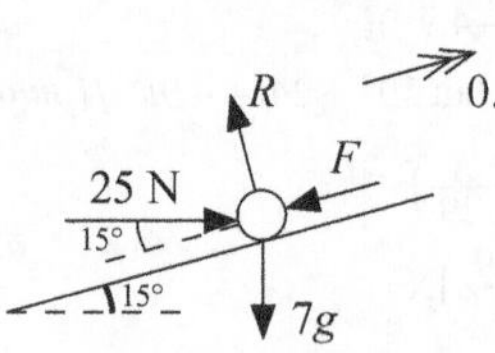

Resolving parallel to the plane (↗):
$F_{net} = ma$
$25\cos 15° - F - 7g\sin 15° = 7 \times 0.2$ ***[1 mark]***
$F = 25\cos 15° - 7g\sin 15° - 1.4$
$F = 4.993...$ N ***[1 mark]***
Resolving perpendicular to the plane (↖):
$F_{net} = ma$
$R - 25\sin 15° - 7g\cos 15° = 7 \times 0$ ***[1 mark]***
$R = 25\sin 15° + 7g\cos 15° = 72.732...$ N
Using $F = \mu R$: ***[1 mark]***
$4.993... = \mu \times 72.732...$ ***[1 mark]***
$\Rightarrow \mu = 0.0686... = 0.069$ (2 s.f.) ***[1 mark]***

b)

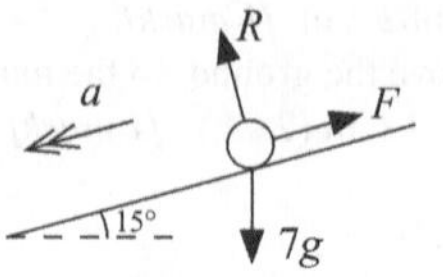

Resolving perpendicular to the plane (↖):
$R = 7g\cos 15°$ ***[1 mark]***
$F = \mu R$ ***[1 mark]***
$F = 0.0686... \times 7g\cos 15°$
Resolving parallel to the plane (↙):
$7g\sin 15° - F = 7a$ ***[1 mark]***
$7g\sin 15° - (0.0686... \times 7g\cos 15°) = 7a$
$a = 1.88...$ ms^{-2} ***[1 mark]***
$s = 3$, $u = 0$, $a = 1.88...$, $t = ?$
$s = ut + \frac{1}{2}at^2$
$3 = \frac{1}{2} \times 1.88... \times t^2$ ***[1 mark]***
$t^2 = 3.18...$
$t = 1.8$ s (2 s.f.) ***[1 mark]***

6

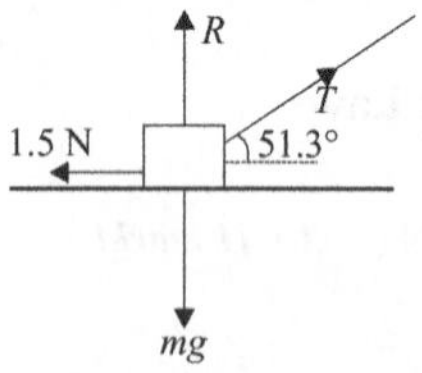

Resolving horizontally:
$1.5 = T\cos 51.3°$ ***[1 mark]***
so $T = \frac{1.5}{\cos 51.3°} = 2.399... = 2.4$ N (2 s.f.) ***[1 mark]***
Resolving vertically:
$mg = R + T\sin 51.3°$ ***[1 mark]***
$R = \frac{F}{\mu} = 1.5 \div 0.6 = 2.5$ N ***[1 mark]***
so $mg = 2.5 + 2.399... \sin 51.3°$
and $m = 0.4461...$ kg $= 0.45$ kg (2 s.f.) ***[1 mark]***

7

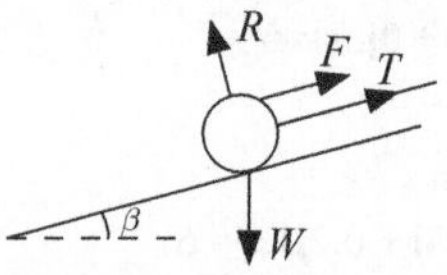

Resolving the forces parallel to the plane (↙):
$W\sin\beta = F + T$ ***[1 mark]***
As the system is in limiting equilibrium, $F = \mu R$, so
$W\sin\beta = \mu R + T$ ***[1 mark]***
Resolving forces perpendicular to the plane (↖):
$W\cos\beta = R$ ***[1 mark]***
Substitute this in for R in the above equation:
$W\sin\beta = \mu W\cos\beta + T$ ***[1 mark]***
$\Rightarrow \mu W\cos\beta = W\sin\beta - T \Rightarrow \mu = \frac{W\sin\beta}{W\cos\beta} - \frac{T}{W\cos\beta}$
$= \tan\beta - \frac{T}{W}\sec\beta$
[1 mark for using trig identities to rearrange into required form]

8 Call the mass of the woman W.
Drawing two force diagrams will really help:

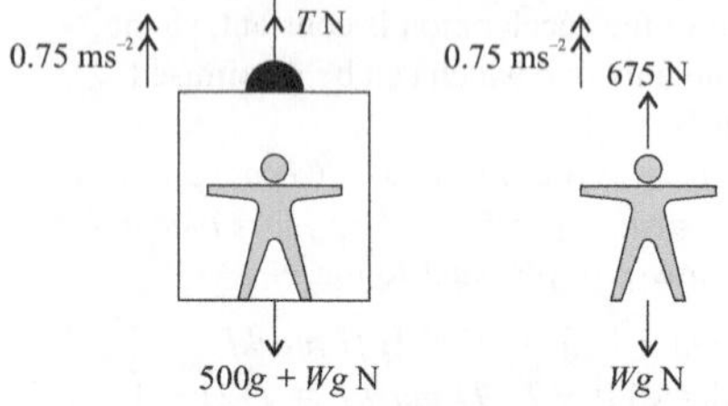

First, use $F = ma$ for the woman in the lift to find her mass:
$675 - Wg = 0.75W \Rightarrow 675 = 0.75W + Wg \Rightarrow W = 63.920...$ kg
Now use $F = ma$ for the whole connected system:
$T - (500 + 63.920...)g = 0.75(500 + 63.920...) \Rightarrow T = 5960$ N (3 s.f.)
[4 marks available — 1 mark for using F = ma for the woman, 1 mark for finding the mass of the woman, 1 mark for using F = ma on the whole system, 1 mark for finding the correct answer]

9 a) The system is at rest, so equating the forces acting on A gives:
$35g - T = 0 \Rightarrow T = 35g$ ***[1 mark]***
Now do the same for forces acting on B:
$Mg + K - T = 0 \Rightarrow K = T - Mg$
Substitute in the value of T to get:
$K = 35g - Mg = g(35 - M)$ ***[1 mark]***

b) i) $v = 1$, $u = 0$, $a = ?$ and $t = 3$. Using $v = u + at$:
$1 = 3a \Rightarrow a = \frac{1}{3}$ ms^{-2} ***[1 mark]***
Using $F = ma$ for A: ***[1 mark]***
$35g - T = 35 \times \frac{1}{3} \Rightarrow T = 35g - \frac{35}{3} = 331.68...$ ***[1 mark]***
Using $F = ma$ for B:
$T - Mg = M \times \frac{1}{3} \Rightarrow T = M(g + \frac{1}{3})$ ***[1 mark]***
$\Rightarrow M = 331.68... \div (g + \frac{1}{3}) = 32.7$ kg (3 s.f.) ***[1 mark]***

ii) E.g. The string is very long, B doesn't reach the pulley, A doesn't reach the ground, acceleration is constant.
[1 mark for a sensible assumption]

10 a)

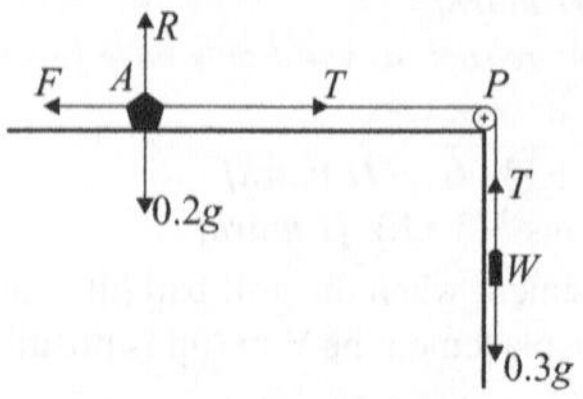

If mass of $A = 0.2$ kg, mass of $W = 1.5 \times 0.2 = 0.3$ kg
For W, $F_{net} = ma$:
$0.3g - T = 0.3(4)$ ***[1 mark]***
$T = 2.94 - 1.2 = 1.74$ ***[1 mark]***
For A, $F_{net} = ma$:
$T - F = 4(0.2) = 0.8$ ***[1 mark]***
$F = \mu R$, but resolving vertically: $R = 0.2g = 1.96$ ***[1 mark]***
So $F = 1.96\mu$, ***[1 mark]***
so $T - 1.96\mu = 0.8$,
$\Rightarrow 1.74 - 1.96\mu = 0.8$
So $\mu = 0.479... = 0.48$ (2 s.f.) ***[1 mark]***

b) Speed of A at h = speed of W at h (where it impacts ground).
Calculate speed of A at h using $v^2 = u^2 + 2as$:
$v^2 = 0^2 + 2(4 \times h)$ ***[1 mark]***
$v^2 = 8h$ ①
Distance travelled by A beyond $h = \frac{3}{4}h$
Calculate frictional force slowing A after h using $F_{net} = ma$:
$F = \mu R$ and $R = mg = 0.2g = 1.96$ ***[1 mark]***
so $F = 0.479... \times 1.96 = 0.94$
so $a = -0.94 \div 0.2 = -4.7$ ms^{-2} ***[1 mark]***
Speed of A at h using $u^2 = v^2 - 2as$:
$u^2 = 3^2 - 2(-4.7 \times \frac{3}{4}h) = 9 + 7.05h$ ***[1 mark]*** ②
Substituting ① into ② (where $v^2 = u^2$):
$8h = 9 + 7.05h$ so $h = 9.473... = 9.5$ m (2 s.f.) ***[1 mark]***
Tricky. The thing to realise is that when W has moved a distance of h and hits the ground, A has also moved a distance of h. A then carries on moving, but is slowed down by friction, so you can calculate the speed of A when it's moved a distance of h in two different ways. This gives you two simultaneous equations that you can solve to find h.

c) Time taken to reach h using $s = ut + \frac{1}{2}at^2$:
$9.473... = (0 \times t) + \frac{1}{2}(4 \times t^2) = 2t^2$ ***[1 mark]***
so $t^2 = 4.736...$ and $t = 2.2$ s (2 s.f.) ***[1 mark]***

d) E.g. The tension is the same throughout the string — so A and W have the same acceleration when W is falling.
[1 mark for a sensible comment]

11 a) Start by adding values to the diagram:

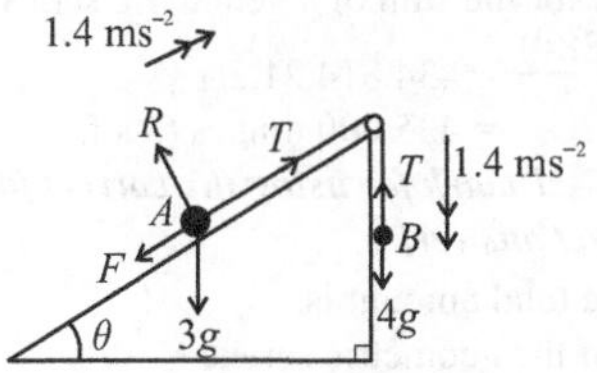

$\tan\theta = \frac{3}{4}$, so you can use the 3-4-5 Pythagorean triple:

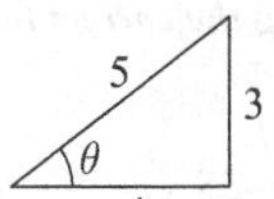

So $\cos\theta = \frac{4}{5}$.
Resolving forces around A perpendicular to the plane (↖):
$R = 3g\cos\theta = 3 \times 9.8 \times \frac{4}{5} = 23.52$ N ***[1 mark]***
Use $F_{net} = ma$ for the vertical motion of B: ***[1 mark]***
$(4 \times 9.8) - T = 4 \times 1.4$
So, $T = 33.6$ N ***[1 mark]***
Use $F_{net} = ma$ for A parallel to the plane:
$T - F - (3 \times 9.8 \sin\theta) = 3 \times 1.4$ ***[1 mark]***
Using the Pythagorean triple again, you know that $\sin\theta = \frac{3}{5}$.
Substitute in values of T and $\sin\theta$:
$33.6 - F - 17.64 = 4.2$
So, $F = 11.76$ N ***[1 mark]***
The system's moving, so friction is 'limiting', i.e. $F = \mu R$ ***[1 mark]***
Rearranging and substituting values in gives:
$\mu = \frac{F}{R} = \frac{11.76}{23.52} = 0.5$ ***[1 mark]***

b) Motion of B: $u = 0$, $a = 1.4$, $s = ?$, $t = 2$
Use $s = ut + \frac{1}{2}at^2$: ***[1 mark]***
$s = 0 + \left(\frac{1}{2} \times 1.4 \times 4\right) = 2.8$ m ***[1 mark]***
Particle B moves 2.8 m before the string breaks.

c) While A and B are attached, they move together at the same speed. So you can use the information given to find the speed of (both) A and B when the string breaks:
$v = u + at = 0 + 1.4 \times 2 = 2.8$ ms^{-1} ***[1 mark]***
Draw a diagram to show the forces on A after the string breaks:

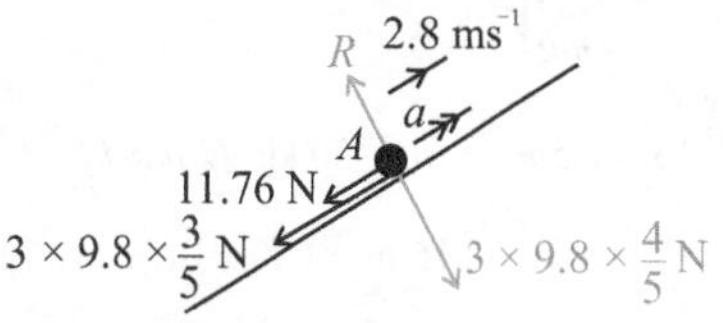

Use $F_{net} = ma$ parallel to the plane to find a:
$-11.76 - \left(3 \times 9.8 \times \frac{3}{5}\right) = 3a$ ***[1 mark]***
So, $a = -9.8$ ms^{-2} ***[1 mark]***
Calculate the distance A travels using $v^2 = u^2 + 2as$ ***[1 mark]***
$u = 2.8$, $v = 0$, $a = -9.8$, $s = ?$, $t = ?$
$s = \frac{v^2 - u^2}{2a} = \frac{0 - 2.8^2}{2 \times -9.8} = 0.4$ m ***[1 mark]***
So particle A moves 0.4 m from the instant the string breaks until it comes to rest.

Pages 105-106: Moments

1

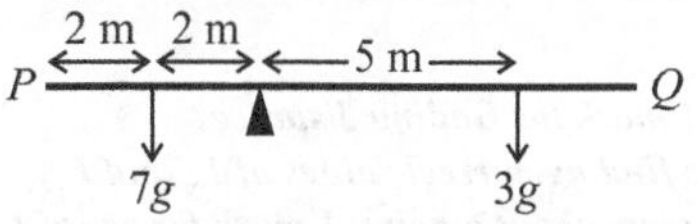

Take moments about the centre of mass, taking clockwise as positive:
Resultant moment = $(3g \times 5) - (7g \times 2) = 15g - 14g = g$
This is positive, so there is a resultant clockwise moment. ***[1 mark]***

2 a) Start by drawing a diagram:

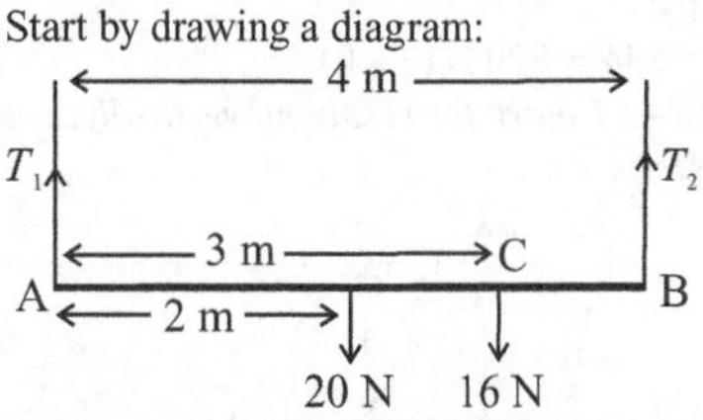

Take moments about A and B, using moments clockwise = moments anticlockwise
A: $(20 \times 2) + (16 \times 3) = T_2 \times 4$
So, $T_2 = 88 \div 4 = 22$
B: $4 \times T_1 = (20 \times 2) + (16 \times 1)$
So, $T_1 = 56 \div 4 = 14$
[3 marks available — 1 mark for taking moments about a point, 1 mark for correct value of T_1, 1 mark for correct value of T_2]
You might've resolved forces vertically or taken moments about other points — if you get the same answers, and show full correct working, then you're fine.

b) Start by drawing a new diagram:

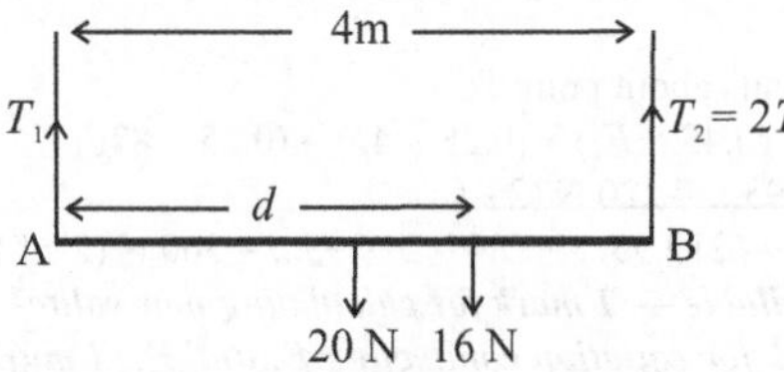

Take moments about A and B:
A: $(20 \times 2) + 16d = 4 \times 2T_1$
So, $T_1 = 5 + 2d$
B: $4T_1 = (20 \times 2) + (4 - d) \times 16$
So, $T_1 = 10 + 16 - 4d = 26 - 4d$
Set the two equations in T_1 equal to each other and solve for d:
$5 + 2d = 26 - 4d \Rightarrow 6d = 21 \Rightarrow d = 3.5$ m
[3 marks available — 1 mark taking moments about a point, 1 mark for attempting to solve simultaneous equations, 1 mark for correct value of d]

3 Let m be the mass of the attached particle. The rod is on the point of tilting about C, so the only reaction force is at C.

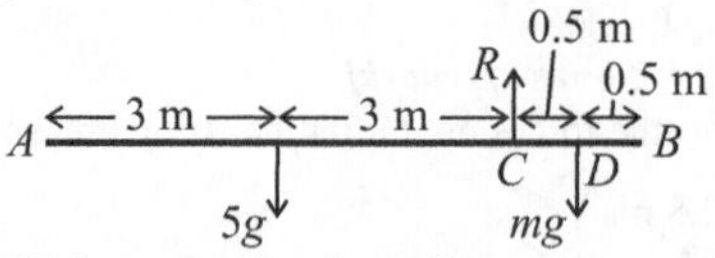

Taking moments about C:
$5g \times 3 = mg \times 0.5 \Rightarrow 15 = 0.5m \Rightarrow m = 30$ kg ***[1 mark]***

4 a)

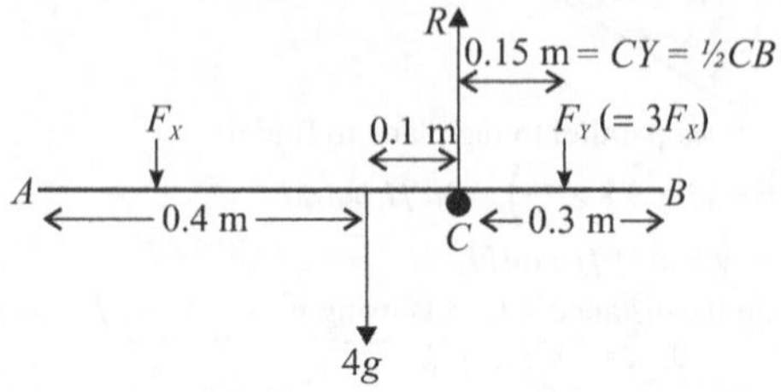

$CY = ½CB = ½(0.3) = 0.15$ m
$F_X + F_Y = 80g$, $F_Y = 3 \times F_X$,
so, $4F_X = 80g$, $F_X = 20g$ and $F_Y = 60g$
Taking moments about C:
$F_Y \times CY = (4g \times 0.1) + (F_X \times CX)$
so $(60g \times 0.15) = (4g \times 0.1) + (20g \times CX)$
and $CX = \dfrac{9g - 0.4g}{20g} = 0.43$ m

$AX = 0.5 - CX = 0.07$ m
[5 marks available — 1 mark for finding distances CB and CY, 1 mark for finding correct values of F_X and F_Y, 1 mark for taking moments about a point, 1 mark for correct workings, 1 mark for correct value of AX]

b) $F_X + F_Y = 80g$
Resolving vertically:
$R = F_X + F_Y + 4g = 84g = 820$ N (2 s.f.)
[2 marks available — 1 mark for resolving vertically, 1 mark for correct value of R]

c)

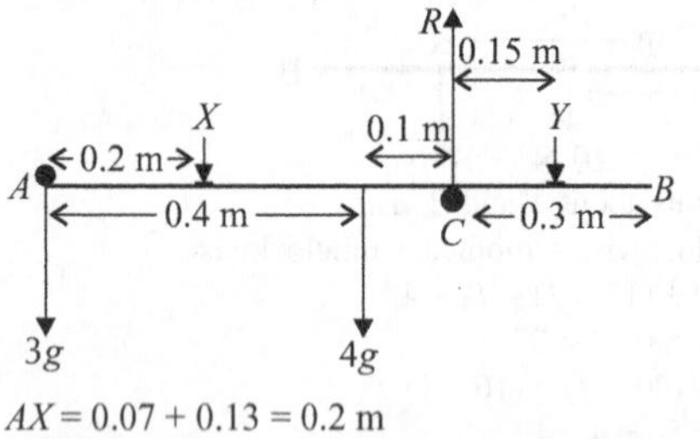

$AX = 0.07 + 0.13 = 0.2$ m
$F_X + F_Y = 80g$
Resolving vertically:
$R = 3g + F_X + 4g + F_Y = 87g$
Taking moments about point X:
$(0.2 \times 3g) + (0.3 \times 87g) = (0.2 \times 4g) + (0.45 \times F_Y)$
so $F_Y = 564.04... = 560$ N (2 s.f.)
and $F_X = 80g - 564.04... = 784 - 564.04... = 220$ N (2 s.f.)
OR:
Taking moments about point Y:
$(0.65 \times 3g) + (0.45 \times F_X) + (0.25 \times 4g) = (0.15 \times 87g)$
so $F_X = 219.95... = 220$ N (2 s.f.)
and $F_Y = 80g - 219.95... = 784 - 219.95... = 560$ N (2 s.f.)
[5 marks available — 1 mark for calculating new value of AX, 1 mark for equation connecting F_X and F_Y, 1 mark for taking moments around a point, 1 mark for correct value of F_X, 1 mark for correct value of F_Y]

5

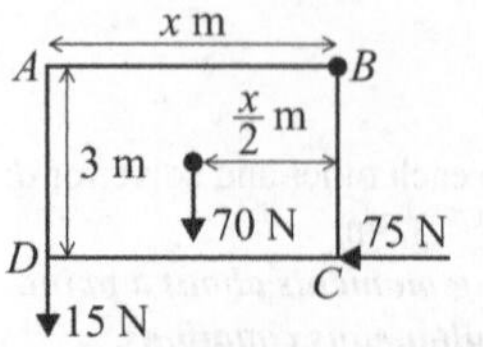

The centre of mass is at the centre of the lamina,
so the horizontal distance between the centre of mass and B is $\frac{x}{2}$ m.
Taking moments about B:
$(15 \times x) + \left(70 \times \frac{x}{2}\right) = 75 \times 3$ ***[1 mark]***
$\Rightarrow 50x = 225 \Rightarrow x = 4.5$ m ***[1 mark]***

Section Four — Problem Solving

Pages 107-110: Problem Solving — 1

1 Position vector of point C is:
Position vector of point $A + \overrightarrow{AB} + \overrightarrow{BC}$
$= (p\mathbf{i} + 4\mathbf{j} + (p-3)\mathbf{k}) + (-2\mathbf{i} - (p-1)\mathbf{j} + \mathbf{k}) + (\mathbf{i} - \mathbf{j} - \mathbf{k})$
$= (p - 2 + 1)\mathbf{i} + (4 - p + 1 - 1)\mathbf{j} + (p - 3 + 1 - 1)\mathbf{k}$
$= (p-1)\mathbf{i} + (4-p)\mathbf{j} + (p-3)\mathbf{k}$ ***[1 mark]***
Then $\sqrt{(p-1)^2 + (4-p)^2 + (p-3)^2} = \sqrt{10}$ ***[1 mark]***
$\Rightarrow p^2 - 2p + 1 + 16 - 8p + p^2 + p^2 - 6p + 9 = 10$
$\Rightarrow 3p^2 - 16p + 26 = 10 \Rightarrow 3p^2 - 16p + 16 = 0$
$\Rightarrow (3p-4)(p-4) = 0 \Rightarrow p = \frac{4}{3}$ or $p = 4$ ***[1 mark for both]***
$p = \frac{4}{3}$ gives a negative $\mathbf{k}$ component, which is impossible as this would put the robot outside of the pool. So $p = 4$, giving the position vector of point A: $4\mathbf{i} + 4\mathbf{j} + (4-3)\mathbf{k} = (4\mathbf{i} + 4\mathbf{j} + \mathbf{k})$ m ***[1 mark for both correct value of p and correct position vector of A]***

2 a) The amount of CO_2 emitted each year is $1 - 0.12 = 0.88$ times the amount of the previous year, so this is a geometric progression. The first term is $A = 56\,000$ for $y = 2020$. So the amount emitted in the year y will be approximately $A = 56\,000 \times 0.88^{y-2020}$.
[2 marks available — 1 mark for 0.88, 1 mark for the correct answer]

b) (i) The total amount of CO_2 emitted follows a geometric series with $r = 0.88$ and $a = 56\,000$.
The emissions for the years 2020-2040 are the first 21 terms, so using the formula for the sum of a geometric series gives:
$S_{21} = \dfrac{56\,000(1 - 0.88^{21})}{1 - 0.88} = 434\,814.21...$
$= 435\,000$ tonnes (3 s.f.)
[2 marks available — 1 mark for using the correct formula, 1 mark for the correct answer]

(ii) The greatest possible total amount is the sum to infinity of the geometric series:
$S_\infty = \dfrac{56\,000}{1 - 0.88} = 466\,666.66... = 467\,000$ tonnes (3 s.f.)
[2 marks available — 1 mark for using the correct formula, 1 mark for the correct answer]

3 For C, when $x = 1$, $2t - 3 = 1 \Rightarrow t = 2$ ***[1 mark]***
So $y = 2 = M(2)^2 + 34(2) + N - 8 \Rightarrow 4M + N = -58$ ①
For D, when $x = 1$, $u + 2 = 1 \Rightarrow u = -1$ ***[1 mark]***
So $y = 2 = 3(-1)^2 + N(-1) - M - 11 \Rightarrow M + N = -10$ ②
[1 mark for a correct method to find M and N]
① – ② gives: $3M = -48 \Rightarrow M = -16$ ***[1 mark]***
Substituting this into ②: $-16 + N = -10 \Rightarrow N = 6$ ***[1 mark]***

4 a) Find the value of k: $f(2) = 0 \Rightarrow k(2)^3 - 49(2)^2 + 70(2) - k = 0$
$\Rightarrow 7k = 56 \Rightarrow k = 8$ ***[1 mark]***, so $f(x) = 8x^3 - 49x^2 + 70x - 8$ ①
By the Factor Theorem, $(x - 2)$ is a factor of $f(x)$. ***[1 mark]***
So $f(x) = (x-2)(ax^2 + bx + c)$, where a, b and c are constants.
So $f(x) = ax^3 + bx^2 + cx - 2ax^2 - 2bx - 2c$
$= ax^3 + (-2a + b)x^2 + (-2b + c)x - 2c$ ②
Equating coefficients of x^3 in ① and ② gives $a = 8$.
Then coefficients of x^2 give $-2 \times 8 + b = -49 \Rightarrow b = -33$.
And the constant terms give $-2c = -8 \Rightarrow c = 4$.
[1 mark for a correct method to find the quadratic factor]
So $f(x) = (x-2)(8x^2 - 33x + 4)$ ***[1 mark]***
$= (x-2)(x-4)(8x-1)$ ***[1 mark]***

b) $70 - 8 \operatorname{cosec} x = 49 \sin x - 8 \sin^2 x$
$\Rightarrow 70 \sin x - 8 = 49 \sin^2 x - 8 \sin^3 x$
$\Rightarrow 8(\sin x)^3 - 49(\sin x)^2 + 70(\sin x) - 8 = 0$ ***[1 mark]***
Using the result from part a) gives:
$(\sin x - 2)(\sin x - 4)(8 \sin x - 1) = 0$ ***[1 mark]***
$\sin x - 2 = 0 \Rightarrow \sin x = 2$, which has no solutions.
$\sin x - 4 = 0 \Rightarrow \sin x = 4$, which has no solutions.
$8 \sin x - 1 = 0 \Rightarrow \sin x = \frac{1}{8} \Rightarrow x = \sin^{-1} \frac{1}{8} = 0.1253...$
So one solution is $x = 0.125$ (3 s.f.) ***[1 mark]***. A second solution is $\pi - 0.1253... = 3.016... = 3.01$ (3 s.f.) ***[1 mark]***

5 a) $\dfrac{4x^2 - 2x - 18}{4x^2 - 9} = \dfrac{(4x^2 - 9) + (-2x - 9)}{4x^2 - 9} = 1 + \dfrac{-2x - 9}{4x^2 - 9}$
So $A = 1$, $p = -2$ and $q = -9$.
[2 marks available — 2 marks for all three correct values, otherwise 1 mark for at least one correct value]

b) $\int_3^4 \frac{4x^2-2x-18}{4x^2-9}\,dx = \int_3^4 1+\frac{-2x-9}{4x^2-9}\,dx$

$\frac{-2x-9}{4x^2-9} = \frac{-2x-9}{(2x+3)(2x-3)}$

Splitting this into partial fractions:

$\frac{-2x-9}{(2x+3)(2x-3)} \equiv \frac{B}{2x+3}+\frac{C}{2x-3}$ ***[1 mark]***

$\Rightarrow -2x-9 = B(2x-3)+C(2x+3)$

When $x=-\frac{3}{2}$, $3-9=B(-3-3) \Rightarrow -6=-6B \Rightarrow B=1$

When $x=\frac{3}{2}$, $-3-9=C(3+3) \Rightarrow -12=6C \Rightarrow C=-2$

[1 mark for a correct method to find B and C]

So $\int_3^4 1+\frac{-2x-9}{4x^2-9}\,dx = \int_3^4 1+\frac{1}{2x+3}+\frac{-2}{2x-3}\,dx$

$= \left[x+\frac{1}{2}\ln|2x+3|-\ln|2x-3|\right]_3^4$ ***[1 mark]***

$= \left[4+\frac{1}{2}\ln(2\times4+3)-\ln(2\times4-3)\right]$

$- \left[3+\frac{1}{2}\ln(2\times3+3)-\ln(2\times3-3)\right]$ ***[1 mark]***

$= 4+\frac{1}{2}\ln 11-\ln 5-3-\frac{1}{2}\ln 9+\ln 3$

$= 1+\ln\sqrt{11}-\ln 5-\ln 3+\ln 3$

[1 mark for the correct use of a log law]

$= 1+\ln\frac{\sqrt{11}}{5}$ ***[1 mark]***

6 $C=\frac{3^t+3^{3t}}{9^t}=\frac{3^t+3^{3t}}{3^{2t}}=3^{-t}+3^t$ ***[1 mark]***

The rate of change of the concentration is given by $\frac{dC}{dt}$.

$\frac{dC}{dt}=\frac{d}{dt}(3^{-t}+3^t)=-3^{-t}\ln 3+3^t\ln 3=(3^t-3^{-t})\ln 3$ ***[1 mark]***

$\frac{dC}{dt}=5\ln 3 \Rightarrow (3^t-3^{-t})\ln 3=5\ln 3 \Rightarrow 3^t-3^{-t}=5$

$\Rightarrow (3^t)^2-1=5(3^t) \Rightarrow (3^t)^2-5(3^t)-1=0$ ***[1 mark]***

Using the quadratic formula:

$3^t=\frac{5\pm\sqrt{(-5)^2-4(1)(-1)}}{2\times1} \Rightarrow 3^t=\frac{5\pm\sqrt{29}}{2}$ ***[1 mark]***

3^t can't be negative, so reject $\frac{5-\sqrt{29}}{2}$. ***[1 mark]***

$3^t=\frac{5+\sqrt{29}}{2} \Rightarrow t=\log_3\left(\frac{5+\sqrt{29}}{2}\right)$

So the rate of change is $(5\ln 3)$ ppms^{-1} at $t=\log_3\left(\frac{5+\sqrt{29}}{2}\right)$ s. ***[1 mark]***

7 a) $\frac{\sin\theta}{1+\sin 2\theta}+\frac{1}{\sec\theta+2\sin\theta}=\frac{\sin\theta}{1+\sin 2\theta}+\frac{1}{\frac{1}{\cos\theta}+2\sin\theta}$

$=\frac{\sin\theta}{1+\sin 2\theta}+\frac{\cos\theta}{1+2\sin\theta\cos\theta}$ ***[1 mark]***

Using the double angle formula $\sin 2\theta \equiv 2\sin\theta\cos\theta$:

$\frac{\sin\theta}{1+\sin 2\theta}+\frac{\cos\theta}{1+2\sin\theta\cos\theta}$

$=\frac{\sin\theta}{1+2\sin\theta\cos\theta}+\frac{\cos\theta}{1+2\sin\theta\cos\theta}=\frac{\sin\theta+\cos\theta}{1+2\sin\theta\cos\theta}$ ***[1 mark]***

Using the identity $1\equiv\sin^2\theta+\cos^2\theta$:

$\frac{\sin\theta+\cos\theta}{1+2\sin\theta\cos\theta}=\frac{\sin\theta+\cos\theta}{\sin^2\theta+\cos^2\theta+2\sin\theta\cos\theta}$ ***[1 mark]***

$=\frac{\sin\theta+\cos\theta}{(\sin\theta+\cos\theta)^2}=\frac{1}{\sin\theta+\cos\theta}$ ***[1 mark]***

b) Using the sine rule: $\frac{\sin\frac{\pi}{6}}{3}=\frac{\sin\alpha}{5}$ ***[1 mark]***

$\Rightarrow \frac{1}{6}=\frac{\sin\alpha}{5} \Rightarrow \sin\alpha=\frac{5}{6}$ ***[1 mark]***

Using the identity $\sin^2\alpha+\cos^2\alpha\equiv1$: $\cos\alpha=\pm\sqrt{1-\sin^2\alpha}$

Since α is obtuse, $\cos\alpha$ is negative, so $\cos\alpha=-\sqrt{1-\sin^2\alpha}$.

So $\cos\alpha=-\sqrt{1-\left(\frac{5}{6}\right)^2}=-\sqrt{\frac{11}{36}}=-\frac{\sqrt{11}}{6}$ ***[1 mark]***

Then $f(\alpha)=\frac{1}{\sin\alpha+\cos\alpha}=\frac{1}{\frac{5}{6}-\frac{\sqrt{11}}{6}}$ ***[1 mark]***

$=\frac{6}{5-\sqrt{11}}=\frac{6(5+\sqrt{11})}{25-11}=\frac{3(5+\sqrt{11})}{7}=\frac{15}{7}+\frac{3}{7}\sqrt{11}$ ***[1 mark]***

Pages 111-114: Problem Solving — 2

1 a) For $1\le x\le m$, $P(X=x)=F(x)-F(x-1)=\frac{x}{m}-\frac{x-1}{m}=\frac{1}{m}$.

For $x=0$, $P(X\le 0)=F(0)=0$, so $P(X=0)$ must be 0.

So $P(X=x)=\frac{1}{m}$ for $1\le x\le m$, and $P(X=x)=0$ otherwise.

[2 marks available — 1 mark for a correct method, 1 mark for the correct answer]

b) E.g. the probability of success (observing the outcome $X=7$) is the same in each trial. ***[1 mark]***

$Y\sim B\left(20,\frac{1}{m}\right)$. ***[1 mark]***

c) $P(Y\ge 5)<0.029 \Rightarrow P(Y\le 4)>1-0.029=0.971$ ***[1 mark]***

$p=\frac{1}{m}$, so find $P(Y\le 4)$ for different values of m:

For $m=10$, $p=\frac{1}{10}$ and $P(Y\le 4)=0.9568...<0.971$

For $m=11$, $p=\frac{1}{11}$ and $P(Y\le 4)=0.9698...<0.971$

For $m=12$, $p=\frac{1}{12}$ and $P(Y\le 4)=0.9784...>0.971$

[1 mark for both 0.9698... and 0.9784...]

The lowest value of m that gives $P(Y\le 4)>0.971$ is 12, so the minimum number of possible outcomes is 12. ***[1 mark]***

2 a) $P(F'\cap T\mid L')=\frac{P(F'\cap T\cap L')}{P(L')}=\frac{y}{0.2+z+y+0.115}=0.2$ ①

$P((F\cup T)\cap L')=0.2+z+y=0.56$ ②

$P(F'\cap L\cap T):P(F\cap L\cap T)=x:w=2:1 \Rightarrow x=2w$ ③

All of the probabilities in the Venn diagram must add up to 1, so:

$0.2+0.075+0.1+z+w+x+y+0.115=1$

$\Rightarrow z+w+x+y=0.51$ ④

Substituting ② into ①: $\frac{y}{0.56+0.115}=0.2 \Rightarrow y=0.135$

②: $0.2+z+0.135=0.56 \Rightarrow z=0.225$

Substituting ③ into ④: $0.225+w+2w+0.135=0.51$

$\Rightarrow w=\frac{0.15}{3} \Rightarrow w=0.05$

③: $x=2\times0.05=0.1$

[5 marks available — 1 mark for a correct method to find y or z, 1 mark for each of y and z correct, 1 mark for a correct method to find w and x, 1 mark for both w and x correct]

b) P('at least 2 traits') $=0.075+0.225+0.1+0.05=0.45$.

So there are $90\div0.45=200$ plants in total.

P('none of the traits') $=0.115$, so $0.115\times200=23$ of the plants have none of the traits.

[2 marks available — 1 mark for a correct method, 1 mark for the correct answer]

3 a) (i) $a=\frac{dv}{dt}=\frac{d}{dt}[(2t+1)\ln(t+1)]$

Use the product rule with $p=2t+1$ and $q=\ln(t+1)$:

$\frac{dp}{dt}=2$ and $\frac{dq}{dt}=\frac{1}{t+1}$ ***[1 mark]***,

so $\frac{dv}{dt}=\frac{2t+1}{t+1}+2\ln(t+1)$ ***[1 mark]***

When $t=0.5$, $\frac{dv}{dt}=\frac{2(0.5)+1}{0.5+1}+2\ln(0.5+1)$

$=2.144...=2.14$ ms^{-2} (3 s.f.) ***[1 mark]***

(ii) The fly moves from A to B in the first second, so the distance between A and B is $\int_0^1 v\,dt=\int_0^1(2t+1)\ln(t+1)\,dt$.

Let $p=\ln(t+1)$, so $\frac{dp}{dt}=\frac{1}{t+1}$.

Let $\frac{dq}{dt}=2t+1$, so $q=t^2+t$.

Using integration by parts,

$\int_0^1(2t+1)\ln(t+1)\,dt=[(t^2+t)\ln(t+1)]_0^1-\int_0^1\frac{t^2+t}{t+1}\,dt$

$=(1^2+1)\ln(1+1)-(0^2+0)\ln(0+1)-\int_0^1\frac{t(t+1)}{t+1}\,dt$

$=2\ln 2-\int_0^1 t\,dt=2\ln 2-\left[\frac{1}{2}t^2\right]_0^1=2\ln 2-\left(\frac{1}{2}(1)^2-\frac{1}{2}(0)^2\right)$

$=2\ln 2-\frac{1}{2}=0.8862...=0.886$ m (3 s.f.)

[5 marks available — 1 mark for correct choice of p and dq/dt, 1 mark for correct differentiation and integration to obtain dp/dt and q, 1 mark for correct integration by parts method, 1 mark for substituting in the limits, 1 mark for the correct answer]

b) In the first model, the initial velocity was:
$(2 \times 0 + 1)\ln(0 + 1) = \ln 1 = 0$
So the initial velocity in the simplified model is also 0. ***[1 mark]***
Then for the first second, $s = s$, $u = 0$, $a = 2$ and $t = 1$.
Using $s = ut + \frac{1}{2}at^2$: $s = (0 \times 1) + \left(\frac{1}{2} \times 2 \times 1^2\right) = 1$ m ***[1 mark]***
Percentage error $= \left|\frac{0.8862... - 1}{0.8862...}\right| \times 100$ ***[1 mark]***
$= 12.82... = 12.8\%$ (1 d.p.) ***[1 mark]***

4 a) The plank is on the point of tilting about the edge of the cliff, so the reaction force at any other point will be zero. Start by working out the missing lengths needed to take moments about the edge of the cliff:

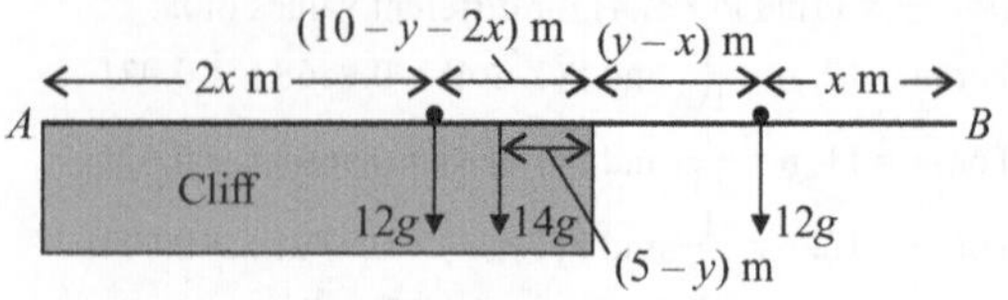

Taking moments about the edge of the cliff:
$(12g \times (10 - y - 2x)) + (14g \times (5 - y)) = 12g \times (y - x)$
$\Rightarrow 120 - 12y - 24x + 70 - 14y = 12y - 12x$
$\Rightarrow 190 - 38y = 12x \Rightarrow x = \frac{95 - 19y}{6}$, as required.
[4 marks available — 1 mark for using the fact that the plank is on the point of tilting, 1 mark for taking moments, 1 mark for a fully correct moments equation, 1 mark for rearranging into the required form]

b) The plank is uniform. ***[1 mark for a valid assumption]***

5 a)

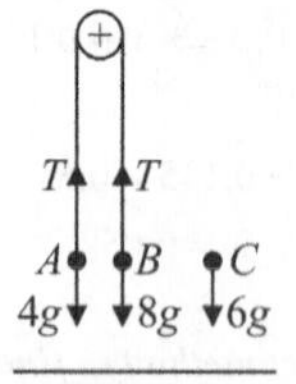

$F_{net} = ma$, so taking up as positive gives:
A: $T - 4g = 4a_{AB}$ ①
B: $T - 8g = -8a_{AB}$ ②
[1 mark for correct expressions for A and B]
① – ② gives: $4g = 12a_{AB} \Rightarrow a_{AB} = \frac{g}{3}$ ***[1 mark]***
C: No other forces acting on C except gravity, so $a_C = -g$
So C will be the first particle to hit the ground.
$u = 0$, $v = -1.96$ and $a = -g$. Using $v = u + at$: $-1.96 = 0 - gt$
$\Rightarrow t = 0.2$ s, so C hits the ground after 0.2 s. ***[1 mark]***
Using $v^2 = u^2 + 2as$: $(-1.96)^2 = 0^2 - 2gs \Rightarrow s = -0.196$ m,
so the starting height of all three particles was 0.196 m. ***[1 mark]***
A is the only one moving upwards, so will have the greatest height at this time. $u = 0$, $a = \frac{g}{3}$ and $t = 0.2$.
Using $s = ut + \frac{1}{2}at^2$:
$s = (0 \times 0.2) + \left(\frac{1}{2} \times \frac{g}{3} \times 0.2^2\right) = 0.0653...$ m ***[1 mark]***
So the height of A when C hits the ground is:
$0.196 + 0.0653... = 0.2613... = 0.26$ m (2 s.f.) ***[1 mark]***

b) The string is taut until B hits the ground. Using results from part a), while B is falling, $s = -0.196$, $u = 0$, $v = v$ and $a = -\frac{g}{3}$.
Using $v^2 = u^2 + 2as$:
$v^2 = 0^2 + \left(2 \times -\frac{g}{3} \times -0.196\right) \Rightarrow v = -1.131...$ ms^{-1} ***[1 mark]***
When B hits the ground, speed of A = speed of B = 1.131... ms^{-1}.
A then continues to rise, momentarily stops and then falls freely under gravity. The string isn't taut again until the displacement of $A = 0$. So while the string is slack, A has $s = 0$, $u = 1.131...$, $a = -g$ and $t = t$. ***[1 mark]***
Using $s = ut + \frac{1}{2}at^2$: $0 = (1.131... \times t) + \left(\frac{1}{2} \times -g \times t^2\right)$
$\Rightarrow 0 = t\left(1.131... - \frac{g}{2}t\right) \Rightarrow t = 0$ or $t = 0.2309...$
[1 mark for a correct method to solve for t]
So the string is not taut for 0.23 s (2 s.f.). ***[1 mark]***

c) E.g. it was assumed that the string's mass didn't affect the acceleration of the masses. ***[1 mark for a sensible answer]***

6 Transform to the standard normal distribution.
$\frac{X - \mu}{\sigma} = Z$, so $P(X - \mu > 7) = P\left(\frac{X - \mu}{\sigma} > \frac{7}{\sigma}\right) = P\left(Z > \frac{7}{\sigma}\right)$
[1 mark for attempting to transform to Z]
So $P\left(Z > \frac{7}{\sigma}\right) = 0.24 \Rightarrow P\left(Z \leq \frac{7}{\sigma}\right) = 1 - 0.24 = 0.76$ ***[1 mark]***
Using the inverse normal function with area 0.76 gives $z = 0.7063...$
$\Rightarrow \frac{7}{\sigma} = 0.7063... \Rightarrow \sigma = 9.910... = 9.9$ (1 d.p.) ***[1 mark]***
The graph of the distribution changes between concave and convex at its points of inflection, which are at $x = \mu - \sigma$ and $x = \mu + \sigma$. It changes from concave to convex at the point with the larger x-value, so:
$x = \mu + \sigma \Rightarrow 34.5 = \mu + 9.910...$
$\Rightarrow \mu = 24.589... = 24.6$ (1 d.p.) ***[1 mark]***

7

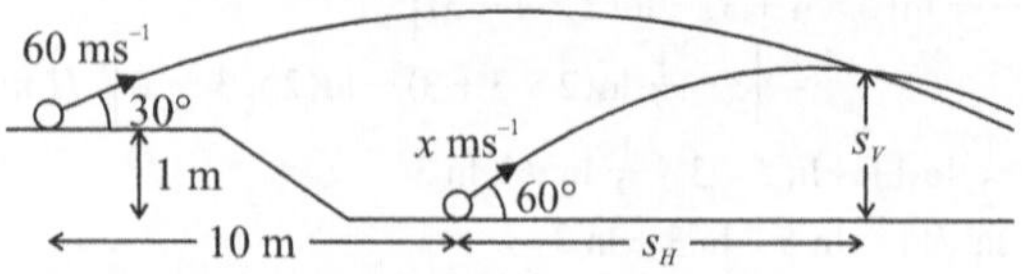

Let t be the time between the balls being struck and colliding.
Considering horizontal motion:
First ball: $s = s_H$, $u = x\cos 60°$, $a = 0$, $t = t$
Using $s = ut + \frac{1}{2}at^2$: $s_H = (x\cos 60°\ t) + \left(\frac{1}{2} \times 0 \times t^2\right) \Rightarrow s_H = \frac{1}{2}xt$
Second ball: $s = s_H + 10$, $u = 60\cos 30°$, $a = 0$, $t = t$
$s_H + 10 = (60\cos 30° \times t) + \left(\frac{1}{2} \times 0 \times t^2\right)$
$\Rightarrow s_H = 30\sqrt{3}t - 10$
[1 mark for correct use of a suvat equation to get two correct expressions for s_H from the horizontal motion of the balls]
Equating these gives: $\frac{1}{2}xt = 30\sqrt{3}t - 10$
$\Rightarrow t = \frac{10}{30\sqrt{3} - \frac{1}{2}x} = \frac{20}{60\sqrt{3} - x}$ ***[1 mark]***

Considering vertical motion, taking up as positive:
First ball: $s = s_V$, $u = x\sin 60°$, $a = -g$, $t = t$
Using $s = ut + at^2$: $s_V = (x\sin 60° \times t) - \frac{g}{2}t^2 \Rightarrow s_V = \frac{\sqrt{3}}{2}xt - \frac{g}{2}t^2$
Second ball: $s = s_V - 1$, $u = 60\sin 30°$, $a = -g$, $t = t$
$s_V - 1 = (60\sin 30° \times t) - \frac{g}{2}t^2 \Rightarrow s_V = 30t - \frac{g}{2}t^2 + 1$
[1 mark for correct use of a suvat equation to get two correct expressions for s_V from the vertical motion of the balls]
Equating these gives: $\frac{\sqrt{3}}{2}xt - \frac{g}{2}t^2 = 30t - \frac{g}{2}t^2 + 1$
$\Rightarrow t(60 - \sqrt{3}x) = -2$ ***[1 mark]***
Substituting in $t = \frac{20}{60\sqrt{3} - x}$:
$\frac{20}{60\sqrt{3} - x}(60 - \sqrt{3}x) = -2 \Rightarrow 600 - 10\sqrt{3}x = x - 60\sqrt{3}$ ***[1 mark]***
$\Rightarrow x(1 + 10\sqrt{3}) = 600 + 60\sqrt{3}$
$\Rightarrow x = \frac{600 + 60\sqrt{3}}{1 + 10\sqrt{3}}$
$\Rightarrow x = 38.422... = 38.4$ (3 s.f.) ***[1 mark]***

Practice Exam Paper 1

1 $0 = x^2 - 8x + 7 \Rightarrow x = 1$ or $x = 7$. The stationary point is halfway between these roots, so $x = 4$. $y = 4^2 - 8(4) + 7 = -9$. So the stationary point is $(4, -9)$. ***[1 mark]***

2 $2 \log a^3b - \log ab = \log (a^3b)^2 - \log ab$
$= \log a^6b^2 - \log ab$
$= \log \frac{a^6b^2}{ab} = \log a^5b$ ***[1 mark]***

3 a) $\frac{x^3 - 9x^2 + 14x}{x^2 - 4} \times \frac{x+2}{x} = \frac{x^3 - 9x^2 + 14x}{(x+2)(x-2)} \times \frac{x+2}{x}$
$= \frac{x^3 - 9x^2 + 14x}{x(x-2)} = \frac{x^2 - 9x + 14}{(x-2)} = \frac{(x-2)(x-7)}{(x-2)}$
$= x - 7$
[3 marks available — 1 mark for factorising the numerator, 1 mark for factorising the denominator, 1 mark for fully simplified expression]

b) The points of intersection occur when $|x - 7| = -\frac{1}{2}x + 5$.
When $x > 7$:
$x - 7 = -\frac{1}{2}x + 5$ ***[1 mark]*** $\Rightarrow \frac{3}{2}x = 12 \Rightarrow x = 8$
When $x = 8$, $y = 8 - 7 = 1$
When $x < 7$: $7 - x = -\frac{1}{2}x + 5$ ***[1 mark]*** $\Rightarrow \frac{1}{2}x = 2 \Rightarrow x = 4$
When $x = 4$, $y = 7 - 4 = 3$
So the lines intersect at $(4, 3)$ ***[1 mark]*** and $(8, 1)$ ***[1 mark]***.

4 a) $y = \frac{2x+7}{3x-5} \Rightarrow y(3x - 5) = 2x + 7 \Rightarrow 3xy - 5y = 2x + 7$
$\Rightarrow 3xy - 2x = 7 + 5y \Rightarrow x(3y - 2) = 7 + 5y$
$\Rightarrow x = \frac{7+5y}{3y-2}$
So $f^{-1}(x) = \frac{7+5x}{3x-2}$
[2 marks available — 1 mark for a correct method, 1 mark for the correct answer]

b) $f(2) = \frac{2(2)+7}{3(2)-5} = \frac{4+7}{6-5} = \frac{11}{1} = 11$
$g(11) = 11^2 - k$, so $120 = 121 - k \Rightarrow k = 1$
[3 marks available — 1 mark for correct method for finding f(2), 1 mark for correct value of f(2), 1 mark for the correct value of k]

c) $gh(x) = (\cos x)^2 - 1 = \cos^2 x - 1$ ***[1 mark]***
The range of $\cos^2 x$ is $0 \le \cos^2 x \le 1$,
so the range of $gh(x)$ is $-1 \le gh(x) \le 0$ ***[1 mark]***
$hg(x) = \cos(x^2 - 1)$ ***[1 mark]***
So the range of $hg(x)$ is the range of cos,
i.e. $-1 \le hg(x) \le 1$ ***[1 mark]***

5 $\tan 3\theta \approx 3\theta$, $\cos 4\theta \approx 1 - \frac{16\theta^2}{2} = 1 - 8\theta^2$ and $\sin \theta^2 \approx \theta^2$, so:
$$\frac{1 - \tan 3\theta}{\cos 4\theta - \sin \theta^2} \approx \frac{1 - 3\theta}{1 - 8\theta^2 - \theta^2} = \frac{1 - 3\theta}{1 - 9\theta^2} = \frac{1 - 3\theta}{(1 + 3\theta)(1 - 3\theta)}$$
$$= \frac{1}{1 + 3\theta} \text{ as required}$$
[3 marks available — 1 mark for substituting the correct small angle approximations into the given function, 1 mark for factorising the denominator, 1 mark for correct answer]

6 Proof by contradiction: assume that $\sqrt{2}$ is rational and can be written $\frac{a}{b}$, where a and b are both non-zero integers and have no common factors ***[1 mark]***.
$\sqrt{2} = \frac{a}{b} \Rightarrow \sqrt{2}b = a \Rightarrow 2b^2 = a^2$ ***[1 mark]***
a^2 must be even, so a must also be even, which means it can be written as $2k$, where k is an integer:
$2b^2 = (2k)^2 = 4k^2 \Rightarrow b^2 = 2k^2$ ***[1 mark]***
This means that b^2 is even, which means that b is also even so can be written as $2l$, where l is an integer. This shows that a and b have a common factor of 2, which contradicts the initial assumption, so $\sqrt{2}$ must be an irrational number ***[1 mark]***.

7 a) At intersection with the x-axis, $y = 0$:
$0 = xe^x \Rightarrow x = 0$ or $e^x = 0$
e^x is never zero, so $x = 0$ only. ***[1 mark]***
When $x = 0$, $y = 0 \times e^0 = 0$
So the graph crosses the x-axis at $(0, 0)$ ***[1 mark]***

b) (i)

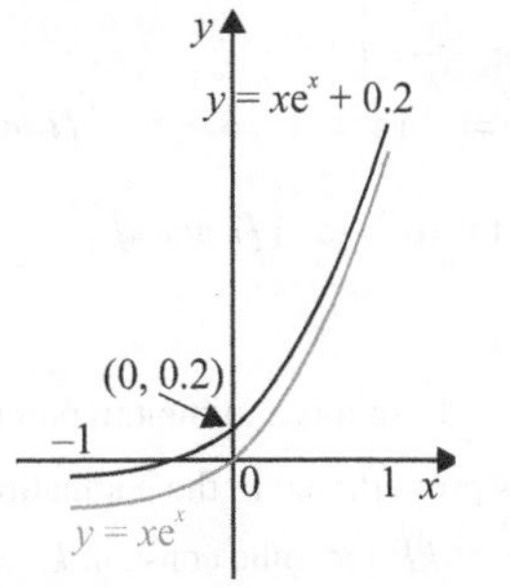

[2 marks available — 1 mark for a vertical translation, 1 mark for the correct y-intercept (0, 0.2)]

(ii)

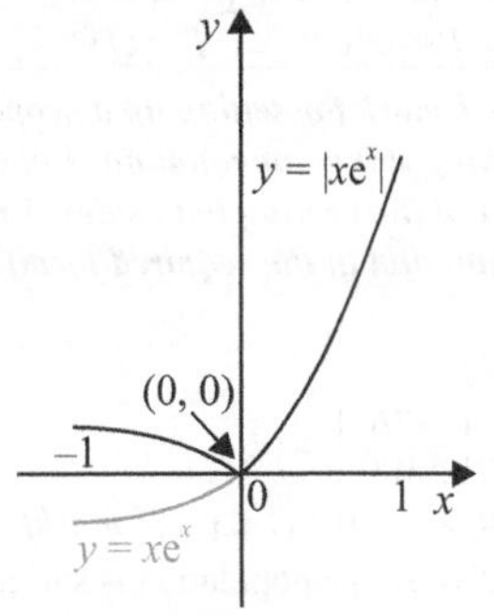

[2 marks available — 1 mark for reflecting the part of the graph below the x-axis in the x-axis, 1 mark for the correct y-intercept (0, 0)]

8 a) $t = 1 \Rightarrow x = 1^3 + 2 = 3$ and $y = 1^2 + 2 = 3$,
so the coordinates of P are $(3, 3)$ ***[1 mark]***.

b) $\frac{dx}{dt} = 3t^2$, $\frac{dy}{dt} = 2t$ ***[1 mark for both]***
Using the chain rule: $\frac{dy}{dx} = \frac{dy}{dt} \div \frac{dx}{dt} = \frac{2t}{3t^2} = \frac{2}{3t}$ ***[1 mark]***.
At P, $t = 1$, so $\frac{dy}{dx} = \frac{2}{3}$ ***[1 mark]***.
Using the equation of a straight line formula at P $(3, 3)$:
$y - 3 = \frac{2}{3}(x - 3) \Rightarrow y = \frac{2}{3}x + 1$ ***[1 mark]***.

9 Differentiate the equation:
$2x - y - x\frac{dy}{dx} = 6y^2\frac{dy}{dx} \Rightarrow \frac{dy}{dx} = \frac{2x - y}{x + 6y^2}$
To find the gradient, substitute $x = 2$ and $y = 1$ into the expression for $\frac{dy}{dx}$:
$\frac{dy}{dx} = \frac{2(2) - 1}{2 + 6(1)^2} = \frac{3}{8}$
[5 marks available — 1 mark for attempting implicit differentiation, 1 mark for differentiating all terms correctly, 1 mark for the correct expression for dy/dx, 1 mark for substituting x = 2 and y = 1, 1 mark for the correct answer]

10 a) $\int_0^{2\pi} 2\cos\frac{x}{4}\,dx$ is the area under the curve between $x = 0$ and $x = 2\pi$. The area of a rectangle with vertices $(0, 0)$, $(0, 2)$, $(2\pi, 0)$ and $(2\pi, 2)$ would have area $2\pi \times 2 = 4\pi$.
The area beneath the curve and between $x = 0$ and $x = 2\pi$ fits inside this rectangle and has an area less than the rectangle, so Lily's answer must be too big ***[1 mark]***.

b) $\int_0^{2\pi} 2\cos\frac{x}{4}\,dx = \left[8\sin\frac{x}{4}\right]_0^{2\pi} = \left[8\sin\frac{\pi}{2}\right] - [8\sin 0] = 8$
[3 marks available — 1 mark for integrating correctly, 1 mark for correct handling of the limits, 1 mark for correct answer]

11 a) Use the product rule: $u = x \Rightarrow \frac{du}{dx} = 1$

$v = \ln x \Rightarrow \frac{dv}{dx} = \frac{1}{x}$ ***[1 mark for both correct]***

$\frac{dy}{dx} = x\left(\frac{1}{x}\right) + \ln x = 1 + \ln x$ ***[1 mark]***

At the stationary point, $\frac{dy}{dx} = 0$

$1 + \ln x = 0$ ***[1 mark]*** $\Rightarrow \ln x = -1 \Rightarrow x = e^{-1}$ ***[1 mark]***

$y = e^{-1} \times \ln e^{-1} = -e^{-1}$

So the stationary point is $(e^{-1}, -e^{-1})$ ***[1 mark]***

b) $\frac{d^2y}{dx^2} = \frac{1}{x}$ ***[1 mark]***

At $(e^{-1}, -e^{-1})$, $\frac{d^2y}{dx^2} = e > 0$, so it is a minimum point ***[1 mark]***

12 a) If the rate of change is proportional to the population, then $\frac{dP}{dt} \propto P \Rightarrow \frac{dP}{dt} = kP$ for some constant k.

Separate the variables and integrate:

$\int \frac{1}{P}\, dP = \int k\, dt \Rightarrow \ln P = kt + \ln Q \Rightarrow P = e^{kt + \ln Q}$

$\Rightarrow P = e^{kt} e^{\ln Q} \Rightarrow P = Qe^{kt}$

[3 marks available — 1 mark for setting up a proportionality statement and converting it into an equation, 1 mark for separating variables and integrating both sides, 1 mark for rearranging to give function in the required form]

b) $Q = 5300$ ***[1 mark]***

$876 = 5300e^{6k}$ ***[1 mark]***

$\Rightarrow \frac{876}{5300} = e^{6k} \Rightarrow \ln\left|\frac{876}{5300}\right| = 6k$

$\Rightarrow 6k = -1.8000... \Rightarrow k = -0.3$ (1 d.p.) ***[1 mark]***

c) The value of k is negative so the population is shrinking ***[1 mark]***.

13 a) $\frac{dH}{dt} = -2\left(\frac{4\pi}{25}\right)\sin\left(\frac{4\pi t}{25}\right) = -\frac{8\pi}{25}\sin\left(\frac{4\pi t}{25}\right)$ ***[1 mark]***

b) $\frac{dH}{dt}$ is the rate of change of the height of the buoy.

So when $t = 7$, $\frac{dH}{dt} = -\frac{8\pi}{25}\sin\left(\frac{4\pi \times 7}{25}\right)$ ***[1 mark]***

$= 0.37007... = 0.370$ m/h (3 s.f.) ***[1 mark]***

c) As $-1 \le \cos\left(\frac{4\pi t}{25}\right) \le 1$, the minimum value that $\cos\left(\frac{4\pi t}{25}\right)$ can take is -1 ***[1 mark]***, and this occurs in the interval $0 < t < 12$.

So the minimum height is $2(-1) + 4 = 2$ m ***[1 mark]***.

14 a) The number of minutes of practice on the nth day is given by

$u_n = a + (n - 1)d = 60 + (n - 1)10 = 50 + 10n$ ***[1 mark]***

4 hours 40 minutes is 280 minutes, so

$50 + 10n = 280$ ***[1 mark]*** $\Rightarrow n = 23$, i.e. day 23 ***[1 mark]***

b) The number of minutes of practice on the nth day is given by

$u_n = ar^{n-1} = 100 \times 1.04^{n-1}$ ***[1 mark]***

$100 \times 1.04^{n-1} > 280 \Rightarrow 1.04^{n-1} > 2.8$ ***[1 mark]***

Taking logs gives: $\log 1.04^{n-1} > \log 2.8$

$\Rightarrow (n - 1)\log 1.04 > \log 2.8$ ***[1 mark]***

$\Rightarrow n - 1 > \frac{\log 2.8}{\log 1.04} \Rightarrow n > 27.3$ (3 s.f.)

So day 28 ***[1 mark]***

c) Pianist: $\frac{1}{2} \times 30[(2 \times 60) + (29 \times 10)] = 6150$ minutes ***[1 mark]***

Violinist: $\frac{100(1.04^{30} - 1)}{1.04 - 1} = 5608.5$ minutes ***[1 mark]***

The pianist will practise for longer over the 30 days ***[1 mark]***.

15 a) Let M be the midpoint of AB. Then angle $DMB = \frac{\pi}{2}$ radians as $BCDM$ is a rectangle.

Using trigonometry, $DM = 5\sin x$ and $AM = 5\cos x$

$\Rightarrow BC = DM = 5\sin x$ and $AM = MB = CD = 5\cos x$

Perimeter of trapezium, $P = AB + BC + CD + DA$

$= (2 \times 5\cos x) + 5\sin x + 5\cos x + 5$

$= 15\cos x + 5\sin x + 5$

Let $15\cos x + 5\sin x = R\sin(x + \alpha)$

$= R(\sin x\cos\alpha + \cos x\sin\alpha)$

So $R\cos\alpha = 5$ and $R\sin\alpha = 15$

$\Rightarrow \tan\alpha = \frac{15}{5} = 3 \Rightarrow \alpha = \tan^{-1}3 = 1.249...$

$R = \sqrt{15^2 + 5^2} = \sqrt{250} = 5\sqrt{10}$

So $15\cos x + 5\sin x = 5\sqrt{10}\sin(x + 1.249...)$

$\Rightarrow P = 5\sqrt{10}\sin(x + 1.249...) + 5$

So $R = 5\sqrt{10}$ and $\alpha = 1.249...$

[7 marks available — 1 mark for finding an expression for DM, 1 mark for finding an expression for AM, 1 mark for perimeter of trapezium in terms of x, 1 mark for expanding R sin (x + α), 1 mark for the correct value of α, 1 mark for finding the value of R, 1 mark for a correct substitution into the expression for P]

b) The perimeter is 17, so $17 = 5\sqrt{10}\sin(x + 1.249...) + 5$

$\Rightarrow 5\sqrt{10}\sin(x + 1.249...) = 12$

$\Rightarrow \sin(x + 1.249...) = \frac{12}{5\sqrt{10}}$ ***[1 mark]***

As x is acute, $0 \le x \le \frac{\pi}{2}$. So you need to find solutions for $1.249... \le x + 1.249... \le 2.819...$:

$x + 1.249... = \sin^{-1}\left(\frac{12}{5\sqrt{10}}\right)$ ***[1 mark]***

$\Rightarrow x + 1.249... = 0.8616...$ (outside range),

$x + 1.249... = \pi - 0.8616... = 2.279...$ ***[1 mark]***

$\Rightarrow x = 2.279... - 1.249... = 1.030... = 1.03$ radians (3 s.f.) ***[1 mark]***

16 Use integration by parts:

$u = \ln x$, $\frac{dv}{dx} = x^{-5}$ ***[1 mark for both]***,

$\frac{du}{dx} = \frac{1}{x}$, $v = \frac{1}{-4}x^{-4}$ ***[1 mark for both]***

$\int \frac{\ln x}{x^5}\, dx = \ln x \times \frac{1}{-4}x^{-4} - \int \frac{1}{-4}x^{-4} \times \frac{1}{x}\, dx$ ***[1 mark]***

$= \frac{-1}{4x^4}\ln x + \frac{1}{4}\int x^{-5}\, dx$

$= \frac{-1}{4x^4}\ln x - \frac{1}{16x^4} + c$ ***[1 mark]***

17 a) Volume $= x^3$, so the price of concrete is $65x^3$ ***[1 mark]***

Surface area $= 6x^2$, so the price of gold leaf is $900x^2$ ***[1 mark]***

Total cost of materials is £250, so $65x^3 + 900x^2 = 250$ ***[1 mark]***

So $900x^2 = 250 - 65x^3 \Rightarrow x^2 = \frac{250 - 65x^3}{900}$

$\Rightarrow x = \sqrt{\frac{250 - 65x^3}{900}}$

[1 mark for correct rearrangement]

b) Let $f(x) = x - \sqrt{\frac{250 - 65x^3}{900}}$

If x, the length of the cube, is between 0.5 and 1, there will be a root of $f(x) = 0$ in the interval $0.5 < x < 1$, and a change of sign for $f(x)$ between 0.5 and 1.

$f(0.5) = 0.5 - \sqrt{\frac{250 - 65(0.5)^3}{900}} = -0.018...$

$f(1) = 1 - \sqrt{\frac{250 - 65(1)^3}{900}} = 0.546...$ ***[1 mark for both]***

There is a change of sign and the function is continuous over this interval, so there is root in the interval $0.5 < x < 1$ ***[1 mark]***.

c) $x_2 = \sqrt{\frac{250 - 65(0.75)^3}{900}} = 0.49730... = 0.4973$ (4 d.p.) ***[1 mark]***

$x_3 = 0.51855...$

$x_4 = 0.51740...$

$x_5 = 0.51746... = 0.5175$ (4 d.p.) ***[1 mark]***

d) Using x_5, concrete costs $65 \times (0.51746...)^3 = £9.0067...$ ***[1 mark]***

Cost of cube = £250

$\frac{9.0067...}{250} = 0.0360...$

So concrete is 3.6% (1 d.p.) of the total cost ***[1 mark]***.

e)

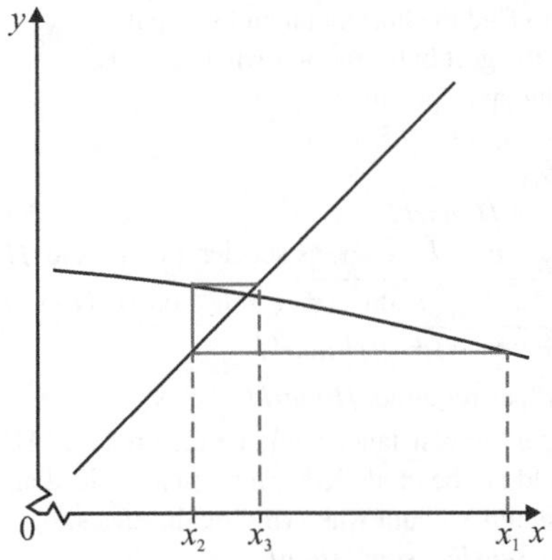

[1 mark for positions of x_2 and x_3 correct]

This is a convergent cobweb diagram.

Practice Exam Paper 2

1 $y = ax^b \Rightarrow \log y = \log (ax^b) \Rightarrow \log y = \log a + \log x^b$
$\Rightarrow \log y = \log a + b \log x$ ***[1 mark]***

2 There is a sign change in the interval (–1, 1) and the function is continuous, so there must be at least one root in the interval. So the answer is 'There are no roots in the interval (–1, 1)'. ***[1 mark]***

3 a) If $(x + 1)$ is a factor of $f(x)$, then $f(-1) = 0$:
$f(-1) = (-1)^3 - 2(-1)^2 - 13(-1) - 10 = -1 - 2 + 13 - 10 = 0$
[1 mark], so $(x + 1)$ is factor of $f(x)$ by the factor theorem ***[1 mark]***.

b) $(x + 1)(x^2 - 3x - 10) = 0$ ***[1 mark]***
$(x + 1)(x + 2)(x - 5) = 0$ ***[1 mark]***
$\Rightarrow x = -2, -1$ and 5 ***[1 mark]***

4 a) $5u_2 - 2 = 38 \Rightarrow 5u_2 = 40 \Rightarrow u_2 = 8$, so
$5u_1 - 2 = 8 \Rightarrow 5u_1 = 10 \Rightarrow u_1 = 2$.
[2 marks available — 1 mark for correct working, 1 mark for correct answer]

b) For a decreasing sequence, $5u_n - 2 < u_n$ for all integer n
$\Rightarrow 4u_n < 2$ for all integer $n \Rightarrow u_n < \frac{1}{2}$ for all integer n.
This has to hold for $n = 1$, so $u_1 < \frac{1}{2}$.
[2 marks available — 1 mark for correct working, 1 mark for correct answer]

c) $\sum_{n=1}^{r} u_n = \frac{1}{2}r$, means that every value of u_n must be $\frac{1}{2}$, including u_1, so $u_1 = \frac{1}{2}$ ***[1 mark]***.

5 $\frac{d}{dx}(5x^3 + 2x^2 + 6) = 15x^2 + 4x$, and $45x^2 + 12x = 3(15x^2 + 4x)$

So $\int \frac{45x^2 + 12x}{5x^3 + 2x^2 + 6}\,dx = \int \frac{3f'(x)}{f(x)}\,dx = 3\ln|f(x)| + C$
$= 3\ln|5x^3 + 2x^2 + 6| + C$

[3 marks available — 1 mark for recognising that the numerator is 3 × the derivative of the denominator, 1 mark for integrating using the correct rule, 1 mark for the correct answer, including the constant]

6 Use the identity $\cot^2 x + 1 \equiv \operatorname{cosec}^2 x$ and substitute it into the equation:
$2(\cot^2 x + 1) + 5\cot x = 9 \Rightarrow 2\cot^2 x + 5\cot x - 7 = 0$ ***[1 mark]***
Factorising gives $(2\cot x + 7)(\cot x - 1) = 0$ ***[1 mark]***

$\cot x = -\frac{7}{2}$ or $\cot x = 1$ ***[1 mark]***
$\Rightarrow \tan x = -\frac{2}{7}$ or $\tan x = 1$ ***[1 mark]***

$x = -15.9°$ (1 d.p.) ***[1 mark]*** and $x = 45°$ ***[1 mark]***.

7 a) Use the chain rule on the e^{x^2} term:
If $y = e^{x^2}$, then let $u = x^2$, so that $y = e^u$.
Then $\frac{du}{dx} = 2x$ and $\frac{dy}{du} = e^u$, which means

$\frac{dy}{dx} = \frac{dy}{du} \times \frac{du}{dx} = e^u \times 2x = 2xe^{x^2}$

So for $f(x) = 4x^3 + e^{x^2}$, $f'(x) = 12x^2 + 2xe^{x^2}$

[2 marks available — 1 mark for using the chain rule to differentiate e^{x^2}, 1 mark for the correct final answer]

b) Differentiate again to find the second derivative:
$\frac{d}{dx}12x^2 = 24x$
Use the product rule to differentiate $2xe^{x^2}$:
Let $u = 2x$, then $\frac{du}{dx} = 2$
Let $v = e^{x^2}$, then $\frac{dv}{dx} = 2xe^{x^2}$ (from part a)).
$\frac{dy}{dx} = u\frac{dv}{dx} + v\frac{du}{dx} = 2x(2xe^{x^2}) + e^{x^2}(2) = 4x^2e^{x^2} + 2e^{x^2}$
[1 mark for using the product rule correctly]
So $f''(x) = 24x + 4x^2e^{x^2} + 2e^{x^2}$
[1 mark for correct second derivative]
The curve is convex when $f''(x) > 0$,
i.e. when $24x + 4x^2e^{x^2} + 2e^{x^2} > 0$ ***[1 mark]***
$e^{x^2} > 0$ and $4x^2 \geq 0$ for all x ***[1 mark]***. If $x > 0$, $24x > 0$.
So for $x > 0$, $f''(x) > 0$, so the curve is convex when $x > 0$ ***[1 mark]***.

8 a) Rearrange the parametric equations:
$x - 1 = 5\cos t \Rightarrow (x - 1)^2 = 25\cos^2 t$ ***[1 mark]***
$y - 2 = 5\sin t \Rightarrow (y - 2)^2 = 25\sin^2 t$ ***[1 mark]***
$(x - 1)^2 + (y - 2)^2 = 25\cos^2 t + 25\sin^2 t$
$= 25(\sin^2 t + \cos^2 t) = 25$ ***[1 mark]***

b) Gradient of the radius from the centre (1, 2) to (4, 6):
$\frac{6 - 2}{4 - 1} = \frac{4}{3}$ ***[1 mark]***
So the gradient of the tangent at P is $-1 \div \frac{4}{3} = -\frac{3}{4}$ ***[1 mark]***
Using the equation of a straight line:
$y - 6 = -\frac{3}{4}(x - 4)$ ***[1 mark]*** $\Rightarrow 3x + 4y - 36 = 0$ ***[1 mark]***
(so $a = 3$, $b = 4$ and $c = -36$)

9 a) Use the distance between two points A and B:
$(2 - 9)^2 + (4 - 8)^2 + (1 - z)^2$ ***[1 mark]*** $= 5^2$ or 9^2
However, as $(2 - 9)^2 + (4 - 8)^2 > 25$ and $(1 - z)^2 \geq 0$,
it cannot be 5^2, so $(2 - 9)^2 + (4 - 8)^2 + (1 - z)^2 = 9^2$ ***[1 mark]***
$49 + 16 + (1 - z)^2 = 81 \Rightarrow (1 - z)^2 = 16$
$\Rightarrow 1 - z = \pm 4$
so $z = 5$ ***[1 mark]*** or $z = -3$ ***[1 mark]***

b) $|\overrightarrow{BC}| = 5$, since this is the other side length of the parallelogram.
So $\overrightarrow{BC} = 5(0.8\mathbf{j} + 0.6\mathbf{k})$ ***[1 mark]***
$= 4\mathbf{j} + 3\mathbf{k}$ ***[1 mark]***
$\overrightarrow{OC} = \overrightarrow{OB} + \overrightarrow{BC} = (9\mathbf{i} + 8\mathbf{j} + 5\mathbf{k}) + (4\mathbf{j} + 3\mathbf{k})$
So C has coordinates $(9, 8 + 4, 5 + 3) = (9, 12, 8)$ ***[1 mark]***
You have to use z = 5 from part a).

c) $\overrightarrow{AC} = \overrightarrow{OC} - \overrightarrow{OA} = (9\mathbf{i} + 12\mathbf{j} + 8\mathbf{k}) - (2\mathbf{i} + 4\mathbf{j} + \mathbf{k})$ ***[1 mark]***
$|\overrightarrow{AC}| = \sqrt{(9 - 2)^2 + (12 - 4)^2 + (8 - 1)^2}$ ***[1 mark]***
$= \sqrt{7^2 + 8^2 + 7^2}$
$= \sqrt{162} = 9\sqrt{2}$ ***[1 mark]***

10 a)

x	0	0.5	1	1.5
y (3 d.p.)	1	**0.627**	0.415	0.270
y (5 d.p.)	1	**0.62671**	0.41497	0.26953

[1 mark for both values correct]

b) $\int_0^{1.5} \frac{e^{\sin x} + x}{(x + 1)^3}\,dx \approx \frac{0.5}{2}(1 + 2(0.627 + 0.415) + 0.270)$
$= 0.8385$
[3 marks available — 1 mark for correct value of h (0.5), 1 mark for using the trapezium rule correctly, 1 mark for correct answer]

c) E.g. Sophie is correct that rounding will have contributed to the error, but as the graph is convex, this will have also contributed to the error ***[1 mark for any comment about the graph being convex]***.

11 $F_{net} = ma = 0.12 \times 6 = 0.72$ N ***[1 mark]***

12 a) $\mathbf{v} = \dot{\mathbf{r}} = (3t^2 - 12t + 4)\mathbf{i} + (7 - 8t)\mathbf{j}$
At $t = 5$:
$\mathbf{v} = (3(5^2) - 12(5) + 4)\mathbf{i} + (7 - 8(5))\mathbf{j} = 19\mathbf{i} - 33\mathbf{j}$ as required.
[3 marks available — 1 mark for attempting to differentiate the position vector, 1 mark for a correct expression for velocity at time t, and 1 mark for substituting t = 5 into this expression to obtain the correct velocity]

b) When P is moving south, component of velocity in direction of **i** will be zero, i.e. $3t^2 - 12t + 4 = 0$ ***[1 mark]***
So $t = 0.36700...$ or $3.63299...$ ***[1 mark]***
When P is moving south, the component of velocity in the direction of **j** will be negative, so find the velocity of P at the two values of t above, and see which is negative:
$\mathbf{v}(0.36700...) = (7 - 8(0.36700...))\mathbf{j} = 4.063...\mathbf{j}$
(so P is moving due north)
$\mathbf{v}(3.63299...) = (7 - 8(3.63299...))\mathbf{j} = -22.06...\mathbf{j}$
[1 mark for checking which t-value gives a negative j-component]
So P is moving due south when $t = 3.63$ s (3 s.f.) ***[1 mark]***
Also, when P is moving due south, 7 – 8t must be negative, so $7 - 8t < 0 \Rightarrow t > \frac{7}{8}$, *so t cannot be 0.3670...*

c) To find force on P, will need to use $\mathbf{F} = m\mathbf{a}$, so first find **a**:
$\mathbf{a} = \dot{\mathbf{v}} = (6t - 12)\mathbf{i} - 8\mathbf{j}$ ***[1 mark]***
When $t = 3$, $\mathbf{a} = (18 - 12)\mathbf{i} - 8\mathbf{j} = 6\mathbf{i} - 8\mathbf{j}$ ***[1 mark]***
So, $\mathbf{F} = m\mathbf{a} = 2.5(6\mathbf{i} - 8\mathbf{j}) = 15\mathbf{i} - 20\mathbf{j}$ ***[1 mark]***
Magnitude of $\mathbf{F} = \sqrt{15^2 + (-20)^2}$ ***[1 mark]***
$= 25$ N ***[1 mark]***

13 a) Resolving forces vertically: $R_P + R_Q = 6g + 4g$
$R_P = R_Q$, so: $2R = 98 \Rightarrow R = 49$ N ***[1 mark]***
Taking moments about A: clockwise = anticlockwise
$(6g \times 3) + (4g \times x) = (49 \times 1) + (49 \times 4)$ ***[1 mark]***
$\Rightarrow 176.58 + 39.24x = 245 \Rightarrow x = 1.74$ (3 s.f.) ***[1 mark]***
You could take moments about any point — as long as your working and answer are correct, you'll get all the marks.

b) For the maximum value of M, the rod will be on the point of tipping about Q, so R_P will be 0. ***[1 mark]***
Taking moments about Q: clockwise = anticlockwise
$(Mg \times 2) = (6g \times 1) + (4g \times 2.25)$
$\Rightarrow 2M = 6 + 9 = 15 \Rightarrow M = 7.5$ ***[1 mark]***

14 a) $\mathbf{u} = (40\mathbf{i} + 108\mathbf{j})$ kmh^{-1}, $\mathbf{a} = (4\mathbf{i} + 12\mathbf{j})$ kmh^{-2}, $t = \frac{1}{2}$ h,
Use $\mathbf{s} = \mathbf{u}t + \frac{1}{2}\mathbf{a}t^2$:
$\mathbf{s} = \frac{1}{2}(40\mathbf{i} + 108\mathbf{j}) + \left[\frac{1}{2} \times \left(\frac{1}{2}\right)^2 \times (4\mathbf{i} + 12\mathbf{j})\right]$ ***[1 mark]***
$\mathbf{s} = (20.5\mathbf{i} + 55.5\mathbf{j})$ km ***[1 mark for 20.5i, 1 mark for 55.5j]***
Make sure you keep track of the units you're using — you have to convert the time from minutes to hours to match the units of the velocity and acceleration.

b) $\mathbf{u} = (60\mathbf{i} + 120\mathbf{j})$, $t = \frac{1}{4}$,
$\mathbf{s} = (20.5\mathbf{i} + 55.5\mathbf{j}) - (2.5\mathbf{i} + 25.5\mathbf{j}) = (18\mathbf{i} + 30\mathbf{j})$ ***[1 mark]***
Use $\mathbf{s} = \mathbf{u}t + \frac{1}{2}\mathbf{a}t^2$:
$(18\mathbf{i} + 30\mathbf{j}) = \frac{1}{4}(60\mathbf{i} + 120\mathbf{j}) + \frac{1}{2} \times \left(\frac{1}{4}\right)^2 \times \mathbf{a}$ ***[1 mark]***
$\Rightarrow \frac{1}{32}\mathbf{a} = (18\mathbf{i} + 30\mathbf{j}) - (15\mathbf{i} + 30\mathbf{j})$
$\Rightarrow \mathbf{a} = 32(3\mathbf{i} + 0\mathbf{j}) = 96\mathbf{i}$
So the magnitude of the acceleration is 96 kmh^{-2} ***[1 mark]***.

c) $\mathbf{u} = (30\mathbf{i} - 40\mathbf{j})$, $\mathbf{a} = (5\mathbf{i} + 8\mathbf{j})$, $\mathbf{v} = \mathbf{v}$, $t = ?$, $\mathbf{s} = ?$,
Use $\mathbf{v} = \mathbf{u} + \mathbf{a}t$ to find the time that G is moving parallel to **i** (the unit vector in the direction of east):
$\mathbf{v} = (30\mathbf{i} - 40\mathbf{j}) + t(5\mathbf{i} + 8\mathbf{j})$ ***[1 mark]***
When G is moving parallel to **i**, the **j**-component of its velocity is zero, so: $0 = -40 + 8t$ ***[1 mark]*** $\Rightarrow t = 5$
Check that the **i**-component is positive: $30 + 5(5) = 55$, so G is moving due east at $t = 5$ ***[1 mark]***.
Now use $\mathbf{s} = \frac{1}{2}(\mathbf{u} + \mathbf{v})t$ to find the position of G at this time:
$\mathbf{s} = \frac{1}{2}(30\mathbf{i} - 40\mathbf{j} + (30\mathbf{i} - 40\mathbf{j}) + 5(5\mathbf{i} + 8\mathbf{j})) \times 5$ ***[1 mark]***
$\mathbf{s} = \frac{5}{2}(85\mathbf{i} - 40\mathbf{j}) = (212.5\mathbf{i} - 100\mathbf{j})$ km ***[1 mark for 212.5i, 1 mark for –100j]***.

15 a) Consider vertical motion, taking up as positive:
$a = -g$, $u = U\sin\alpha$ ***[1 mark]***, $v = 0$, $s = ?$:
Use $v^2 = u^2 + 2as$:
$0 = U^2\sin^2\alpha - 2gs$ ***[1 mark]*** $\Rightarrow s = \frac{U^2\sin^2\alpha}{2g}$ ***[1 mark]***.
The golf ball is initially 0.5 m above the ground, so the maximum height, h, it reaches is:
$h = \frac{1}{2} + \frac{U^2\sin^2\alpha}{2g} = \frac{g + U^2\sin^2\alpha}{2g}$ m, as required ***[1 mark]***.

b) You first need to find the horizontal and vertical components of the golf ball's motion when it lands.
Vertically, taking up as positive:
$u = U\sin\alpha$, $a = -g$, $s = -0.5$, $v = v_V$.
Use $v^2 = u^2 + 2as$:
$v_V^2 = U^2\sin^2\alpha + g$ ***[1 mark]***.
Horizontally, $v_H = u_H = U\cos\alpha$, as acceleration is zero ***[1 mark]***.
So, $V = \sqrt{v_V^2 + v_H^2} = \sqrt{U^2\sin^2\alpha + g + U^2\cos^2\alpha}$ ***[1 mark]***
$= \sqrt{U^2(\sin^2\alpha + \cos^2\alpha) + g}$ ***[1 mark]***
$= \sqrt{U^2 + g}$ ms^{-1}, as required ***[1 mark]***.

c) E.g. The effects of air resistance could be factored in. / The beach ball should not be modelled as a particle — its diameter should be taken into account when finding distances.
[1 mark for any sensible suggestion]

16 a) $\theta = \tan^{-1}\left(\frac{3}{4}\right)$ so $\tan\theta = \frac{3}{4}$. This means that the opposite and adjacent sides of a right-angled triangle are 3 and 4, so the hypotenuse is $\sqrt{3^2 + 4^2} = 5$.
This gives $\sin\theta = \frac{3}{5} = 0.6$ and $\cos\theta = \frac{4}{5} = 0.8$
Resolving forces parallel to the plane (↗) for A, where T is the tension in the string:
$F_{net} = ma \Rightarrow T - mg\sin\theta = ma$
$\Rightarrow ma = T - 5.88m$ ① ***[1 mark]***
Resolving forces perpendicular to the plane (↗) for B:
$R - 2mg\cos 70° = 0 \Rightarrow R = 19.6m\cos 70°$ ***[1 mark]***
Friction is limiting, so:
$F = \mu R = 0.45 \times 19.6m\cos 70° = 8.82m\cos 70°$ ***[1 mark]***
Resolving forces parallel to the plane (↘) for B:
$F_{net} = ma \Rightarrow 2mg\sin 70° - T - F = 2ma$ ② ***[1 mark]***
Now consider ① + ②:
$3ma = T - 5.88m + 2mg\sin 70° - T - F$
$= 2mg\sin 70° - 5.88m - 8.82m\cos 70°$ ***[1 mark]***
Divide through by $3m$ to find a:
$a = \frac{2g\sin 70° - 5.88 - 8.82\cos 70°}{3}$
$= 3.1737... = 3.2$ ms^{-2} (2 s.f.) ***[1 mark]***

b) A is on the point of sliding down the plane, so both particles are in equilibrium.
Resolving forces parallel to the plane (↙) for A:
$10g\sin\theta - T = 0 \Rightarrow T = 58.8$ N ***[1 mark]***
Resolving forces perpendicular to the plane (↗) for B:
$R - 2mg\cos 70° = 0 \Rightarrow R = 2mg\cos 70°$
Again, friction is limiting, so:
$F = \mu R = 0.45 \times 2mg\cos 70°$ ***[1 mark]***
Resolving forces parallel to the plane (↖) for B (where the friction now acts down the plane):
$T - F - 2mg\sin 70° = 0$
$\Rightarrow 58.8 - 0.45 \times 2mg\cos 70° - 2mg\sin 70° = 0$ ***[1 mark]***
$\Rightarrow m = \frac{58.8}{2(0.45g\cos 70° + g\sin 70°)} = 2.7$ kg (2 s.f.) ***[1 mark]***

Practice Exam Paper 3

1 $x = t - 3 \Rightarrow -7 = t - 3 \Rightarrow t = -4$
$y = (t + k)^2 \Rightarrow 0 = (-4 + k)^2 \Rightarrow k = 4$ ***[1 mark]***

2 $\frac{dy}{dx} \neq 0$, so P is not a maximum point, minimum point or stationary point of inflection. $\frac{d^2y}{dx^2} = 0$ and changes sign at P, so P is a point of inflection. ***[1 mark]***

3 Start with the LHS:
$\sec 2\theta \equiv \frac{1}{\cos 2\theta}$
Use the double angle formula $\cos 2\theta \equiv \cos^2\theta - \sin^2\theta$:
$\equiv \frac{1}{\cos^2\theta - \sin^2\theta}$ ***[1 mark]***
Divide the numerator and denominator by $\cos^2\theta$:
$\equiv \frac{\sec^2\theta}{1 - \tan^2\theta}$ ***[1 mark]***
Use the trig identity $\tan^2\theta \equiv \sec^2\theta - 1$:
$\equiv \frac{\sec^2\theta}{1 - (\sec^2\theta - 1)}$
$\equiv \frac{\sec^2\theta}{2 - \sec^2\theta}$ as required ***[1 mark for correct rearrangement]***

4

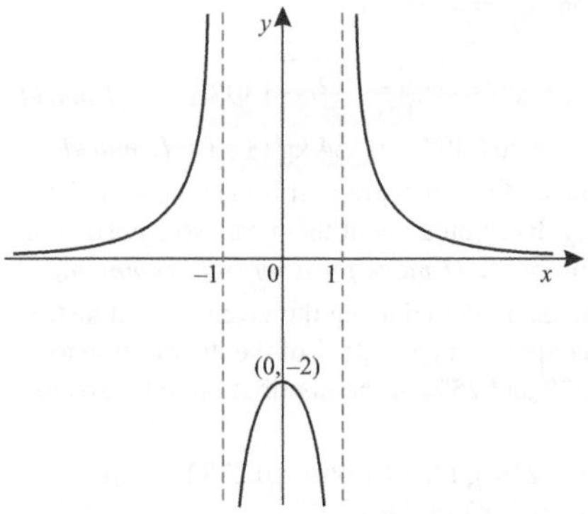

[1 mark for the correct shape]
Asymptotes at $x = 1$, $x = -1$ ***[1 mark]*** and $y = 0$ ***[1 mark]***,
y-intercept at $(0, -2)$ ***[1 mark]***

5 a) $\frac{11x - 7}{(2x - 4)(x + 1)} \equiv \frac{A}{2x - 4} + \frac{B}{x + 1}$ ***[1 mark]***
$\Rightarrow 11x - 7 \equiv A(x + 1) + B(2x - 4)$ ***[1 mark]***
Putting in $x = -1$ gives: $-18 = -6B \Rightarrow B = 3$
Putting in $x = 2$ gives: $15 = 3A \Rightarrow A = 5$
So $\frac{11x - 7}{(2x - 4)(x + 1)} \equiv \frac{5}{2x - 4} + \frac{3}{x + 1}$.
[1 mark for each correct fraction]

b) $\frac{11x - 7}{(2x - 4)(x + 1)} \equiv 5(2x - 4)^{-1} + 3(x + 1)^{-1}$ ***[1 mark]***
$5(2x - 4)^{-1} = 5\left((-4)^{-1}\left(-\frac{x}{2} + 1\right)^{-1}\right)$
$= 5\left(-\frac{1}{4}\left(1 + -1\left(-\frac{x}{2}\right) + \frac{-1 \times -2}{1 \times 2}\left(-\frac{x}{2}\right)^2 + \ldots\right)\right)$ ***[1 mark]***
$= -\frac{5}{4} - \frac{5}{8}x - \frac{5}{16}x^2 + \ldots$
$3(x + 1)^{-1} = 3\left(1 + -1(x) + \frac{-1 \times -2}{1 \times 2}x^2 + \ldots\right)$ ***[1 mark]***
$= 3 - 3x + 3x^2 + \ldots$
$\frac{11x - 7}{(2x - 4)(x + 1)} \equiv -\frac{5}{4} - \frac{5}{8}x - \frac{5}{16}x^2 + 3 - 3x + 3x^2 + \ldots$
$\equiv \frac{7}{4} - \frac{29}{8}x + \frac{43}{16}x^2 + \ldots$
[1 mark for each correct term]

6 a) The dog's range is a sector, bounded by the edge of the pen, the fence and the arc that is formed by the limit of its rope.
The angle of the sector is the exterior angle of the regular hexagon:
$360° \div 60° = \frac{\pi}{3}$ radians ***[1 mark]***
So the area is $\frac{1}{2} \times 2^2 \times \frac{\pi}{3}$ ***[1 mark]*** $= \frac{2\pi}{3}$ m² ***[1 mark]***

b) The hexagon is made up of 6 equilateral triangles of side length 2 m. Area of one of these triangles:
$\frac{1}{2} \times 2 \times 2 \times \sin\left(\frac{\pi}{3}\right)$ ***[1 mark]*** $= 2 \times \frac{\sqrt{3}}{2} = \sqrt{3}$ m²
So the hexagon's area is $6\sqrt{3}$ m² ***[1 mark]***
This means the cat can go in an area of
$(20 \times 8) - \frac{2\pi}{3} - 6\sqrt{3}$ ***[1 mark]*** $= 148$ m² (3 s.f.) ***[1 mark]***

7 Use the quotient rule: $u = 3 + \sin x \Rightarrow \frac{du}{dx} = \cos x$ ***[1 mark]***
$v = (2x + 1)^4 \Rightarrow \frac{dv}{dx} = 4(2)(2x + 1)^3 = 8(2x + 1)^3$ ***[1 mark]***
$f'(x) = \frac{(2x + 1)^4\cos x - 8(3 + \sin x)(2x + 1)^3}{(2x + 1)^8}$
$= \frac{(2x + 1)\cos x - 8(3 + \sin x)}{(2x + 1)^5}$
[1 mark for use of quotient rule, 1 mark for correct answer]

8 $u = \sqrt{x - 1} \Rightarrow \frac{du}{dx} = \frac{1}{2\sqrt{x - 1}}$
$\Rightarrow 2\sqrt{x - 1}\,du = dx \Rightarrow dx = 2u\,du$ ***[1 mark]***
Change the limits: $x = 10 \Rightarrow u = \sqrt{10 - 1} = \sqrt{9} = 3$
$x = 5 \Rightarrow u = \sqrt{5 - 1} = \sqrt{4} = 2$ ***[1 mark for both limits]***
$u^2 = x - 1 \Rightarrow x = u^2 + 1$
$\int_5^{10} \frac{2x}{\sqrt{x - 1}}\,dx = \int_2^3 \frac{2(u^2 + 1)}{u} \times 2u\,du$ ***[1 mark]*** $= \int_2^3 (4u^2 + 4)\,du$
$= \left[\frac{4u^3}{3} + 4u\right]_2^3$ ***[1 mark]***
$= \left(\frac{4}{3}(3^3) + 4(3)\right) - \left(\frac{4}{3}2^3 + 4(2)\right)$
$= 48 - \frac{56}{3} = \frac{88}{3}$ ***[1 mark]***

9 a) Set the equations equal to each other and rearrange:
$\frac{1}{x^3} = x + 3 \Rightarrow 1 = x^4 + 3x^3$
$\Rightarrow x^4 + 3x^3 - 1 = 0$ ***[1 mark]***

b) Let $f(x) = x^4 + 3x^3 - 1$, then $f'(x) = 4x^3 + 9x^2$ ***[1 mark]***
Using the Newton-Raphson formula
$x_{n+1} = x_n - \frac{f(x_n)}{f'(x_n)} = x_n - \frac{x_n^4 + 3x_n^3 - 1}{4x_n^3 + 9x_n^2}$ ***[1 mark]***
$x_1 = 0.6$
$x_2 = 0.6 - \frac{0.6^4 + 3(0.6^3) - 1}{4(0.6^3) + 9(0.6^2)}$ ***[1 mark]***
$= 0.65419... = 0.6542$ (4 d.p.) ***[1 mark]***
$x_3 = 0.65419... - \frac{0.65419...^4 + 3(0.65419...^3) - 1}{4(0.65419...^3) + 9(0.65419...^2)}$
$= 0.64955... = 0.6496$ (4 d.p.) ***[1 mark]***

10 a) $\frac{dT}{dt}$ is the rate of heat loss with respect to time.
The difference in temperature is $(T - 15)$ °C.
$\frac{dT}{dt} \propto (T - 15)$, so $\frac{dT}{dt} = -k(T - 15)$, with the negative sign indicating that the temperature is decreasing ***[1 mark]***.

b) Rearrange and integrate both sides of the equation from a)
$\int \frac{1}{T - 15}\,dT = \int -k\,dt$
$\ln|T - 15| = -kt + C$ ***[1 mark]***
$T - 15 = e^{-kt + C}$ ***[1 mark]*** $= Ae^{-kt}$ (where $A = e^C$)
Put in the initial condition $t = 0$, $T = 95$ to find A:
$95 - 15 = Ae^0 \Rightarrow A = 80$
$T = 80e^{-kt} + 15$ ***[1 mark]***

c) Put in the given condition $t = 10$, $T = 55$ to find k:
$55 = 80e^{-10k} + 15$ ***[1 mark]*** $\Rightarrow e^{-10k} = 0.5$
$\Rightarrow -10k = \ln 0.5 \Rightarrow k = -\frac{\ln 0.5}{10}$ ***[1 mark]***
$T = 80e^{\frac{\ln 0.5}{10} \times t} + 15$ ***[1 mark]*** $= 80(e^{\ln 0.5})^{\frac{t}{10}} + 15$
$\Rightarrow T = 80(0.5)^{\frac{t}{10}} + 15$ ***[1 mark]***

d) E.g. the model assumes that the temperature in the kitchen remains constant ***[1 mark for any sensible assumption]***.

11 a) She picked a random starting point and then moved through the population using a regular interval, so she has used systematic sampling. ***[1 mark]***

b) $n = 50$ and $p = 0.4$, so she should use $N(np, np(1 - p))$
$= N(50 \times 0.4, 50 \times 0.4 \times (1 - 0.4)) = N(20, 12)$. ***[1 mark]***

12 a) The data from the graph, in ascending order, is:
0.15, 0.20, 0.21, 0.21, 0.21, 0.35, 0.38

$\frac{7}{4} = 1.75$, so Q_1 is the 2nd value. $Q_1 = 0.20$

$\frac{3 \times 7}{4} = 5.25$, so Q_3 is the 6th value. $Q_3 = 0.35$

[1 mark for both Q_1 and Q_3]

IQR $= Q_3 - Q_1 = 0.35 - 0.20 = 0.15$ ***[1 mark]***

Outliers: $Q_1 - (1.5 \times \text{IQR}) = 0.20 - (1.5 \times 0.15) = -0.025$
$Q_3 + (1.5 \times \text{IQR}) = 0.35 + (1.5 \times 0.15) = 0.575$
[1 mark for the upper fence correct]

There can't be any data values less than –0.025, and there aren't any greater than 0.575, so there are no outliers ***[1 mark]***.

b) The average of H will be somewhere between the average of E and the average of F, so $0.35 < h < 0.38$.
The averages of the six groups in ascending order are now:
0.15, 0.20, 0.21, 0.21, 0.21, h

$\frac{6}{4} = 1.5$, so Q_1 is still the 2nd value: $Q_1 = 0.20$

$\frac{3 \times 6}{4} = 4.5$, so Q_3 is the 5th value: $Q_3 = 0.21$. ***[1 mark]***

So IQR $= 0.21 - 0.20 = 0.01$
$Q_3 + (1.5 \times \text{IQR}) = 0.21 + (1.5 \times 0.01) = 0.225$,
and $h > 0.225$, so body type H is an outlier. ***[1 mark]***
E.g. No, the data values shouldn't be excluded. The data for hatchbacks make up too significant a portion of the data and so excluding them would give results that are not representative of the majority of vehicles. ***[1 mark for a sensible explanation]***

c) E.g. Yes, the general pattern of emissions by body type in London and the South West will be similar. /
No, the distribution of body types registered in London is different to those registered in the South West, which will affect the overall distribution of emissions.
[1 mark for a sensible explanation]

13 a) Using the conditional probability formula:

$P(R|S) = \frac{P(R \cap S)}{P(S)} = \frac{4}{9} \Rightarrow P(R \cap S) = \frac{4}{9}P(S)$ ***[1 mark]***

$P(S|R) = \frac{P(R \cap S)}{P(R)} = \frac{4}{11} \Rightarrow P(R \cap S) = \frac{4}{11}P(R)$ ***[1 mark]***

So $\frac{4}{9}P(S) = \frac{4}{11}P(R) \Rightarrow P(S) = \frac{9}{11}P(R)$ ***[1 mark]***

Now, using the addition law:
$P(R \cup S) = P(R) + P(S) - P(R \cap S)$

$\frac{8}{10} = P(R) + \frac{9}{11}P(R) - \frac{4}{11}P(R)$ ***[1 mark]***

$\frac{8}{10} = \frac{16}{11}P(R) \Rightarrow P(R) = \frac{11}{20} = 0.55$

And $P(S) = \frac{9}{11}P(R) = \frac{9}{11} \times \frac{11}{20} = \frac{9}{20} = 0.45$

[1 mark for both P(R) and P(S)]

b) $P(R \cap S) = \frac{4}{9}P(S) = \frac{4}{9} \times \frac{9}{20} = \frac{1}{5} = 0.2$

$P(R) \times P(S) = \frac{11}{20} \times \frac{9}{20} = \frac{99}{400} = 0.2475$

[1 mark for both probabilities]

So $P(R \cap S) \neq P(R) \times P(S)$, meaning that the events R and S are not independent ***[1 mark]***.

There are other ways to check whether or not these are independent events — for example, you could show that $P(R) \neq P(R | S)$.

c) $P(S \cap T) = P(S) \times P(T) = 0.45 \times 0.15 = 0.0675$
Now work everything out using the known probabilities:

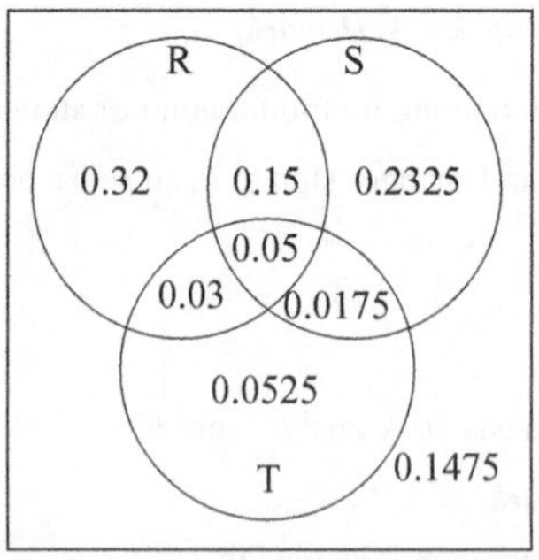

[4 marks for a completely correct Venn diagram, otherwise 1 mark for a correct method to find $P(S \cap T)$, 1 mark for $P(S \cap T) = 0.0675$, 1 mark for $P(R \cap S \cap T')$ or $P(R \cap T \cap S')$ correct]

14 a) mean $= \frac{\sum fx}{\sum f} = \frac{557\,250}{400} = 1393.125 = 1390$ kg (3 s.f.) ***[1 mark]***

standard deviation $= \sqrt{\frac{\sum fx^2}{\sum f} - \bar{x}^2}$

$= \sqrt{\frac{804\,302\,500}{400} - 1393.125^2}$ ***[1 mark]***

$= 264.497... = 264$ kg (3 s.f.) ***[1 mark]***

b) E.g. From the shape of the histogram, it is clear that the data is not symmetrically distributed about the mean, so a normal model would not be appropriate ***[1 mark for a sensible comment]***.

c) If the data, X, can be modelled using the given normal distribution, you would expect approximately 25% of the distribution to be less than $Q_1 = 1399$ and 25% of the distribution to be greater than $Q_3 = 1786$.
Using $X \sim N(1597, 278^2)$, $P(X < 1399) = 0.2382$ (4 d.p.)
and $P(X > 1786) = 0.2483$ (4 d.p.).
Both of these probabilities are close to 0.25, so this normal distribution seems like a suitable model.
[3 marks available — 1 mark for finding $P(X < 1399)$, 1 mark for finding $P(X > 1786)$, 1 mark for a sensible conclusion]
You could have done this one slightly differently — e.g. by finding Q_1 and Q_3 for the given normal distribution and comparing them to the values Leanne calculated.

15 a) Let V be the number of vehicles in the sample with particulate emissions of less than 0.04 g/km, then, using Lara's model:
$V \sim B(15, 0.80)$.
The probability needed is:
$P(5 \leq V < 10)$ ***[1 mark]*** $= P(V < 10) - P(V < 5)$
$= P(V \leq 9) - P(V \leq 4)$ ***[1 mark for a correct method]***
$= 0.0610514... - 0.00001246...$
$= 0.0610$ (4 d.p.) ***[1 mark]***

b) E.g. Data in the large data set is only for 2002 and 2016 so is not up to date. / The large data set only contains data for five makes of cars, whereas the service station is likely to contain different makes. ***[1 mark for a sensible comment]***.

c) E.g. Lara has assumed that each vehicle in the sample is independent of all the others. / She has assumed that the probability is the same for all the vehicles. ***[1 mark for a correct assumption]***

16 a) $P(J < 493) = 0.05$ and $P(J > 502) = 0.025$ ***[1 mark]***

$P(J < 493) = 0.05 \Rightarrow P\left(Z < \frac{493 - \mu}{\sigma}\right) = 0.05$

$\Rightarrow \frac{493 - \mu}{\sigma} = -1.6449 \Rightarrow \mu - 493 = 1.6449\sigma$ ***[1 mark]***

$P(J > 502) = 0.025 \Rightarrow P(J < 502) = 0.975$

$\Rightarrow P\left(Z < \frac{502 - \mu}{\sigma}\right) = 0.975$

$\Rightarrow \frac{502 - \mu}{\sigma} = 1.9600 \Rightarrow 502 - \mu = 1.9600\sigma$ ***[1 mark]***

Solve these simultaneously:

$(\mu - 493) + (502 - \mu) = 1.6449\sigma + 1.9600\sigma$

$\Rightarrow 9 = 3.6049\sigma \Rightarrow \sigma = 2.4966... = 2.50$ (3 s.f.) ***[1 mark]***

$\mu = 493 + 1.6449 \times 2.4966... = 497.10...$

$= 497$ (3 s.f.) ***[1 mark]***

b) From part a), $J \sim N(497, 2.50^2)$ ***[1 mark]***.
The probability that a carton fails to meet the manufacturer's standards is $P(J < 492)$. From your calculator, this is $0.02275... = 0.0228$ (4 d.p.) ***[1 mark]***

c) $H_0: \mu = 497$, $H_1: \mu \neq 497$ ***[1 mark for both]***
— so this is a 2-tail test.
Under H_0, $J \sim N(497, 2.50^2)$, so the sample mean,

$\bar{J} \sim N(497, \frac{2.50^2}{20})$ ***[1 mark]***, and $Z = \frac{\bar{J} - 497}{\frac{2.50}{\sqrt{20}}} \sim N(0, 1)$.

$\bar{j} = 498.7$, so $z = \frac{498.7 - 497}{\frac{2.50}{\sqrt{20}}} = 3.0410...$ ***[1 mark]***

This is a 2-tail test, and as $z > 0$, you're interested in the upper tail — so you need to find z such that $P(Z > z) = 0.005$. From your calculator, $P(Z > 2.5758) = 0.005$, so the critical value is 2.5758 and the critical region is $Z > 2.5758$. Since $3.0410... > 2.5758$, the result is significant ***[1 mark]***, so there is evidence at the 1% level of significance to reject H_0 in favour of the alternative hypothesis that the mean volume of juice in a carton has changed ***[1 mark]***.

You could have found $P(Z > 3.0410...)$ instead — you get a value of 0.00117..., which is less than 0.005 so is significant. You'd get the marks for either method — use whichever one you prefer.

17 a) Amira's result shows moderately strong positive correlation, which suggests that the number of bacteria tends to be higher in deeper ponds ***[1 mark]***.
Ben's result is greater than 1, which is not a valid answer, so he must have made an error in his calculation ***[1 mark]***.

b) While the results suggest that they are linked, they do not mean that deeper ponds cause higher numbers of bacteria. There could be a third variable linking them, or it could just be coincidence ***[1 mark]***.

c) $H_0: \rho = 0$, $H_1: \rho > 0$ ***[1 mark]***, so this is a 1-tail test.
The test statistic is $r = 0.71$. The critical value is 0.6215.
Since $0.71 > 0.6215$, the result is significant.
There is evidence at the 5% significance level to reject H_0 and to support the alternative hypothesis that the depth of a pond and the number of this type of bacteria in the pond are positively correlated ***[1 mark]***.

Formula Sheet

These formulas are the ones you'll be given in the exam, but make sure you know exactly **when you need them** and **how to use them**.

Series

Arithmetic Series:

$$S_n = \frac{1}{2}n(a+l) = \frac{1}{2}n[2a+(n-1)d]$$

Geometric Series:

$$S_n = \frac{a(1-r^n)}{1-r} \qquad S_\infty = \frac{a}{1-r} \text{ for } |r|<1$$

Binomial Series:

$$(a+b)^n = a^n + \binom{n}{1}a^{n-1}b + \binom{n}{2}a^{n-2}b^2 + \ldots + \binom{n}{r}a^{n-r}b^r + \ldots + b^n \quad (n \in \mathbb{N})$$

$$\text{where } \binom{n}{r} = {}^nC_r = \frac{n!}{r!(n-r)!}$$

$$(1+x)^n = 1 + nx + \frac{n(n-1)}{1\times 2}x^2 + \ldots + \frac{n(n-1)\ldots(n-r+1)}{1\times 2\times \ldots \times r}x^r + \ldots \quad (|x|<1, n\in\mathbb{Q})$$

Trigonometry

$$\sin(A \pm B) \equiv \sin A\cos B \pm \cos A \sin B$$

$$\cos(A \pm B) \equiv \cos A\cos B \mp \sin A \sin B$$

$$\tan(A \pm B) \equiv \frac{\tan A \pm \tan B}{1 \mp \tan A \tan B} \quad (A \pm B \neq (k+\tfrac{1}{2})\pi)$$

Small Angle Approximations:

For small angle θ, measured in radians:

$$\sin\theta \approx \theta \qquad \cos\theta \approx 1 - \frac{1}{2}\theta^2 \qquad \tan\theta \approx \theta$$

Differentiation

First Principles:

$$f'(x) = \lim_{h\to 0}\frac{f(x+h)-f(x)}{h}$$

For $y = \frac{f(x)}{g(x)}$,

$$\frac{dy}{dx} = \frac{f'(x)g(x) - f(x)g'(x)}{(g(x))^2}$$

f(x)	f'(x)
$\tan x$	$\sec^2 x$
$\sec x$	$\sec x \tan x$
$\cot x$	$-\text{cosec}^2 x$
$\text{cosec}\, x$	$-\text{cosec}\, x \cot x$

Integration

$$\int u\frac{dv}{dx}dx = uv - \int v\frac{du}{dx}dx$$

$$\int \frac{f'(x)}{f(x)}dx = \ln|f(x)| + C$$

f(x)	$\int f(x)\,dx$
$\tan x$	$\ln\lvert\sec x\rvert + C$
$\cot x$	$\ln\lvert\sin x\rvert + C$

Numerical Methods

The Newton-Raphson iteration for solving f(x) = 0: $x_{n+1} = x_n - \frac{f(x_n)}{f'(x_n)}$

Trapezium rule: $\int_a^b y\,dx \approx \frac{1}{2}h[(y_0+y_n)+2(y_1+y_2+\ldots+y_{n-1})]$, where $h = \frac{b-a}{n}$

Mechanics

Constant acceleration equations:

$s = ut + \frac{1}{2}at^2$	$\mathbf{s} = \mathbf{u}t + \frac{1}{2}\mathbf{a}t^2$
$s = vt - \frac{1}{2}at^2$	$\mathbf{s} = \mathbf{v}t - \frac{1}{2}\mathbf{a}t^2$
$v = u + at$	$\mathbf{v} = \mathbf{u} + \mathbf{a}t$
$s = \frac{1}{2}(u+v)t$	$\mathbf{s} = \frac{1}{2}(\mathbf{u}+\mathbf{v})t$
$v^2 = u^2 + 2as$	

Probability

$$P(A\cup B) = P(A) + P(B) - P(A\cap B)$$

$$P(A\cap B) = P(A)\times P(B|A)$$

Standard Deviation

$$\sqrt{\frac{\sum(x-\bar{x})^2}{n}} = \sqrt{\frac{\sum x^2}{n} - \bar{x}^2}$$

The Binomial Distribution

If $X \sim B(n, p)$, then

$$P(X=x) = \binom{n}{x}p^x(1-p)^{n-x}$$

Mean of $X = np$

Variance of $X = np(1-p)$

Sampling Distributions

For a random sample of n observations from $N(\mu, \sigma^2)$:

$$\frac{\bar{X}-\mu}{\sigma/\sqrt{n}} \sim N(0,1)$$

MAO72